St Antony's Series

General Editor: **Richard Clogg** (1999–), Fellow of St Antony's College, Oxford

Recent titles include:

Karen Jochelson
THE COLOUR OF DISEASE
Syphilis and Racism in South Africa, 1880–1950

Julio Crespo MacLennan
SPAIN AND THE PROCESS OF EUROPEAN INTEGRATION, 1957–85

Enrique Cárdenas, José Antonio Ocampo and Rosemary Thorp (*editors*)
AN ECONOMIC HISTORY OF TWENTIETH-CENTURY LATIN AMERICA
Volume 1: The Export Age
Volume 2: Latin America in the 1930s
Volume 3: Industrialization and the State in Latin America

Jennifer G. Mathers
THE RUSSIAN NUCLEAR SHIELD FROM STALIN TO YELTSIN

Marta Dyczok
THE GRAND ALLIANCE AND UKRAINIAN REFUGEES

Mark Brzezinski
THE STRUGGLE FOR CONSTITUTIONALISM IN POLAND

Suke Wolton
LORD HAILEY, THE COLONIAL OFFICE AND THE POLITICS OF RACE AND
EMPIRE IN THE SECOND WORLD WAR
The Loss of White Prestige

Junko Tomaru
THE POSTWAR RAPPROCHEMENT OF MALAYA AND JAPAN, 1945–61
The Roles of Britain and Japan in South-East Asia

Eiichi Motono
CONFLICT AND COOPERATION IN SINO-BRITISH BUSINESS, 1860–1911
The Impact of the Pro-British Commercial Network in Shanghai

Nikolas K. Gvosdev
IMPERIAL POLICIES AND PERSPECTIVES TOWARDS GEORGIA, 1760–1819

Bernardo Kosacoff
CORPORATE STRATEGIES UNDER STRUCTURAL ADJUSTMENT IN ARGENTINA
Responses by Industrial Firms to a New Set of Uncertainties

Ray Takeyh
THE ORIGINS OF THE EISENHOWER DOCTRINE
The US, Britain and Nasser's Egypt, 1953–57

Derek Hopwood (*editor*)
ARAB NATION, ARAB NATIONALISM

Judith Clifton
THE POLITICS OF TELECOMMUNICATIONS IN MEXICO
Privatization and State–Labour Relations, 1928–95

Cécile Laborde
PLURALIST THOUGHT AND THE STATE IN BRITAIN AND FRANCE, 1900–25

Craig Brandist and Galin Tihanov (*editors*)
MATERIALIZING BAKHTIN

C. S. Nicholls
THE HISTORY OF ST ANTONY'S COLLEGE, OXFORD, 1950–2000

Anthony Kirk-Greene
BRITAIN'S IMPERIAL ADMINISTRATORS, 1858–1966

Laila Parsons
THE DRUZE BETWEEN PALESTINE AND ISRAEL, 1947–49

M. K. Flynn
IDEOLOGY, MOBILIZATION AND THE NATION
The Rise of Irish, Basque and Carlist Nationalist Movements in the
Nineteenth and Early Twentieth Centuries

Karina Sonnenberg-Stern
EMANCIPATION AND POVERTY
The Ashkenazi Jews of Amsterdam, 1796–1850

Shane O'Rourke
WARRIORS AND PEASANTS
The Don Cossacks in Late Imperial Russia

St Antony's Series
Series Standing Order ISBN 978–0–333–71109–5
(*outside North America only*)

You can receive future titles in this series as they are published by placing a standing order.
Please contact your bookseller or, in case of difficulty, write to us at the address below with
your name and address, the title of the series and the ISBN quoted above.

Customer Services Department, Macmillan Distribution Ltd, Houndmills, Basingstoke,
Hampshire RG21 6XS, England

The Colour of Disease

Syphilis and Racism in South Africa, 1880–1950

Karen Jochelson

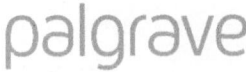

in association with
St Antony's College, Oxford

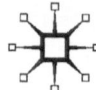

First published 2001 by
PALGRAVE
Houndmills, Basingstoke, Hampshire RG21 6XS and
175 Fifth Avenue, New York, N. Y. 10010
Companies and representatives throughout the world

PALGRAVE is the new global academic imprint of
St. Martin's Press LLC Scholarly and Reference Division and
Palgrave Publishers Ltd (formerly Macmillan Press Ltd).

ISBN 978-0-333-74044-6

This book is printed on paper suitable for recycling and made from fully managed and sustained forest sources.

A catalogue record for this book is available from the British Library.

Library of Congress Cataloging-in-Publication Data
Jochelson, Karen, 1963–
    The colour of disease : syphilis and racism in South Africa, 1880–1950 / Karen Jochelson.
        p. cm. — (St. Antony's)
    Includes bibliographical references and index.
    ISBN 978-0-333-74044-6
    1. Syphilis—Social aspects—South Africa. 2 Racism—South Africa. 3. South Africa—Race relations. I. Title. II. St. Antony's/Macmillan series (London, England)
    RA644.V4 J63 2000
    362.1'969513'00968—dc21
                                                                00–048355

10   9   8   7   6   5   4   3   2   1
10   09   08   07   06   05   04   03   02   01

For the best things in my life
David, **Sam** *and* **Sophie**

Contents

List of Tables

Acknowledgements

I first thought of writing a history of venereal disease in 1988 while I was working on a research project on AIDS and migrant labour in South Africa. I found that there was no South African historical work to back up my arguments about the socioeconomic determinants of AIDS. I was also challenged by questions about race and stereotyping provoked by this research. These issues provided the root of the idea for my doctoral thesis, which I then extended for this book.

In the process of researching and writing the thesis and the book I incurred several debts of thanks. The benefactors and trustees of the Patrick and Margaret Flanagan Scholarship (administered by the University of the Witwatersrand) funded three years of full-time study at the University of Oxford, which enabled me to undertake the doctoral thesis. The Beit Fund of the University of Oxford twice awarded me grants that covered the costs of archival research trips. The Wellcome Foundation awarded me a two-year postdoctoral fellowship at the Institute of Commonwealth Studies at the University of London, which enabled me to research the nineteenth-century history of syphilis and turn the thesis into a book. Megan Vaughan, Shula Marks and Terence Ranger offered me insightful criticisms of the thesis and asked questions I found hard to answer, thus making me think more carefully about my argument and conclusions. My publishers, Macmillan, were patient about the endless but inevitable delays resulting from the birth of two children and a career change.

Finally, I want to thank David Bodanis for lox, bagels and his endless optimism about The Problem Chapter of the moment. We certainly found that there was Life After the Thesis, in the form of Sam and Sophie, who made the time I spent writing the book extremely joyful. You two can now scribble over my notes and unsort my record cards in whatever way you wish and without comment from me – or will that take the fun out of it?

Abbreviations

ANC	African National Congress
AIDS	Acquired immuno-deficiency syndrome
CDA	Contagious Diseases Act
CDC	Contagious Diseases Commission (1906)
CDPA	Contagious Diseases Prevention Act
DPH	Department of Public Health
HIV	Human immuno-deficiency virus
ICU	Industrial and Commercial Workers' Union
MOH	Medical Officer of Health
NAD	Native Affairs Department
NCCVD	National Council for Combating Venereal Diseases
NEC	Native Economic Commission
NUAA	Native Urban Areas Act
PHA	Public Health Act
RCSCH	Red Cross Social Hygiene Committee
RWS	Race Welfare Society
SAIRR	South African Institute of Race Relations
SHC	Social Hygiene Council
STDs	Sexually transmitted diseases
VD	Venereal disease
WNLA	Witwatersrand Native Labour Association
ZAR	Zuid Afrikaansche Republiek (South African Republic)

Introduction

During the early 1980s reports began to flood the press and medical journals about an epidemic of a new disease: acquired immune deficiency syndrome (AIDS). While the disease initially seemed to be confined to the male homosexual population in Europe and North America, cases were soon reported in Africa, where the disease seemed to be spreading through heterosexual sexual contact. Medical researchers speculated that the human immuno-deficiency virus (HIV), which eventually causes AIDS, had originated in Africa and then infected Europe. Some researchers suggested that the virus had jumped species due to Africans' closer proximity to wild animals, bizarre food habits and exotic initiation ceremonies or sexual customs involving monkey blood. Other doctors felt that Africans might have a racial predisposition to AIDS or were naturally more promiscuous than Europeans, resulting in the disease spreading rapidly.[1]

These popular and medical explanations of AIDS and HIV resonate with the colonial image of Africa as a sick and dying continent, harbouring deadly disease and inhabited by an essentially promiscuous people who are part of a dangerous, wild, natural world and bound by primitive traditions and superstitions. This portrayal of AIDS in Africa makes it evident that empirically based, scientific medical knowledge can be shaped by racist assumptions, and can authoritatively affirm perceptions that Africa and Africans are different from whites in Europe and North America.[2]

This racism resonates with similar reactions to venereal disease (VD) between 1880 and 1950 in South Africa, when 'half-castes', poor whites and Africans were regarded as responsible for spreading VD. VD usually referred to syphilis, which seemed to be more widespread than other sexually transmitted diseases and is the focus of this book. (I have

1

retained the term VD as more apt for an historical study of moral connotations of disease than the modern clinical term: sexually transmitted diseases, or STDs).

My intention is not simply to present a history of a disease, its causes and cure, but rather to restore syphilis to its social and historical environment. This involves, firstly, examining the way in which broader economic, political and social forces disrupted communities and made individuals vulnerable to a range of new diseases, including STDs, associated with conquest, poverty, urbanisation and industrialisation. Secondly, I also look at the social construction of disease and its carriers. VD is a prism through which to examine anxieties about changing relations of gender, race and class in periods of social change and the way in which particular groups come to represent social disorder. It is a prism that reflects changing meanings about masculinity and femininity, and 'being' African or white. Those doctors and administrators who tried to define the identity and origin of the VD carrier, drew on broader theories in psychology, sociology and anthropology about the nature of 'the poor white' or 'the African', and frequently confirmed these ideas. Finally, VD is a prism through which to examine the nature of colonial power and the regulation of social relationships by means other than legislative edict. Racial and gendered categories regulated sexual and racial relationships in broader society by defining what was normal behaviour. These differences also structured the type of VD medical services established for whites and Africans and their gradual segregation. This Introduction explores these three themes, demonstrating the theoretical premises underlying the study.

Epidemiology and political economy

An historian venturing to study the history of disease in Southern Africa enters relatively uncharted territory. Some studies of health and disease in Africa or Southern Africa focus on the medical conquest of disease and the benefits of European colonial rule. Medicine is assumed to be a neutral, progressive, scientific influence that gradually supplanted indigenous, traditional, non-scientific remedies.[3] This approach has been widely criticised. It ignores the existence of African systems of disease control, which were disrupted by colonial conquest. It overrates the benefits of medicine since many chemotherapeutic remedies only began to emerge in the late nineteenth and early twentieth centuries. The improvement in the health status of the general population in Europe has been associated more with a healthier environment and better nutrition than with scientific cures. Finally, this model removes the study of health and disease from its social and political context.

Historians critical of this heroic model began to investigate a political economy of health and disease in former colonies. They showed how colonial conquest, coercive labour recruitment, disruption of subsistence production and harsh industrial working conditions led to a decline in African health. This model has been influential in South African studies showing how epidemiology is shaped by cleavages of race and class. Migrant labour, social dislocation and poverty in the countryside and towns helped create environments in which diseases proliferated, a situation aggravated by the acute lack of medical facilities for Africans. State officials, the mining industry and whites frequently only expressed concern about ill-health in the African population when this threatened labour supplies or threatened to spread into white areas of town.[4] The political economy approach has also influenced studies of HIV and AIDs in Africa and Southern Africa. Researchers have shown how landlessness, poverty, migrancy, urbanisation and the disruption of family relationships and sexual mores have moulded behaviour and susceptibility to HIV.[5]

I have been influenced by the political economy approach in reconstructing a history of the epidemiology of syphilis and relating it to broader socioeconomic transformation. Sexually transmitted syphilis was introduced into South Africa by European settlers, sailors and soldiers. Initially the disease was confined to port and garrison towns, but it began to move inland following the army in its conquest of African kingdoms, and then the railways and labour markets as thousands of people flooded into the new diamond and gold mining towns in the interior. The migrant labour system proved a particularly effective way for STDs to spread. It undermined stable social and sexual relationships in rural and urban areas, predisposing many men and women to enter transient sexual relationships and it spread STDs from urban to distant rural areas.

The focus of the political economy model is on the impact of large-scale forces, while the role of ordinary people in shaping their own lives is underplayed. The model implicitly assumes that male or female migrants are free of family constraints and able to indulge every sexual whim. This feeds into racist assumptions about African sexuality. Thus I also show how migrant associations and rural communities tried to control men's relationships with town women and their exposure to STDs, emphasising the obligations and future these men had in their home areas. Despite the pressures of migrant and urban life, men and women still made their own choices and shaped their own lives, and were not simply victims of large-scale socioeconomic forces.[6]

Disease and the moral order

Fears about an epidemic of STDs and blaming a particular segment of a population for its spread may reflect wider fears about social and moral disorder, rather than a real increase in the incidence of disease. I have drawn on the insights of a social constructionist approach to examine how disease may act as a powerful metaphor for social and moral disorder.

Groups or individuals existing on the margins of the social structure, who threaten social norms or blur social hierarchy, come to embody the essence of disease and social corruption. Where a 'social type' seems to exist on the boundaries of what is socially acceptable, it becomes a 'folk devil', suggests Stanley Cohen – 'visible reminders of what we should not be'. In periods of moral panic the social type comes to be 'defined as a threat to societal values and interests'.[7] This approach is useful in alerting one to the symbolic aspect of a disease and to the possibility that a group identified as responsible for spreading a disease may in fact represent a range of fears and anxieties arising in a period of social change, and that calls for stricter moral or political regulation are a way to restore social consensus.

Since the nineteenth century in Europe and North America, VD has been a sign of a society corrupted by deviant sexuality and a decaying social order that threaten the idealised values of society. In Britain in the early twentieth century VD became a metaphor that condensed political and eugenic fears about the physical and moral deterioration of civilians, and the decay of family, race and empire.[8] In North America, at different times VD encapsulated fears about class, race, ethnicity and the family, as women's social and economic roles changed. New immigrants arrived in the cities, threatening political disorder and racial dilution, and politicians and doctors tried to understand how blacks were fundamentally different from whites.[9] When AIDs emerged in Europe and North America in the early 1980s conservative moralists, doctors and politicians were quick to depict it as retribution for a 'permissive' and 'unnatural' gay lifestyle. The gay and women's liberation movements had thrown into question what was 'normal' and 'natural' about masculinity, femininity and the family. AIDs came to signify the decline of moral society and justified calls for the preservation of marriage, monogamy and heterosexuality.[10]

In South Africa, concerns about wider social changes were reflected in the focus on VD. In the late nineteenth century 'half-castes' were blamed for spreading syphilis and this reflected contemporary fears about increasing racial interaction in towns and the dangers of the cultural assimilation of Africans. The 1920s and 1930s were turbulent years as whites and Africans left failing rural economies for the city and established new lives. White women moved into the industrial labour force, while African women relied on beer brewing, prostitution or domestic work and seemed beyond the control of African men, employers and municipal authorities. White 'amateur prostitutes' and African 'loose town women' were blamed for VD, mirroring wider anxieties about the instability of the social, political and moral order.

Race and the social construction of biomedical knowledge

New studies on the emergence of racism in the nineteenth-century Cape Colony,[11] the emergence of segregationism in the 1920s[12] and the development of racial science in South Africa[13] show that conceptions of race in the political and policy-making arena change over time. Historians are also questioning the obviousness of racial categories. Though skin colour is an obvious determining factor, in the late nineteenth and early twentieth centuries there was much concern about how 'white' were poor whites and how 'African' were educated blacks. Recent studies on the emergence of segregation in prisons, reformatories, hospitals and asylums have looked at the way in which racial difference was constructed in gender and class terms, and gender difference in racial terms.[14] Notions of white identity were built up against notions of what 'the African' represented.

Historians looking at the social construction of medicine argue that medical knowledge is not just a reflection of an empirical, biological reality independent of a social context. Rather they suggest that medicine exists as a distinct discourse – it is deeply embedded in moral values, social attitudes and political prejudices of the time and structures these ideas too.

Historians looking at the construction of femininity and homosexuality have shown how medical ideas have helped to define the social categories used to understand gender and sexual identity.[15] This approach has also emerged in the study of colonial medicine, as historians recognise that colonists' perceptions of subject peoples deeply structured the way they explained the causes and effects of and the cures for disease. Medical explanations of Africans' predisposition to disease drew on anthropological or sociological discourses for authority and legitimation, and also helped create knowledge of 'the African'.[16] And in South Africa, medical discourse drew on evolutionary theory, sociology or social anthropology to help explain why 'half-castes', poor whites, white 'amateur prostitutes', Africans and 'loose town women' spread VD, and in doing so confirmed theories about racial difference.

Foucault on Africa

Foucault suggests that the modern state relies on social and scientific discourses to define 'normal' behaviour, through which individuals come to know themselves as subjects.[17] Vaughan questions the value of a Foucauldian approach in the colonial context. She suggests that colonial power was more concerned with defining and pathologising the normal African than with distancing the Other through the notion of the madman or sexual deviant. Colonial medical discourse also attributed Africans – as a group rather than as individuals – with distinctive characteristics. Africans did not necessarily accept the terms in which they were portrayed. Thus while medical discourse construed the African as an object of study, it did not necessarily constitute Africans as subjects.[18]

The state that emerged in early-twentieth-century South Africa increasingly differentiated between its white and African subjects, both in the way in which whites and Africans were constructed as objects and subjects and in the enactment of health and social welfare policy. For whites, moral and medical discourse constructed normal and abnormal gendered sexuality in a way that clearly differentiated white men and women from what were deemed African characteristics. But Africans were already seen as Other on the basis of their skin colour, subjugated status and cultural difference. Immorality seemed to be characteristic of Africans in general, and was a sign of their difference from whites rather than of the abnormal sexuality of particular individuals. Thus while constructs of morality seem to follow Foucault's schema and define 'normality' for whites, for Africans, as Vaughan suggests, moral discourse seems more concerned with specifying racial difference.

Foucault's periodisation of state power shifting from an absolutist, public spectacle of power to a disciplinary technology based on surveillance and normalisation is too simple for the South African context.

State policy and practice was shaped by perceptions of racial difference and attempts to make this concrete through segregation.

Cape legislation did not explicitly differentiate between whites and blacks, but in practice the way in which Acts were implemented paralleled moves to racialise perceptions of poverty and introduce social and institutional segregation. The Public Health Act of 1919 marked a shift towards a more modern, interventionist state. Doctors and welfare workers believed that VD could be controlled if individuals sought outpatient treatment and followed the prescriptions of welfare and education programmes on moral behaviour for men and women. Here lay the beginnings of state power as surveillance – for whites. However detection, treatment and health education for Africans remained coercive. Africans were regarded as a homogeneous, potentially diseased population, and VD was monitored through the pass system and police raids.

Outline

In this book, I try to meld the strengths of the political economy and social constructionist approaches to the study of health and health services. A political economy approach to the study of VD in South Africa reveals how the spread of the disease can be linked to broader historical processes of socioeconomic transformation as land dispossession, migrancy and urbanisation disrupted social networks and stable sexual relationships.

I draw on the insights of a social constructionist approach to examine how blaming a particular group for the spread of VD may reflect a range of anxieties about class, race or gender relationships in a period of social upheaval, rather than being truly indicative of epidemiological patterns. I look at the way in which medical discourse has been shaped by the contemporary intellectual and social milieu and how it has offered social explanations – defining normal and abnormal categories of behaviour – for medical phenomena. The way in which medical discourse has identified the problem of the VD carrier mirrors the way in which racial and gendered identity has been constructed. These perceptions have shaped the implementation of medical policy for VD. Through treatment of and education about VD, the state was able to monitor the mores and health of the white and African populations, while simultaneously emphasising racial difference and creating racial identities. The study of a disease is thus a way to explore the effects of social transformation on health, the symbolic representation of social disorder through disease, and how gendered and racial identities are negotiated and defined through moral prescription, medical discourse and state health policy.

Historical epidemiology and the analysis of epidemics and health care are relatively under-researched in the case of South Africa, and this guided my decision to adopt a national rather than a local perspective. I relied mainly on medical journals, central state archives and the Johannesburg and Durban municipal archives. These sources clearly had limitations as they are places where the voices of the powerless – Africans, poor whites and women – are least likely to be recorded. Recourse to oral history was one possible solution, but this would have orientated the research project differently. This book is largely concerned with the construction of racial identity through objectifying discourses, rather than with poor whites' or Africans' experience of medical institutions, their acceptance of biomedicine or their indigenous medical systems.

Chapter 1 looks at an apparent epidemic of sexually transmitted syphilis in the 1880s. Conquest, land dispossession and migrancy certainly helped create markets for prostitution, encouraged transient sexual relationships and facilitated the spread of VD into the hinterland. However I suggest that the epidemic was an indigenous disease: endemic syphilis, which is related to venereal syphilis but is not transmitted sexually. Unhygienic working and living conditions in towns probably helped the transmission of endemic syphilis to new individuals, who then introduced the disease into their home communities on their return. Doctors regarded the disease as 'African syphilis', and I explore how the development of scientific racial ideas and the decline of assimilationism shaped medical perceptions.

Chapter 2 discusses the Contagious Diseases Act in the Cape Colony and the pass legislation in the Transvaal Republic, showing the roots of racial segregation in the late nineteenth and early twentieth centuries in the provision of health services.

Chapter 3 discusses how the urbanisation of whites, the incorporation of women into the workforce, changing sexual mores and miscegenation were seen as markers of poor white degeneration and a threat to white supremacy. Doctors' and social workers' analyses of the causes of 'amateur prostitution' helped to construct 'abnormal' white behaviour as similar to 'normal' African characteristics, and affirmed the qualities of 'Europeanness' that would ensure the strength of the white polity.

Chapter 4 discusses how the role of the state was recast to include responsibility for the health of its citizens, thus obliging it to offer medical and welfare services. I examine the gradual segregation of medical institutions for the treatment of VD, and the way in which health education defined normal sexuality for men and women and tied normality to white identity.

Chapter 5 analyses the incidence of VD in the African population between 1920 and 1950, focusing particularly on the impact of migration on rural and urban populations. If endemic syphilis provided immunity against cross-infection with venereal syphilis in the late nineteenth century, from the 1920s there is clear evidence of the impact of venereal syphilis in urban and rural communities. I try to temper this analysis with a sensitivity to African controls on migrant sexuality.

Chapter 6 focuses on VD in Africans and 'loose town women'. I suggest that the concern about African women's behaviour reflected a fear that the uncontrolled influx of women into the towns would lead to the collapse of the traditional rural order and male authority, and prevent the creation of a stable moral order in urban areas. I show how medical explanations of Africans' susceptibility to VD drew on anthropological analyses of Africans to suggest that the normal African was pathological and predisposed to disease.

From 1920 Africans were subject to the same health legislation as whites, but as Chapter 7 shows it was implemented differently. African health was initially important only insofar as it affected the labour supply. Africans in urban areas were monitored through the pass system, and those with VD were institutionalised or sent back to rural areas. Medical intervention was largely associated with repressive, public displays of state power, rather than with the normalisation of sexual and moral identity. In the late 1930s and 1940s local urban authorities began to introduce a clinic and education system based on the white model, reflecting their concern about the health of the permanently settled urban population. The new welfarism was still repressive, but some education programmes began to recognise Africans as individuals with a moral conscience.

Finally, Chapter 8 examines the socioeconomic conditions that have facilitated the spread of HIV, and discusses the way in which perceptions of this modern epidemic in the 1980s were shaped by contemporary white fears about the decline of white political and economic supremacy.

1
Tracking Down the Treponema, 1880–1910

'The natives are to be divided in three classes, of which the first has had the disease [syphilis], the second one has got it, and the third one will get it.' So reported the district surgeon of Carnavon in 1886.[1] His view was representative of the Cape Colony district surgeons, Transvaal doctors and administrators of the time. 'A wave of syphilis', remarked another doctor, 'has overtaken the Colony'.[2]

Studies of other colonial societies in Western Canada, Malaysia, Bengal and Australia point to the role of traders, sailors, police, soldiers, slaves and migrant workers in the introduction of STDs.[3] This is true for South Africa as well. Sexually transmitted syphilis was undoubtedly introduced into South Africa by European settlers, sailors and soldiers. It is questionable whether the disease was transmitted widely enough by the early 1880s to create the rural epidemic that doctors believed existed. In this chapter I argue that the symptoms and epidemiology of this disease were more representative of another treponemal disease: endemic syphilis, which is spread though non-sexual contact.

Endemic syphilis was probably indigenous to South Africa, but confined to small or isolated groups. The opening of the mineral fields and the development of mining towns brought together huge numbers of people. Prostitution helped transmit venereal syphilis, and the crowded and dirty living and working conditions at the mines and in the slums provided an ideal environment for endemic syphilis to spread. The migrant labour system then facilitated the transmission of venereal and endemic syphilis to new regions, and into communities without previous exposure to the disease.

Despite the different clinical appearance and epidemiology of venereal syphilis and endemic syphilis, during the late nineteenth and early twentieth centuries doctors continued to insist that the disease they witnessed in patients was transmitted sexually. Their views were shaped by contemporary medical knowledge, but especially by the racial views of the time.

The incidence of syphilis

From the 1880s the governments of the Cape Colony and the Transvaal Republic began specifically to request information from district surgeons about the extent of syphilis. Their reports are impressionistic and anecdotal, but still capture the astonishing incidence of what doctors believed to be venereal syphilis. The Barkly West district surgeon reported in 1883 that he had treated 1140 patients after opening a free dispensary with outstations in the reserve. Patients came from Taungs, Kuruman, Sivonels, Douglas and Hart's River for treatment.[4] The Bedford district surgeon estimated in 1885 that 'one in every three of natives is afflicted' and warned that syphilis was 'ravaging the district in its most malignant and loathsome forms. There is hardly a farm which is not infected.'[5] Two years later, to establish the extent of the disease in the ward of Baviaanse River he examined 2044 Africans, of whom 1122 were found to be syphilitic.[6] Oudtshoorn's district surgeon treated 1074 patients in 1882 and 1003 the following year.[7] In Richmond the district surgeon felt that it was no exaggeration to say that 'two-thirds of the coloured inhabitants are affected with this loathsome disease'.[8] District surgeons claimed that the disease was 'very prevalent' among the Basutho, the Baralongs, Kafirs, Griquas and 'bastards'.[9] The worst affected areas were in the north-western Cape. In 1906 the medical officer of health (MOH) for the colony estimated that in Kuruman over a third of the population had syphilis, in Gordonia 70–80 per cent of the 'bastard' population had it, and in Mafeking, Vryburg and Taungs the statistics were 'scarcely credible'.[10]

Syphilis also affected the rural white population. In Cradock, by 1888 the extent of disease had become 'so serious . . . that many people refused to go to communion because they know people who were suffering from syphilis were there as communicants'.[11] And in Oudtshoorn the district surgeon believed that syphilis 'has circulated to such an extent that it has become dangerous to perform the common acts of everyday life, such as shaking hands, receiving money, etc. etc.'[12] The disease seemed to affect the poorer, white tenant farmers who were small stock owners, rather than landed proprietors, according to the district surgeons in Oudtshoorn and Beaufort West.[13] But the disease had also 'crept now into some of our most respectable families'.[14] There were also numerous cases where the disease had spread from African or coloured nurses to white families. In the south-western districts, which included Oudtshoorn, Mosselbay, George, Somerset East and Graaff-Rienet, 12 per cent of the poor white population was said to have syphilis, compared with 5 per cent in other areas.[15]

The disease was not confined to the Cape Colony. The district surgeon at Herbert claimed in 1885 that he had heard reports of the disease being present in the Transvaal and Orange Free State, and had learned that it had also 'existed for many years amongst the natives in the interior, even as far up the country as the Zambezi'.[16]

The hearsay about the extent of syphilis in the ZAR was confirmed by the replies of landdrosts and mine commissioners to a government circular of 1895 aimed at determining the extent of syphilis in the republic. In most districts syphilis was rare, but in the Waterberg, Zoutpansberg, Nylstroom and Middelburg districts it seemed to be widespread.[17] Medical officers' reports dated 1904 and 1906 indicate that syphilis was widespread in the northern and western Transvaal, but relatively rare in the eastern Transvaal. In the northern Transvaal doctors believed it was extensive among pauper Boers and 90 per cent of Africans.[18] It was also reported to be widespread in the southern regions of Southern Rhodesia (Zimbabwe) at the turn of the century.[19]

The most detailed reports about syphilis come from doctors' evidence to the Contagious Diseases amongst Natives Commission (CDC) of 1906, which tried to determine the extent of VD and suggest measures of control. A doctor from the Elim mission in the Northern Transvaal reported that '[t]he natives tell me that very often most of them in their kraals are infected. . . . In some parts you have one or two per cent, and in other parts eighty per cent.'[20] Pietersburg's district surgeon stated that eight out of ten of his patients consulted him about syphilis, and his colleague from Potgietersrust district estimated that 'nine out of ten patients' were syphilitic.[21] A German missionary who had established a hospital at Bochem in the 1890s especially to treat syphilitics thought that 'not less than 75% of the western tribes (Basuthos and Matabeles) were syphilitics'. He had treated 5000 cases between 1902 and 1906.[22] The CDC concluded that syphilis was 'very common' in the Pretoria, Western, Waterberg and Lydenberg districts, and 'very seriously prevalent' among the Basotho and Ndebele tribes in the west and south-west parts of the Zoutpansberg district. The Shangaan and Bavenda groups were comparatively free of syphilis.[23] This pattern continued during the following decade.[24]

Syphilis seemed to be relatively rare in the eastern Cape and Natal at the turn of the century. In the Native Territories district surgeons either failed to mention syphilis in their reports or stated that they saw only occasional cases. In 1908, cases of syphilis were still infrequently reported but in certain areas such as Idutwya, Libode, Mt Fletcher, Mt Frere, Mquanduli and Xalanga it was thought to be increasing.[25] In Natal, likewise, doctors felt that syphilis was not common. A survey of 37 magistrates and district surgeons in Natal and Zululand in early 1899 showed that 18 thought syphilis was uncommon among Africans, seven felt it was increasing, though they personally had not seen many cases, and 12 stated that they treated cases frequently, though not on the scale experienced in the Cape and Transvaal. A practioner in Ingwavuma, for example, had found only one case among the 7000 Africans he had examined and vaccinated for smallpox. In Umfolozi the district surgeon had seen only three people at his dispensary, while the Eshowe district surgeon saw one case a month.[26]

It is impossible to determine the precise extent of syphilis in the wider population as district surgeons served huge areas and were unlikely to speak the local languages, and Africans probably visited traditional healers in preference to a white doctor. Nevertheless the reports from the Cape and Transvaal reveal a sense of alarm about an emerging epidemic, while those from the Eastern Cape and Natal indicate no anxiety about the incursion of a new disease.

Prostitution, migrant labour and the military

The discovery of diamonds in 1867 in Kimberley and of substantial gold deposits on the Witwatersrand in 1886 marked the beginning of the transition of South Africa from an agricultural backwater to an industrial capitalist economy shaped by the mining industry and its dependence on cheap migrant labour. Roads and railways were built from the mines to agricultural districts and the ports. Thousands of men flooded to the mining camps in search of work.

Initially the Pedi, Shangaan and South Sotho predominated in the mining workforce. These groups had been engaged in voluntary migrancy for several decades – the Pedi and Sotho from the 1840s and the Tsonga from the 1860s – to earn cash for guns, ploughs and bridewealth.[27] However the colonial wars in the late 1870s and early 1880s, the alienation of land, declining peasant production, a series of environmental disasters (droughts, epidemics and the destruction of local game and forests) and the imposition of annual taxes to be paid in cash gradually forced growing numbers of men from southern Mozambique, the eastern Cape and Natal into paid work.

From 1871 to 1875, between 50 000 and 80 000 Africans worked in Kimberley each year.[28] The rapid expansion of the gold industry resulted in the growth of Johannesburg from a tented town of 3000 inhabitants in 1887 to a city of 100 000 by 1896 and over a quarter of a million by 1914.[29] In 1889 almost 10 000 men worked in the mine industry and by 1892 their number had increased to 25 800.[30] In 1903–4 there were 77 600 African mineworkers, rising to 207 900 in 1910.[31]

The mining communities were predominately male. This population imbalance helped create a market for prostitution and ensured that STDs spread fairly rapidly. In Kimberley's white population, in 1877 the ratio of women to men was 3:5, declining to 4:5 by 1891. Among 'all others' the ratio was 17:100 in 1877 and 38:100 in 1891.[32] In Johannesburg an 1896 census reported that the white population consisted of 25 000 men and 14 000 women, a ratio of 1.8:1. In the black population, with 54 000 men and almost 3000 women, the ratio was even more extreme at 18.5:1, rising to 63:1 in the mining areas around Johannesburg and 98:1 in the case of men aged 25 to 39.[33]

The mining towns supported a thriving population of prostitutes. The first prostitutes at the Kimberley diggings were mostly Cape coloured and white women, the residual product of Cape commercial development, who operated alone but attached themselves to canteens and hotels with the support of the owners. When the railway from Cape Town reached Johannesburg in 1892, a stream of prostitutes left Kimberley for Johannesburg and local officials soon appealed for government assistance to deal with these women, whom they believed were spreading VD. From the mid 1890s prostitution in the Witwatersrand was controlled by organised crime, with most women now living in brothels or controlled by pimps.[34] Locally born women were replaced by 'continental women' – victims of the white slave trade and of female unemployment and underemployment in Europe.[35] The brothels catered mainly to white miners, though some accepted black customers.

In Kimberley, black communities quickly grew up on the edge of the diamond mining camps. These settlements were a haven for off-duty workers, offering food, drink, dancing and sex.[36] Many of the women in the camps were Griqua, Kora or of mixed race,[37] whose families had lost their land, either through land speculation or, after a rebellion in 1878, through government confiscation. They were forced into waged labour at the mines, on white farms or as domestic servants.[38] Women of the poorest families or those without kin were most likely to engage in prostitution.

In Johannesburg in 1896, of the 1678 black women residents fewer than 2 per cent were married and few had formal employment because men dominated domestic work. Hence many women turned to brewing beer, which they had learnt in the rural areas, and entered temporary sexual relations with migrants, whose gifts supplemented their informal incomes.[39] Most of the women were recorded as Fingo, AmaXhosa and Zulu, reflecting the impact of a series of natural disasters in the eastern Cape and Transkei from the 1890s, which had also forced many men to migrate. Eales suggests that many of the women had travelled to the Rand in search of their spouses, while others had gone with their husbands and families and set up permanent homes.[40] Many of the women were Basotho. Some were from polygynous households and were probably cowives or junior wives, others had been abandoned by their husbands, who – to avoid inflated bridewealth payments – had seduced or eloped with them and never paid significant bridewealth. By 1911, 3000 women were recorded as absent from Basotholand.[41]

By the end of the century, doctors were drawing attention to the effect of industrial development on the spread of syphilis. District surgeons in Albany and Grahamstown noted that in their districts the disease had started at the ports and military stations and then spread inland, following the extension of the railway line and roads.[42] The district surgeon at Hopetown similarly maintained that among the white population, 'since the nearer approach of the railway works a larger number of primary sores have been seen'.[43]

Doctors increasingly pointed to the growing mining centres as the source of syphilis, and blamed returning migrants for importing the disease into rural areas. The MOH for the Cape Colony regularly reported that syphilis was exceedingly prevalent in Kimberley and large labour centres. The disease, he claimed, was 'spread by the class of coloured and native women engaged in the pursuit of prostitution', and then 'infected natives returning to their kraals, spread the disease, among their families in the native districts'.[44] The primary medical officer of Basutholand reported that 'prior to 1876 the disease was unknown in Basutoland. It was brought there by labourers returning from the Diamond fields', and later from Johannesburg.[45]

Reports from the Transvaal described similar routes of transmission. Even in districts where syphilis was rare, the few cases were usually linked to contact with Johannesburg or Pretoria, or prostitution at mines or along railway lines.[46] One doctor, when giving evidence to the

Contagious Diseases Commission, stated that in the Waterberg 'the tribes who had most to do with the whites were badly infected'. African witnesses from various settlements in Zoutpansberg emphasised the role that Kimberley had played. Lucas Molaba of Mpahlela's Location 'first saw it in 1884. It was brought by a man who came from Kimberley'. Chief Mohlaba of Haenertsburg maintained that the first case in his community was 'a native who came from Kimberley' and the second 'a woman infected by a Basuto from Johannesburg'. The commission concluded that 'its introduction appears to be of comparatively recent date, having usually been brought to the kraals by natives who had been to work at some mining centre, especially Kimberley, where . . . the disease is very prevalent'.[47]

In Natal, too, in almost every case the district surgeons associated the disease with migration and contact with the urban centres. The resident magistrate of Nkandla recalled that 'about two years ago a native who had been working in Johannesburg was reported to have come home infected with the disease and to have conveyed it to his wives and he and the women, three in number, were said to be very bad with it'. The district surgeon of Ngutu had treated very few cases, but in each one the carrier had come from either Johannesburg or Natal.[48] In Upper Tugela the district surgeon had treated two women, one of whom had been infected by a man who had contracted syphilis in Johannesburg, the other by a man infected in Ladismith.[49]

Doctors also blamed the military. The concentration of soldiers in garrison towns or temporary camps created an immediate market for services – fresh food, washing, and of course commercial sex. Garrison and port towns became a focal point for the transmission of STDs in the Cape Colony. Over 13 per cent of troops were hospitalised for VD between 1887 and 1896.[50] As British troops criss-crossed the country during the Boer War of 1899 to 1902, they too spread VD in their wake. British recruits underwent several health checks prior to and after conscription, but the examinations were often cursory. About 7000 men arrived in South Africa only to be immediately hospitalised.[51] About 6 per cent of soldiers (24 775 cases) were also admitted to hospital after contracting VD within South Africa.[52]

These soldiers consorted with women in the coastal towns where they were initially based. When the war began, Cape Town and Durban were flooded with Rand prostitutes, mainly European-born 'continental women' fleeing Johannesburg. Soldiers continued to find sexual partners once in the field. Boer women offered sexual favours to soldiers in return for money, medicine or other goods, or to prevent soldiers commandeering their livestock. Soldiers also sought liaisons with African women who sold beer and fruit to the soldiers or were employed as washerwomen by the army, despite the risk of 25 days' imprisonment.[53] The legacy of the war was not only burnt farms and displaced families, but also, complained local health officials, an increase in VD.[54]

Was the disease syphilis?

Today venereal syphilis, endemic syphilis and yaws coexist in Southern Africa. The agent that causes each syndrome is morphologically similar and the syndromes are largely clinically similar. Hence they are usually differentiated according to their epidemiology and certain clinical symptoms (see Appendix 1).

By the 1880s doctors understood the clinical features of venereal syphilis. A Parisian surgeon, Phillipe Ricord, had identified the three stages of syphilis in 1838 and his work had been translated into English ten years later. In 1858 Rudolf Virchow, a German physician and one of the founders of cell biology, had shown that syphilis was disseminated through the body to different tissues and organs even when it was not evident on the skin surface. Jonathan Hutchinson (1828–1913), an English surgeon, had identified the characteristics of congenital syphilis in 1861. Yaws was only just beginning to be recognised as an aetiological and clinical entity.

In the Cape Colony some doctors doubted that what they were seeing was syphilis as the disease did not follow the accepted stages of venereal syphilis. Most doctors said they never saw patients with the primary chancres or residual scars that were typical of primary syphilis. The district surgeon for Oudtshoorn commented in 1884 that despite his heavy case load of syphilitics, '[d]uring the whole year we did not observe a single primary sore'.[55] Numerous witnesses to the 1906 CDC concurred.[56]

The predominant manifestation of the disease was secondary lesions. These lesions sometimes resembled those of typical venereal syphilis, but the most characteristic symptoms, according to the Barkly West district surgeon, were 'moist sores in the throat and mouth, on the tongue and lips, under the armpits, and on the lower portions of the body', which were typical of endemic syphilis. The lesions could be extremely painful and '[s]ome went about merely covered by a blanket, unable to wear their clothes on account of the sores; others were confined to their huts totally incapacitated for work'.[57] Doctors frequently reported that the lesions destroyed the nasal bones and soft palate. The district surgeon from Herbert reported that ulcerating lesions in the alimentary canal could cause death by haemorrage, as could lesions in the genitals and anus.[58]

The typical tertiary symptoms were also absent. One doctor, recalling his practice in Potgietersrust in the late 1880s, said that tabes and general paralysis were absent in the African population, despite widespread cases of secondary syphilis.[59] Another Cape district surgeon remarked that he had come 'across no symptoms of tertiary syphilis amongst the crowd of Natives I treated some years ago . . . all the young children, who had [it] at the same time, have grown up healthy, with apparently no undermining of the constitution'.[60]

As is characteristic of endemic syphilis, the disease was widespread among children. In Colesberg the disease was 'most prevalent among young children'.[61] Similarly, in Waterberg in 1892 syphilis 'was practically congenital and all the children in the location were syphilised, also all the young girls who went down to carry water'.[62] In Oudtshoorn the district surgeon reported that of the 1839 white and black patients he had treated, 39 per cent were under the age of eight, 19 per cent were between eight and 20, and 42 per cent were over 20.[63] Yet congenital syphilis appeared to be absent. There were no reports of widespread spontaneous abortion, stillbirths or infertility, which might have been expected in cases of venereal syphilis. Rather, doctors frequently commented that healthy children were born to parents who were known to have had syphilis: 'the present generation of babies – there are swarms of them – [do not] suffer in appearance in [the] slightest from the fact that their parents are supposed to have had syphilis'.[64] Conversely, children often seemed to contract the disease even though their parents were healthy.[65]

In case after case, district surgeons agreed, the source of contagion was never 'immoral practices',[66] that is, sexual intercourse, as would be expected with venereal syphilis. The district surgeon of Knysna commented that 'a third of those brought under treatment are virgins, girls whose innocence is beyond doubt and children, some of whom are only a few months old'.[67]

Non-sexual direct or indirect contact with sufferers seemed to spread the disease, another indication of endemic syphilis. Jansenville's district surgeon noticed that 'wherever there are locations of Natives, syphilis spreads rapidly when one case exists, as the children all play together and so contract it from each other'.[68] Similarly, where white and African or coloured children played together, the disease was transmitted between them.[69] Many doctors recounted cases of how infection in one child quickly spread to other children in the family and the parents.[70] There were also endless cases where the disease had been passed on from African or coloured nursemaids or washerwomen to white families through the children.[71]

In the Cape Colony, doctors traced cases to 'kissing, using the same vessels for washing or drinking purposes, drying with the same cloth after washing' and 'using the same cup or spoon, foul linen, sheets, seat of privies'.[72] In country districts in the northern Cape, according to McArthur and Thornton, 'case-to-case infection without sexual intercourse is the method of infection which gives rise to the major portion of the acquired syphilis seen in these districts'. They too suggest that the disease was spread through common use of smoking pipes, eating and drinking utensils, clothing and bedding.[73] The district surgeon of Oudtshoorn suggested that the house tax was to blame, as overcrowding facilitated the spread of the disease.[74] Among poor whites, doctors similarly noted that the disease was transmitted via unclean drinking utensils and by children sharing a bed.[75]

Contemporary medical surveys also offer corroboratory evidence for the existence of indigenous endemic syphilis. Serological sampling in Rhodesia (now Zimbabwe) in the 1950s revealed syphilis positivity rates ranging from 20 per cent to 75 per cent in southern rural areas.[76] At the turn of the century this area had experienced an epidemic of syphilis attributed to the disruption that followed the wars of conquest and rebellion in the 1890s, and to migration to Kimberley and the gold mines.[77] The disease was identified as endemic syphilis, with characteristics similar to those which doctors had witnessed in the Cape Colony and the Transvaal in the late nineteenth and early twentieth centuries. In the late 1950s the World Health Organisation conducted a survey and mass treatment programme in the Bakwena Reserve in Bechuanaland Protectorate (Botswana). There the seropositivity rates ranged from 25 per cent to 64 per cent in the southern regions. The clinical manifestations of the disease were again similar to those described in South Africa 70 years before.[78] Between the 1950s and 1970s four outbreaks were reported in the eastern and northern Cape, numerous Karoo towns and an area outside Bloemfontein.[79] Yet again the characteristics of the disease were the same. Belatedly a pathologist, coauthor of the report on Bechuanaland, reevaluated the historical evidence for the Cape and concluded that the disease had been endemic syphilis.[80]

Paleopathologists have also identified signs of a yaws-like disease in skeletal remains dating from AD 1000–1300 at Iron Age sites close to the borders with Botswana and Zimbabwe.[81] Another study found evidence of yaws in collections of Bechuana-Tswana, Zulu and Griqua skeletons from the eighteenth and nineteenth centuries.[82] Endemic syphilis was probably indigenous to a region stretching from what is now southern Zimbabwe and southern Botswana, through the northern and north-western Transvaal and the northern Cape and Cape interior.

There is also linguistic evidence that African communities were well aware of the difference between venereal and endemic syphilis. A district surgeon from Hebron commented in 1889 that '[t]he Natives themselves do not look upon the disease as venereal. They have a word meaning venereal disease, which they apply to gonorrhoea and chancres on the penis, but they do not apply it to mucous tubercle, but another word signifying "the sores".'[83] Likewise a doctor in the Mount Fletcher area reported that 'if you were to say to Natives that "ukwekwe" and syphilis are the same disease, they would probably smile at "the white doctor's ignorance" and would point out ... [t]hat syphilis is quite a comparatively recent imported disease, whereas "ukwekwe" has been with them for generations'.[84]

African communities where endemic syphilis was widespread were easily able to tell the difference between that and venereal syphilis, suggesting a long acquaintance with endemic syphilis. One doctor's African informants told him that 'syphilis is a disease more prevalent amongst grown-up people than children, whilst "ukwekwe" is the contrary; ... that syphilis is hereditary – not so "ukwekwe" [and] ... that syphilis is a serious disease, difficult to cure, whilst "ukwekwe" is a benign disease, which is cured by them'.[85] The district surgeon of Hebron reported that Africans 'look upon "the sores" much as they do upon measles, that once the disease is cured it is over and done with'[86] – an observation also made by a missionary near Zoutpansberg.[87] The CDC reported that Africans did not associate the disease with 'impure sexual connection'.[88]

In Natal the records seem to suggest that venereal syphilis predominated and that the disease was connected with the incorporation of Zulu speakers into the migrant labour force. A Natal district surgeon reported that 'Native words interpreted by some to mean syphilis describe evils popularly supposed to befall those indulging in illicit or impure intercourse.'[89] Syphilis was called *isifo sabelungu* (disease of white men) or *isifo sedolopi* (disease of the town), which captured the connection between migration, sex in towns and venereal disease.[90] Doctors' descriptions of syphilis in Natal are typical of venereal syphilis, and several reports describe the treatment provided for the initial chancre of primary syphilis and to the wives of infected men, and also mention the stillbirth or death of infants with congenital syphilis.[91] Cases of endemic syphilis are mentioned less often, and are usually related to the arrival at a kraal of a child from outside Natal, in one case from Johannesburg, or to the infection of white children by their African male nurses.[92] In Natal, venereal and endemic syphilis probably coexisted, but the Zulu-speaking inhabitants may not have recognised this, perhaps because cases of endemic syphilis were infrequent.

Doctors' failure to differentiate between endemic and venereal syphilis makes it difficult to assess the extent of the latter in the African population, but some idea may be gained from a comparison with the incidence of gonorrhoea. In the Waterberg area, where endemic syphilis was widespread, the district surgeon of Louis Trichardt reported that gonorrhoea was 'not so common amongst the natives', an opinion shared by his colleague in Nylstroom. Many district surgeons felt that syphilis – that is, endemic syphilis – was the only STD evident in the rural African population.[93]

Gonorrhoea also seemed to be infrequent among Africans in urban areas. The medical superintendent of Rietfontein Lazaretto believed that 'compared with syphilis, soft chancres and gonorrhoea are of comparatively infrequent occurrence'.[94] Between 1904 and 1906, admissions of Africans to the lazaretto for treatment for gonorrhoea averaged around 2 per cent of the total hospital population, compared with 25–50 per cent for syphilis, and these rates were well below those for whites.[95] One medical officer at the Witwatersrand Native Labour Association (WNLA), who was responsible for examining jobseekers at several mines, likewise thought that gonorrhoea was practically non-existent.[96] Doctors did identify cases of primary syphilis, but the incidence was low. Another medical officer for the WNLA thought that he had stopped 0.5 per cent of jobseekers because of syphilis.[97] The medical attendant for the compounds of the Johannesburg Municipality reported that he had identified eight primary cases in 1904–5 out of a population of 11 363 (0.07 per cent), and the following year he had diagnosed 26 primary and early secondary cases of syphilis in a population of 14 965 (0.17 per cent).[98] Of course the mines were more concerned about the quantity than the quality of labour, so these statistics are likely to be far from accurate.[99] However the low incidence of primary syphilis and gonorrhoea among several institutional populations (the mines, the compounds and in the lazaretto) contrasts strikingly with the reports of a syphilis epidemic, and seems to suggest that the incidence of

sexually transmitted diseases in the African population was still relatively low.

Endemic syphilis and migrant labour

Researchers studying endemic syphilis in the trans-Kalahari populations
have concluded that the disease has been present for a long time, and
that desert dwellers act as a reservoir from where the disease filters
into the settled agricultural populations.[100] A similar process may have
occurred a century ago. When the district surgeon of Swellendam
discovered a few isolated cases of syphilis in 1887 he attributed it to
servants who had been brought in from the Karoo, which seems to
suggest that the disease already existed in the hinterland.[101] The district
surgeon at Herbert similarly believed the disease had been 'brought
from the interior by natives seeking employment, or by refugees'.[102]

When population movement was limited, endemic syphilis remained
localised in hunter-gatherer groups or isolated villages. The opening of
the mineral fields and the development of mining towns brought huge
numbers of people together, some of them carriers of venereal syphilis,
others of endemic syphilis and others – those from the northern tropical areas – of yaws. Previous exposure to endemic syphilis or yaws
among Africans from areas in which the diseases were indigenous gave
them cross-immunity to venereal syphilis, and thus prevented its spread
regardless of their involvement in casual sexual relations. Africans from
areas untouched by endemic syphilis would have been susceptible to
both venereal and endemic syphilis.

Historical epidemiologists cite urbanisation as the key factor in the
transition from endemic to venereal syphilis. Urbanisation, they argue,
was accompanied by improved community and personal hygiene, and
the emergence of new social habits such as separate sleeping quarters
and the wearing of clothes that covered more of the body. These acted
as barriers to casual body contact among children, resulting in the
decline of endemic syphilis and yaws, the emergence of a virgin adult
population and the development of a strain of syphilis dependent on
sexual intercourse for transmission.[103]

However in the early colonial context urbanisation did not necessarily result in better community and personal hygiene. Slums were overcrowded, filthy and lacked any sanitation system. The living conditions
in compounds at the mines were also extremely poor. In Kimberley,
miners were crowded together in barracks that were sometimes so
overcrowded that workers slept on the floor or outside, and shifts

shared beds. On the Rand, barracks in the early compounds were so inadequately heated that on cold nights the occupants slept closely together.[104]

Although those Africans who were in closest contact with whites began to adopt European clothing, working miners were usually scantily dressed. The transmission of endemic syphilis was more likely in a group where much of the body was exposed, as was the case among children. Photographs of workers in Kimberley and the Witwatersrand show them wearing loin clothes. Between 1882 and 1886 the Kimberley mines forced Africans to work naked to prevent them from stealing diamonds and hiding them about their person.[105]

Conditions underground may also have facilitated the spread of endemic syphilis. Workers laboured closely together in narrow, poorly ventilated stopes for long hours. In 1931 Robinson Deep Mine experienced an outbreak of yaws among underground workers. The mine medical officer believed that the most probable point of infection was in the cages (closely packed lifts taking workers from the surface to the workface), and noted that abrasions were easily infected by contact with contaminated clothing. About 10 per cent of the workforce was affected by this outbreak.[106] At Spring Mines and Rand Gold Mines in the early 1940s workers developed florid treponematosis in the heat and humidity underground. Many of the infections began on workers' arms and backs, and the researcher attributed this to the drilling position, where two men braced themselves back to back in the stope. The incidence at these mines ran to 17 per cent.[107]

Medical authorities note that population density and the crowded, unsanitary conditions of village life have been conducive to the spread of endemic syphilis and yaws, both historically and currently. Similarly the sheer number of people living in the slums and compounds, and workers' close physical contact in their barracks and at work, might have enabled the skin-to-skin transmission of endemic syphilis. As with venereal syphilis, the migrant labour system may then have facilitated the spread of endemic syphilis into regions and communities without previous exposure to the disease. Certainly among the yaws cases occurring at Robinson Deep Mine, 19 men (7 per cent of the original 254 cases) returned home even though they were still potentially infectious.[108]

In many areas, especially in the Cape Colony, doctors described the disease as an epidemic, appearing suddenly, infecting many people virulently and then gradually dying out – a pattern that is typical of a new disease in an isolated virgin population.[109] In Barkly West in 1883 the district surgeon reported that a vast number of Africans were suffering from syphilis,[110] but by 1889 there were very few cases.[111] Likewise in Oudtshoorn, where the disease affected coloureds and poorer white tenant farmers, the district surgeon's reports between 1883 and 1895 describe a sudden outbreak and gradual decline of cases. In 1883 he treated 238 whites, but in 1895 only 12 cases came to his attention.[112] There is less detailed evidence of an endemic syphilis epidemic gradually becoming benign in the Transvaal, but the evidence is suggestive of this.[113] Epidemics of yaws, another form of non-venereal syphilis, have been documented in east, central and southern Africa.[114]

The epidemiological history of syphilis in the late nineteenth and early twentieth centuries is thus more complicated that would at first appear. Conquest, dispossession of land and the emergence of forced migrancy and commercialised sexual relationships certainly created a large population of men and women who were potentially vulnerable to venereal syphilis. But the unhygienic living and working conditions in urban communities may also have provided an opportunity for endemic syphilis to spread, and migrants then passed on the disease to their families and communities on their return home.

The scale of the endemic syphilis epidemic was astonishing, and most doctors recognised the irregular symptoms of the disease, yet they refused to accept the suggestion that the disease was not venereal syphilis. Their perceptions were shaped by limitations of medical knowledge at the time, but especially by prevailing ideas about race, sexuality and susceptibility to disease.

Syphilis versus yaws: the racial foundations of medical perceptions

Doctors seeing yaws for the first time in tropical colonial territories tended to identify it as scrofula, leprosy or, most frequently, syphilis. Medical orthodoxy in Europe and America held that blacks had a racial tendency to syphilis and were 'a notoriously syphilis soaked race'.[115] In this context doctors' confusion about the exact nature of the syphilis epidemic was understandable.

A district surgeon from Herbert thought that the disease was yaws, as occurred in the West Indies.[116] His views were supported by the district surgeon from Barkly West, who noted that the disease both resembled and differed from typical syphilis and yaws and defined the disease as a new one, which he called 'mucous tubercle'.[117] Their conclusions were supported by only a few district surgeons, though the medical officers of health for Basutoland and the Colony accepted that the disease was not spread sexually.[118] The CDC felt 'unable to associate ourselves with this view'.[119] The consensus of the medical profession from the 1880s was that the disease was syphilis.[120] Most doctors' perceptions of the apparent epidemic of syphilis were shaped by the prevailing racial ideas, which in South Africa, as in Europe, had begun to rigidify.

In the Cape, from the early nineteenth century racial ideas were shaped by a liberal and humanitarian optimism about the common humanity of Africans and whites and the belief that acceptance of Christianity and the individual work ethic was the key to the inevitable progress and assimilation of individual Africans into civilised European society.[121]

By the late nineteenth century, recurrent frontier wars had led to a loss of faith in the assimilationist project within the administration, even among the liberal 'negrophilists'. The ascendancy of settler power meant that the reconstruction of the African polity would be based on the administration's alliance with the traditional rather than the assimilated African elite. The new ethos saw in African tradition a source of stability and also, by circumscribing the right to land, facilitated the creation of a labour force for the mineral fields. These policies were shaped not only by the changing socioeconomic terrain, but also by new scientific ideas about the biological basis of race.

The emerging racial 'science' drew its strength from the new sciences of comparative anatomy, physiology and the theory of evolution. Phrenology, the study of skull shape as a determinant of abilities and character, had been taken up by British settlers in the Cape who maintained contact with leading British theorists during the 1820s and 1840s.[122] By the 1880s racial capacities were seen as fixed and as determining social customs, and history was reinterpreted in racial terms. Evolutionism now described how struggle, competition and survival occurred between racial types during their rise from barbarism to civilisation. Applied to European cities, the theory seemed to explain how urbanisation and industrialisation had caused both the natural division into classes and the degeneration of the working class.[123] Applied to the colonies, social Darwinism described the decline of indigenous populations in New Zealand, Australia, Southern Africa and North America. These 'lower races' were the least evolved or least fit in the competition for survival with the 'civilised races', hence their natural extinction unless the civilised races became their perpetual guardians.[124]

In his study of Victorian Cape Town, Vivian Bickford-Smith shows how these ideas seeped into local political and social discourse. The wars against Africans in the eastern Cape and Natal between 1877 and 1879 were reported as a struggle for the supremacy of race, and the colonial victories were seen as proof that the white 'race' was to be the governing class. From the mid 1870s English and Afrikaans journals and newspapers published local articles and reprints from metropolitan journals about inferior African intelligence, the difficulty of inculcating civilised values into barbaric people, and the importance of preserving African customs and limiting interaction between Europeans and Africans.[125]

Racial theories also led to new perceptions of the poor. By the 1880s ethnicity had become the key to defining the difference between the 'deserving poor' and the 'residuum'. The deserving poor were regarded as poor through no moral fault of their own, deserved some relief from the state and were regarded as white. The residuum were believed to be inherently poor due to degeneration during generations of exposure to a debilitating urban environment, were racially inferior and were regarded as coloured or African.[126]

The focus of doctors' blame for syphilis was primarily people of mixed race. In a period in which ideologues and policy makers were turning against assimilation, and ever increasing numbers of whites, Africans and coloureds were heading for the mine-fields and thus coming into greater contact with one another, medical discourse on syphilis highlighted the dangers of intimate racial interaction by pathologising people of mixed race. By the 1880s it was Hottentots, Bushmen and 'half-castes' that doctors blamed again and again for the spread of syphilis.[127] The cause of the preponderance of syphilis and its strange symptoms in this group, doctors believed, was racial degeneration and racial promiscuity. In contrast they frequently noted that syphilis was either absent or less virulent in 'pure' Africans.[128] This probably reflected the relative novelty of large-scale migrancy, but doctors maintained that it was a sign of racial purity. The district surgeon at Cathcart reported in 1886 that he saw few cases of syphilis among Africans. 'This comparative immunity from venereal disease', he explained, was 'due . . . in the first place to the fact that our natives are pure Kafirs, Fingoes and Tembus, not of mixed race'.[129] The district surgeon at Carnavon reported that the 'AmaXhosas are clean, and only intermarry amongst themselves, not mixing up with the bastards, Bushmen and Hottentots who are mostly the bearers of the disease'.[130] When syphilis was found in 'pure' Africans, doctors blamed contact with white towns, assimilation and the social and sexual intermingling of different races. A resident of Ladysmith believed that the few cases of syphilis occurred 'mostly among the more educated part of the native (Kaffir) population' due to their 'being in constant contact with the white and coolie population'.[131]

The conviction that races were biologically different added weight to the earlier theory of 'hybridisation', which held that while similar races could mix beneficially, the social or sexual mixing of different races would cause degeneration.[132] Since at least the 1830s the *South African Quarterly Journal*, the local mouthpiece for phrenologists, had blamed the decay of the Bushman race on interracial mixing and civilised life.[133] By the late nineteenth century, being 'half-caste' was a sign of degeneracy, licentiousness, immorality and racial decay. A series of books published from the 1880s applied Social Darwinist ideas to the Cape context and identified people of mixed race as most likely to become degenerate. One writer described the 'bastard Hottentots' of the western Cape as examples of 'racial retrogression' due to the human tendency to 'absorb the bad and neglect the good'. Olive Schreiner, a novelist with socialist and anti-imperialist sympathies, described in 1896 how 'half-castes' 'unite the vices of all races' and filled the gaols, brothels and lock hospitals of the colony.[134]

In the Cape, many doctors regarded people of mixed race as inherently licentious. From the eighteenth century Hottentots were commonly portrayed as the lowest of the savage races whose skin colour and physique were signs of natural lascivity and sexual degeneration.[135] The district surgeon at Port Nolloth blamed syphilis on 'a system of general and promiscuous sexual intercourse much in vogue amongst the native hottentots'.[136]

Although doctors excluded 'pure' Africans as the origin of syphilis, many still believed that, being lower down the evolutionary scale, Africans were inherently promiscuous, and thus once the disease entered a community it would spread rapidly. A district surgeon in Richmond reported that local inhabitants were 'simply rotten' with syphilis due to a 'system of promiscuous intercourse among the coloured people'.[137] Another district surgeon suggested that although 'as a rule there is no professed prostitution', syphilis nevertheless spread as 'it is all done clandestinely', again defining all Africans as promiscuous and diseased.[138]

Doctors explained the existence of endemic syphilis in the white population differently. Many of the poor whites were Dutch-speaking, and since the turn of the century, the English had tended to view them as a cruel, immoral people who had regressed into barbarism due to their close association with the indigenous inhabitants and too great a distance from civilisation.[139] But doctors did not seem to regard the race of the Boers as an explanatory factor for syphilis. Some doctors held to the general medical wisdom of the time: that the climate in the colonies affected the symptoms of and cures for diseases.[140] Others drew on earlier explanations of poverty whereby the poor were assumed to be morally responsible for their own poverty, choosing to live in dirty, overcrowded homes, refusing to find work because they were workshy, and by implication choosing immorality.[141] Some local authorities, according to the parliamentary member for Malmesbury, believed that 'the loafer, the man who runs about the street . . . is the cause of it all [spreading syphilis]'.[142]

Most frequently doctors associated syphilis in the white population with poverty. The district surgeon of Barkly West reported that only 'white people of dirty habits contract mucous tubercle'.[143] Dirtiness was also significant in the spread of syphilis among Africans. But as the district surgeon at Humansdorp put it, 'their dirty habits and the crowded state in which they live' was a 'condition of the life of the natives', a belief that many also held about coloureds.[144] The implication was that dirty habits were an inherent characteristic of blacks, whereas among whites they were learnt habits that could be corrected. By the 1880s in Cape Town white ethnicity had become a potentially uniting discourse in local politics, and English and Afrikaans journals and books stressed their common whiteness and racial superiority.[145] It was poor whites' poverty rather than their racial heritage that explained why they contracted syphilis, thus fitting in with the new racialised perceptions of poverty.

When white women were blamed for spreading syphilis it was their status as prostitutes, rather than as whites, that was regarded as significant. Prostitutes, both white and black, were part of the residuum – licentious and degenerate. In 1895 the district surgeon and medical inspector of the CDPA Act in Wynberg described prostitutes as a 'class of female' who were 'drunken, dissolute and devoid entirely of all shame'.[146] Women involved in prostitution, reported the *South African Medical Journal* in 1897, are 'the most worthless variety of women, the degenerates or criminals, and the idle, the mercenary and shameless of the working classes'.[147] However by 1906 ethnicity had begun to shape even the definition of a prostitute. One reformer explained that European prostitutes were 'very particular about cleanliness', but among 'coloured women, where the disease originates, it is impossible for the police to draw a line between the coloured prostitutes and other coloured women'.[148] For observers of the time, white prostitutes and respectable poor or middle-class women were worlds apart, but African and coloured women were all promiscuous and potential carriers of syphilis.

Syphilisation and segregation: the beginnings of a new discourse

Fritz Shaudinn and Erich Hoffmann identified the spirochaete in 1905, but this did not clarify the relation between yaws and syphilis. The same year Aldo Castellani discovered that the spirochaete that caused yaws was indistinguishable from that which caused syphilis when examined under the microscope, and later both diseases were found to test positive with the Wasserman test. Medical authorities such as Jonathan Hutchinson continued to define yaws as syphilis modified by race and climate. When he visited South Africa in 1902 he assured the colonial secretary that the cases of yaws he saw were 'nothing but native syphilis'.[149] At the end of the decade his views were still widely accepted by doctors in South Africa.[150]

The debate over whether the widespread syphilis in South Africa was in fact yaws reemerged in the medical community in 1910. Doctors now focused on Africans as a homogeneous group, creating a notion of 'the African' as diseased, and as inherently different from whites. At the medical congress in 1910 an MOH for the Cape Colony (E. N. Thornton) and the district surgeon at Taungs (D. C. McArthur) reported their findings on syphilis in the Taungs–Vryburg–Kuruman region. They noted that 'syphilis in Natives is by no means so typical as in Europeans. . . . There is rarely the usual sequence of symptoms.'[151] All the doctors attending the session agreed with them. Africans, they insisted, experienced 'true syphilis . . . in a mild form'.[152]

Firstly, they noted that skin colour altered the presentation of syphilis. Secondly, they blamed Africans for not seeking medical attention promptly.[153] Thirdly, they increasingly looked to African culture, rather than racial ancestry, to explain the extent of syphilis and the strange symptoms. A doctor in the Transkei rejected the possibility that syphilis could be yaws, as then 'the rarity of syphilis among such an immoral people [would] seem so extraordinary for belief'.[154] A Swiss medical missionary at Elim hospital in the Transvaal thought that in Zoutpansberg, where whole tribes were infected by syphilis, 'the promiscuous and communal habits of the natives' were to blame,[155] while a district surgeon from the western Transvaal similarly stated that 'immorality among these Kaffirs is dreadful' and 'legal marriage almost non-existent'.[156] The government officer in Waterberg and Zoutpansberg likewise blamed the poor morals of Africans.[157]

However McArthur and Thornton did not think that the disease was transmitted by sexual intercourse and did not accept that gross immorality existed among natives, as despite the greater licence enjoyed by wives and unmarried adults than was acceptable by European moral standards, 'examination of many young adult females has shown that virginity is the rule'.[158] In line with the new germ theory of disease, they sought an explanation based on the behaviour of the pathogen in the African body. Africans, they argued, were 'syphilised' and the disease was spreading through 'hereditary taint', transmissible to all generations. The strange manifestations of the disease were thus examples of 'late-heredo syphilis'.[159]

Their theory of 'syphilisation' seems to have been widely accepted. An MOH on tour in Middelburg district reported that '[w]ithout the acceptance of the theory of syphilisation even the healthy and natural lives led by these natives is insufficient to account for the mildness of the symptoms and the low contagiousness of the disease among them'.[160] The MOH for the northern Transvaal reported in 1913 that in Waterberg and Zoutpansberg

The natives seem to be so saturated with the virus of the disease that the toxins seem to have much less action on them than is the case with the white man. I suppose having their fathers and grandfathers as syphilitics and inheriting it, and then again acquiring it when they grow up, the poison has by now gradually decreased in virulence until today it is very mild in action compared with a European.[161]

In Mafeking too, a government officer reported that Africans had 'acquired, in process of time, a certain immunity so that the disease manifests itself in many instances in a mild form'.[162]

The theory of syphilisation resonated with the late-nineteenth-century view that blacks were inherently pathological and diseased.[163] With the decline of assimilationism, it was now more accepted that Africans were experiencing 'racial degeneration' due to contact with European influences and civilisation. McArthur and Thornton noted that even though the Bechuana had had the benefit of 'protective European government and guidance' and therefore 'a marked racial improvement might have been expected', in fact the reverse had occurred. The explanation, the authors concluded, 'clearly is that of a steady syphilisation of the community'.[164]

If Africans were 'syphilised' even in their natural tribal habitat, then exposure to civilisation was especially dangerous, doctors figured. Africans' susceptibility to tuberculosis was attributed by mine doctors to inadequate cultural adaptation to urban life.[165] In a similar vein McArthur and Thornton believed that 'the Town Native of either sex has every inducement to lose restraint, becomes usually thoroughly immoral, and consequently, is frequently affected by sexual disease'.[166] Several of their colleagues agreed.[167] Other doctors believed that contact with civilisation, even through the medium of Christianity, resulted in syphilis, as evident from its apparent prevalence among the educated Christian elite. Alfred John Gregory, MOH for the colony, believed that 'in the Native districts . . . the degree of morality is in inverse ratio to the extent of their civilisation; because when the native becomes Christianised and the native checks to immorality are removed, they become very much more immoral'.[168] These observations did hold some truth. Controls over adolescent sexuality among Christian Africans had begun to break down, and migrants did visit town prostitutes who used sexual relationships to supplement their income from brewing beer.[169] But the belief that Christianity and civilisation resulted in the demoralisation of Africans also reflected the growing idea that the civilised African was an anomaly. Africans were basically tribal, and could only ape the etiquette and polish of civilisation. If they relinquished their tribal customs, then all restraints on sexuality disappeared.

Doctors' new concerns with the nature of African culture, rather than with racial evolution, hybridisation and racial purity, mirrored the emergence of segregationist ideas about native policy during the reconstruction period after the Boer War. In 1903 the South African Native Affairs Commission, which attempted to create a common, federation-wide native policy, concluded that

civilisation has a demoralising tendency as its first effect upon primitive races. It is clear that the Native year by year is becoming familiar with new forms of sexual immorality, . . . and that his naturally imitative disposition, his virility and escape from home and tribal influences provide a too congenial soil for the cultivation of acquired vices.[170]

The Commission thus defined 'the African' as an overly sexual, naturally primitive, tribal and rural being whose exposure to urban life led to racial degeneration. It pinned its hopes for the 'elevation of the

Native races' on extending Christianity, formalising territorial separation and approval of segregated locations for Africans.[171]

Not every doctor accepted the theory of syphilisation, but the
dissidents were very few.[172] A district surgeon in Schweizer Reneke
openly contested the notion that Europeans and Africans experienced
the same diseases differently. He reported that lesions 'as seen here
amongst Europeans . . . differ in no respect from those in the case of
natives'.[173] He concluded emphatically that in 'the whole history of
medicine there is no evidence to prove that any blood disease of Europeans can be altered fundamentally when coloured races are affected by
it. . . . [T]he disease so prevalent in these parts runs precisely the same
course in Europeans as it does in Natives.'[174] A doctor in the Mount
Fletcher district in the Transkei suggested the cause of the disease was
a lack not of morals but of hygiene. He noted that the 'disease is more
prevalent amongst the raw and savage Native than amongst the well-
to-do, which points to the fact that material prosperity and better
hygienic conditions have more power that I.K. [potassium iodide]
in checking the disease'. White communities were free of the disease
except where poor whites were 'to be found squatting amongst
the Natives in their locations' and thus shared the same unhygienic
conditions.[175]

These doctors were correct. However the idea that Africans and whites
were physiologically the same, or that the syphilis-like disease was no
reflection of the state of either African or poor-white culture or morality was difficult for most doctors to accept, given the racial assumptions
of the time. The notion of 'syphilisation' pathologised all Africans as
diseased and justified the growing conviction that 'the native problem'
could only be solved through segregation.

Conclusion

During the 1880s doctors became aware of an epidemic of syphilis in
the Cape interior, the northern Cape and the north-western Transvaal.
The outbreak coincided with the discovery of diamonds and gold and
the enormous increase in migrant labour. Venereal syphilis was
undoubtedly spread within mining towns through prostitution.
Furthermore the unhygienic living and working conditions in the
slums and the mines provided the right environment for endemic
syphilis to spread. And both diseases were introduced to rural areas
when migrants returned home. The epidemic of syphilis in the 1880s
is more likely to be a reflection of the poverty and lack of hygiene in

poor urban and rural communities than of a breakdown of traditional authority and controls over sexuality.

Although doctors recognised that the syphilis they were treating had different symptoms from venereal syphilis, they continued to identify it as the latter, largely because their perceptions of Africans and poor whites were moulded by contemporary ideas about racial difference. In the late nineteenth and early twentieth centuries medical discourse helped reinforce concerns about racial origins and development.

By the early twentieth century the concept of syphilisation had expanded to include all Africans, thus pathologising 'the African' as diseased and inherently different from whites. The construction of racial difference on the basis of culture rather than biology foreshadowed the onset of segregationist ideas and policies in the 1920s, as will be discussed in Chapter 6.

2
From Paupers to Pass Laws: Control of VD in the Cape and Transvaal, 1880–1910

The extent of the apparent syphilis epidemic in the 1880s called for urgent action, and this chapter examines government schemes to control the spread of VD in the Cape and Transvaal. Although these schemes evolved out of different political concerns, they each contributed to the emergence of a segregated society and created systems of detection and treatment that perceived and treated white and black patients differently. The schemes also shared an underlying approach to VD carriers as criminal offenders, rather than defining them as abnormal deviants, as occurred in the 1920s and 1930s.

In the Cape Colony the government introduced a Contagious Diseases Prevention Act (CDPA), modelled on British legislation. The aim of the Act was not simply to control prostitution in port and military towns, as van Heyningen suggests,[1] but also to control the spread of VD among the poor in urban and, especially, rural areas. The legislation did not differentiate between the white and black poor, reflecting the colony's liberal heritage, but in practice the way in which the Act was implemented complemented the move towards social segregation and reflected the emergence of more rigid racial ideas.

The Transvaal Republic also introduced legislation to control the spread of VD among the poor, but from the outset it explicitly differentiated between white and black, and – reflecting the significance of the mining industry in the economy – attempted to link the detection of VD cases to pass controls. By 1910 the Transvaal government had developed a system for the large-scale surveillance of the African population through a combination of missionary hospitals, regular rural and urban tours and pass laws. This was to be the basis of later schemes to detect and treat VD in the African population throughout the Union.

Origins of the Contagious Diseases Prevention Act of 1885

Until the 1880s the Cape Colony state, the parliament and the electorate had been relatively unconcerned about poverty or the need for philanthropy. The assumption was that the poor were to blame for their own plight.[2] The dominant classes were also relatively unconcerned about racial integration among the poor. By 1875 whiteness correlated with economic and political power, but segregation was not formalised in political, social or economic life. The assimilationist ethos that 'civilised' Africans deserved equal treatment meant that segregation had emerged along class rather than colour lines. In large towns such as Cape Town and Kingwilliamstown the poorer areas were racially integrated, and poor white children attended mission school along with African and coloured children. On Robben Island, paupers and lepers were not racially segregated, nor were hospital patients in general. Segregation was considered an unnecessary expense in institutions that wealthy whites were unlikely ever to use.[3]

However, as discussed in the previous chapter, during the 1880s the dominant classes began to differentiate between the 'deserving poor' and the 'residuum' along racial lines. The deserving poor were the respectable working class, and white; the rest were inherently poor due to degeneration and immorality.[4] Despite Robert Koch and Louis Pasteur's discovery in the 1870s that bacteria caused specific diseases, in the Cape disease was still associated with environmental factors such as overcrowding, the absence of sanitation, poverty, 'dirty habits' and implicitly with immorality and race. During the 1890s segregation was introduced in hotels, bars and trains.[5] State intervention was increasingly viewed as the way to improve the conditions of the deserving white poor: unemployment relief, whites-only education and residential segregation could rescue poor whites from their corrupting and dirty environments.[6] Removing Africans from the town, remarked the MOH, was a way to prevent 'uncleanly, half-civilised units' coming into 'intimate contact with the more cleanly and civilised portions of the community'. The metaphoric association between blacks and disease – the 'sanitation syndrome' – provided ready justification for segregation.[7]

It was in this context – in which the poor were increasingly seen as a health and moral threat – that public apathy about VD disappeared. Contagious Diseases Acts (CDAs) were first introduced in British colonial possessions to reduce STDs in the army by controlling the health of prostitutes.[8] The Cape Colony had introduced a CDA in 1868 under duress from the British War Office, but this had been withdrawn in 1872 because of local opposition.[9] By the 1880s the imperial naval and military authorities, local urban and rural medical practioners and the white public were keen to reintroduce a CDA.[10]

In discussions preceeding the CDPA, and in evidence to various select committees examining the Act thereafter, those who advocated the CDPA in port and military towns began with the assumption that prostitution was a 'necessary evil' that could not be prohibited but could be controlled, and so protect the chastity of respectable women.[11] They focused on prostitutes as the source of VD, portraying these women as part of the residuum – licentious and degenerate – while still suggesting, in line with older environmentalist explanations of disease, that removing the prostitute from her environment might redeem her. Regulation and treatment in a lock hospital, with its orderly, moral environment, would give prostitutes 'a chance of social reclamation' away from their 'immoral haunts'.[12] This implied that although prostitutes were part of the residuum, prostitution was still a moral choice that women could abandon for a new life.

In country districts, where, as suggested in Chapter 1, endemic syphilis was widespread, white inhabitants, fearing infection by their servants, petitioned the government to induce syphilitics to submit to treatment.[13] District surgeons were also keen for some kind of government action. The district surgeon at Herschel warned in 1884 that without government action, 'the Colony may become infected as the natives are not only a migratory race, but the labour market through a great part of the Colony is being supplied from Herschel'.[14] Landless peasants were leaving the area to search for work, and their number increased during the droughts and depression of the late 1870s and early 1880s.[15] In a similar vein, the district surgeon at Oudtshoorn complained that 'the coloured people are afflicted in all directions . . . and are allowed to roam about wherever they please, *carrying infection wherever they go*, and so this loathsome disease is allowed to go unchecked year after year'.[16] Doctors also worried about poorer white farmers who hired grazing land, 'and in trekking from place to place, being received into the farmhouses they pass, so spread the disease broadcast'.[17] Syphilis also contributed to pauperism as farmers tended to dismiss infected workers, who then, if obviously disfigured and unable to find work, resorted to theft, and only received medical attention when gaoled.[18]

The anxiety about syphilis did not initially spark off energetic measures to control the disease. The first Public Health Act (PHA) of 1883 placed the burden of responding to epidemics, including dealing with VD, on local boards of health, which were given rudimentary powers by Acts passed in 1881 and 1882.[19] A few local authorities did take their new health responsibilities seriously. For example in Caledon the divisional council and muncipality built a hospital for syphilitics.[20] Some district surgeons offered outpatient treatment, while complaining about the absence of isolation facilities. In Ladismith, for example, the district surgeon gave medicine to dismissed farm workers, but as there was no hospital the syphilitic patients lived on the commonage and wandered about, mixing with their friends working on the farms.[21]

These examples were the exceptions and most boards refused to take any action to control or treat syphilis. The district surgeons at Barkly West, Philipstown, Oudtshoorn and Aliwal North, for example, reported that their local boards were ignoring the problem or refusing to bear the expense of setting up even the most minimal treatment facilities.[22] Local authorities, explained the parliamentary member for Malmesbury, were unwilling for the 'landed proprietors' to bear the cost of funding a treatment scheme 'while the loafer . . . does not contribute'.[23]

In some areas local authority apathy reflected local tensions over land and labour. In the Barkly West district, the Kora and Tlhaping had lost their land after a rebellion in 1878, and by 1880 most were landless, taxed and dependent on waged labour on white farms or in the mines.[24] The district surgeon reported that local ratepayers were reluctant to fund any treatment scheme and 'openly advocate that the natives should be allowed to die off as fast as they possibly can, as a good riddance'.[25] He himself believed that Africans still had too much land and should be resettled 'to make medical access easier', and of course free further land for white settlement.[26] For him, public health measures could complement conquest and offered greater control over the African population.

This reluctance to fund pauper health care was part of the general antipathy to philanthropy that until the 1890s characterised the colony. However, many district surgeons and local authorities now felt that a formalised method of state intervention was necessary. Overwhelmingly the call was for strict legislation to compel syphilitics to place themselves under treatment.[27]

The Contagious Diseases Prevention Act, No. 39 was passed in 1885 without opposition. The CDPA aimed to deal with venereal disease among the poor – both black and white – and not just prostitutes. The 'great tradition' of Cape liberalism, which involved legal equality and colour-blind franchises, as well as the 'small tradition' of liberalism based on local political alliances between whites and wealthier blacks, still meant that despite more rigid racial attitudes, class but not racial legislation was acceptable.[28]

The CDPA was divided into two parts to deal with the problems of prostitution and VD in port towns and widespread apparent syphilis in rural areas. Part I provided for the registration, periodic examination and compulsory lock hospital treatment of prostitutes, and was largely similar to the 1868 Act and the British CDA. Part II empowered magistrates, after enquiry *in camera* and acting on a report by a medical inspector or district surgeon, to place syphilitics, whether male or female, under medical treatment. If they failed to place themselves under treatment, or were paupers, they were consigned to the care of a district surgeon. Local divisional and municipal authorities were responsible for establishing lock hospitals. The decision to apply Part II to men and women was probably due as much to fears that syphilis was epidemic in the African, coloured and pauper communities as to doctors' recognition that the syphilis that prevailed in rural areas seemed to spread quickly through family groups, though they were reluctant to recognise this disease as different from venereal syphilis. The assumption that entire indigenous and poor communities, rather than just prostitutes, were saturated with disease also shaped CDAs in other British colonies, such as India and Singapore.[29]

The cost of implementing the Act deterred the government from taking any action immediately, particularly as the colony had entered a depression in 1881 and government expenditure had dropped by half, only recovering at the end of the decade.[30] As before, some local authorities, especially in areas where endemic syphilis was rampant, acted on the intention of the Act and the PHA of 1883 and continued to fund their own schemes. However most councils continued to refuse to subsidise treatment for the poor.[31]

As the depression lifted, and following a parliamentary enquiry in 1888 into the extent of syphilis in the colony, the government decided to promulgate the Act nationally and transferred the implementation and funding of the Act from local bodies to central government, reflecting a new responsibility for philanthropy and public health. Part I was implemented in the seaports of Cape Town (including Wynberg and Simonstown), Port Elizabeth, East London and Kingwilliamstown, and in 1893 was extended to Uitenhage and Knysna, and in 1904 to Umtata. It was also extended to the Transkei, Griqualand East, Tembuland and St Johns River in 1892, but was never implemented. Part II was applied throughout the colony.

Purely in terms of expenditure and numbers it is too simple to confine examination of the CDPA to the prostitute population in scheduled towns. Though van Heyningen is correct to argue that the colony could not afford 'wholesale hospitalisation' of the rural poor,[32] it still intervened actively in rural areas to control the potential health threat to the poor. Between 1890 and 1920 the government spent between £3000 and £4000 per annum on implementing Part I and on average examined 623 women per year (see Appendix 2, Table A2.1). Government expenditure on Part II of the Act climbed from £8700 in 1891 to over £14000 in 1898. This covered the construction of many small lazarettos and the conversion of existing buildings, as well as in- and outpatient treatment. Expenditure remained at over £10000 per year during the Boer War years, and declined to about £9000 per year only after 1905 with the closure of several lazarettos and the shift to outpatient treatment.[33] The government still retained syphilitic wards or hospitals in 21 districts. The total number treated as inpatients or outpatients hovered around 2170 a year throughout this period (see Appendix 2, Table A2.2).

The CDPA marked a shift towards a more interventionist state, which despite its rudimentary bureacracy was willing to invest in health services. This shift was also reflected in the decision in 1891 to appoint Dr A. J. Gregory as a medical advisor and later medical officer of health to the colony. He virtually single-handedly created a medical department and pushed the PHA of 1897 through parliament to give the colony its first, modern, sanitationist health legislation, which was also used to remove Africans forcibly from Cape Town to a segregated location in 1901.[34]

Medicine and imperialism

The Cape British Medical Association believed that doctors should use their influence to promote 'civilised values', which by the 1880s were tied to an idea of Englishness and respectability.[35] With the medical community keen to emphasise its professional stature and expertise, civilised values, in their eyes, also implied an acceptance of medical authority, scientific medical concepts and treatment.

Doctors complained about 'ignorant persons' in the Dutch community who viewed syphilis as a harmless disease so that 'no notice is taken of it'.[36] This reflected the recognition by Dutch speakers that endemic syphilis in some communities was not particularly virulent, and that an infection generally resolved itself without intervention. District surgeons also reported that many rural whites avoided medical treatment and preferred to rely on home remedies of 'herbs and roots', not simply because it was cheaper and their malady remained hidden from public gossip, but also because they had more faith in these remedies than in professional treatment.[37] Farmers were also reluctant to send their labourers for treatment, preferring to treat them with home remedies.[38] To doctors, who were still diagnosing the disease as venereal syphilis, this opposition and apathy was an indication of the backwardness of the poorer Dutch.

District surgeons reported that as well as refusing 'scientific' treatment, the Dutch were ignoring circulars informing them about the dangers of syphilis and offering free treatment for paupers. The Oudtshoorn district surgeon pointed out that '[a]ny document in English is useless, and only thrown on one side', and recommended that the circulars be printed in Dutch. The Prince Albert district surgeon similarly pointed out that the Dutch 'quite ignore the notices sent to them to place themselves under treatment'.[39] However this may have simply reflected the high illiteracy rates in rural areas. In Cape Town in 1875, for example, a quarter of white children under the age of 15 could not read or write.[40] However linking acceptance of scientific medicine to civilisation and Anglicisation probably aroused antagonism in the Dutch communities, and their refusal to read the notices may have also reflected incipient ethnic nationalism.[41]

In certain areas farmers' unwillingness to report cases or support local treatment schemes was also linked to labour shortages. In many areas, by the 1890s black and white farmers were complaining about labour shortages, as landless peasants and migrants preferred to seek better-paid work in the towns or mines.[42] The district surgeon at Fraserburg complained that 'many of the farmers here . . . do not co-operate sufficiently with the Government. In this district labour is scarce and farmers are not always able to spare a shepherd or replace him.'[43]

Medical care for Africans was also seen in imperialist terms. In the mid-nineteenth century Governor Glen Grey had portrayed medicine as a way to win over frontier African communities.[44] Likewise missionaries, especially those attached to the Free Church of Scotland, valued medical care as a way to attract followers and combat the influence of indigenous healers. Medicine, they believed, complemented evangelism, and both led to the 'civilisation of the natives'.[45] Many doctors saw their role in these terms, and regarded the widespread treatment of syphilis as an opportunity to put their beliefs into action.

Some doctors complained, as they had about the Dutch-speaking poor, that Africans 'don't seem to think seriously of it'.[46] This may have reflected indigenous knowledge about endemic syphilis and many Africans preferred to consult herbalists or *nyangas*.[47] Other doctors reported that Africans tried to avoid hospitalisation. According to one practitioner, after three people died in a lock ward in Grahamstown, Africans 'got frightened, and say the hospital is the place where they kill people'.[48] Again, this was reasonable, since hospitals were unhygienic dumping grounds for the chronically ill, and patients often did succumb to cross-infection.

However in many areas, especially those newly stricken by endemic syphilis, Africans willingly experimented with new treatments. When Barkly West established a dispensary in 1883 the district surgeon hired an African interpreter, and over 1500 people attended his surgery for treatment. Families were willing to travel up to 120 miles for attention.[49] The district surgeons at Bedford, Kingwilliamstown and Taungs similarly mentioned that Africans voluntarily travelled long distances to seek free treatment.[50] The district surgeon at Glen Grey found that 'school natives' were willing to seek treatment but 'red natives' avoided him, fearing imprisonment.[51] This seemed to demonstrate the significance of Christianity and education in converting Africans to Western medicine and 'civilised' ideas. But he also noted that when the initially suspicious saw the benefits of treatment – lesions seemed to react quickly to mercurial ointments – they came willingly. He stressed the importance of avoiding coercion or demanding payment, as this immediately scared patients away.[52] For these administrators, missionaries and doctors, Africans' acceptance of Western medical ideas and treatment signalled their progress towards 'civilisation' and the fruits of assimilation.

Implementation of the CDPA: the criminalisation of VD

The CDPA also reflected new, harsher ideas about how to deal with people infected with VD. Despite the philanthropic intentions of the Act, it helped separate the poor from the wider society and transformed poor VD carriers into criminal offenders. The process of criminalisation was evident in the way in which cases of syphilis were detected and syphilitics were treated.

In many areas, groups of district surgeons, police and farmers swept their districts to cleanse them of infected Africans and coloureds. In Oudtshoorn the district surgeon reported that mounted police were 'occasionally employed in hunting them up', and so people left the district 'to avoid trouble to themselves'.[53] In Albany the district surgeon urgently requested a police inspector 'to hunt up cases from the low slums of towns and from the Hottentot and Native locations'.[54] In Sutherland, farmers organised search parties, which 'hunted out the natives infected and . . . caused them to be brought into the hospital . . . and there properly treated'.[55] Most farmers simply dismissed infected workers.[56] 'Fortunately for this district', reported the district surgeon at Alexandria, 'the landed proprietors in the different localities have taken the initiative and driven away syphilitic natives'.[57]

The state did not have the bureaucratic resources to mount a large-scale, methodical campaign to comb the coloured and African population for syphilitics. Nor did the CDPA grant district surgeons the power to enforce compulsory detention and treatment, as this would have been too expensive. Yet vigilante-like patrols were similar in intent to the sporadic, military campaigns that characterised colonial medical efforts elsewhere to control epidemics.[58]

The burden of medical inspections and registration under Part 1 also seems to have been largely borne by coloured and African rather than European prostitutes, an issue remarked upon by that was a visiting abolitionist but never taken up by Cape abolitionists.[59] It is difficult to assess the racial composition of the prostitute population, but by the turn of the century, with the influx of 'continental women', the prostitute population was regarded in official eyes as predominately white. The commissioner of police in Cape Town reported in 1902 that the city was home to 600 prostitutes, of whom only 100 were coloured. The rest consisted of 75 white women born in the colony, 25 from Britain and 400 'continentals'.[60] However the number of coloured prostitutes examined under the CDPA far outnumbered the white. Medical inspectors may have focused on particularly rowdy, publicly soliciting prostitutes, while those who could blend in with the white town population may have been more discreet and hence were tolerated. In 1891 in East London, for example, the lock hospital medical officer examined 137 women, of whom only 22 were European – the rest he described as Malays, bastards and Hottentots. This was not because few white prostitutes existed. Before the Act, 'white women used to openly solicit in the streets', he admitted, but they had become surreptitious and were more difficult to identify.[61]

The CDPA ruled that lay inspectors rather than the police should be used to find and summon women for inspection, an improvement the abolitionists had strongly urged as befitting a health law. But the legal requirement was not applied to both white and black prostitutes. In 1902 in East London, the notice for European prostitutes to attend an inspection was served by a white medical inspector, but African prostitutes in East London, Kingwilliamstown and Umtata were notified verbally by an African constable. This made the process of medical examination and registration a form of criminal surveillance rather than a medical safeguard.[62] The harsher attitude towards black women reflected the assumption that all poor women, but especially black women, were potential prostitutes and potentially diseased, and so required more stringent control.

The criminalisation of poverty and VD was also reflected in a shift from voluntary treatment in general hospitals to isolation and coerced treatment in lock hospitals. After the 1868 CDA, syphilitic patients continued to be treated in the general hospitals in Cape Town, Port Elizabeth, Grahamstown and Kingwilliamstown. This was the cheapest option favoured by most doctors, but also implied that VD patients were not regarded as outcasts. Only the governor of the colony advocated building separate lock hospitals.[63] He was in line with the trend in Britain, where, since the eighteenth century, general hospitals had gradually excluded various disorders and types of patient to protect the health and moral welfare of the other patients. By the 1880s most general hospitals in Britain had a rule against admitting VD patients, though a few beds were reserved for VD patients who were respectable and had financial support. Female patients, especially poor women and prostitutes, were sent to lock hospitals.[64]

By the 1880s in the Cape, medical opinion had also turned against treating VD cases in general hospitals, fearing, as the East London medical officer explained, that this would deter 'better class' patients from seeking treatment.[65] Wealthier whites who could afford private treatment were regarded by district surgeons as 'very respectable' despite their syphilitic infections.[66] The CDPA and lock hospitals were aimed at the poor – prostitutes and paupers.

The moral and physical reclamation of paupers required their isolation from an unsavoury environment, and discipline as well as treatment. So lock hospitals were usually built within or alongside gaols, reinforcing the association between poverty, criminality and disease. The Cape Town Lock Hospital, built in the late 1880s, was next to the Roeland street gaol and lay within the gaol wall. The Vryburg lock hospital, built in 1899, was near the goal and adjoined a leprosy ward, and both were surrounded by an eight-foot wall.[67] In most country districts paupers treated under Part II of the Act were admitted to gaol to isolate them from the general population, or to crude, temporary buildings alongside the gaol, established as lock hospitals and run by the local gaoler and gaol matron.[68] Some authorities recouped the costs of accommodation by putting syphilitics, when fit enough, to work with the gaol's hard-labour gangs.[69]

Not surprisingly, remarked the district surgeons of Willowmore, Carnavon and Herbert, Africans and coloureds were deterred from seeking treatment because they feared they would lose their liberty.[70] Africans regarded the CDPA as one more authoritarian measure amid the new taxes and laws, rather than as medical altruism. In Herschel in 1888, for example, the district surgeon summoned headmen to a meeting to report on the extent of syphilis in the district. Some headmen never arrived; others were extremely reticent about offering any information. According to the district surgeon:

> Some headmen remarked that the disease I was asking about had existed amongst them for years, that they had been left to treat themselves after their own customs hitherto, therefore why this interference of Government just now? That they had only recently been left to be killed by a fever. Government offered no help. But that, when the white people catch any sickness from us, then measures of relief are introduced all in a hurry. Others said . . . [t]his merely means more taxes. . . . Before we give you the information you ask we want to know who is to pay the costs. If we are to pay, we prefer to employ our own native doctors, as heretofore.[71]

When he began to confine syphilitics to the gaol hospital, he reported that '[s]ome of the natives have been influenced to boycott the lock wards altogether, being under the impression that they are nothing but prison cells, and that as they have not committed any crime through catching the disease they will not willingly give themselves up for detention in these gaol hospitals'.[72]

Lock hospitals and racial segregation

The CDPA criminalised VD among poor whites and blacks by linking treatment to isolation, imprisonment and punishment. Reflecting the gradual racialisation of poverty and philanthropy, government institutions also began to shift from informal segregation along class lines to enforced racial segregation.

In Cape asylums, initially the 'better class' and 'common' patients were housed separately. As class was the determining distinction, a few 'respectable' black patients were housed with white patients, while very violent or troublesome white patients were housed with coloured patients. As racial medical discourses emerged to explain and justify different treatment for white and black patients, segregation was introduced. By the 1890s all whites, regardless of class, were often housed together and received the same privileges, while respectable blacks were pushed into the lower-class black wards. Separate asylums for blacks and whites were built from the 1890s.[73] This shift had also occurred in juvenile reformatories and prisons by the 1890s.[74]

Initially lock hospitals were not racially segregated. In East London all women were confined to a room at the end of the gaol hospital ward.[75] Likewise in the Cape Town Lock Hospital, African, coloured and white women were housed together.[76] By the late 1880s, however, doctors were regarding the committal of the 'poorer class of European' to racially mixed wards as problematic[77] – as were poorer whites. One district surgeon reported that those who were 'too poor to procure medical advice privately . . . dread the reproach of being classed as pauper syphilitic patients along with the coloured persons who constitute the bulk of the Board of Health patients'.[78] By the late 1880s, to be treated as a pauper was a sign not only of moral failure and economic distress but also of being 'low class', and by implication 'not respectable' and similar to the black residuum.

Doctors began to request that wards be racially segregated. By 1904 the Cape Town and Port Elizabeth Lock Hospitals had separate wards for white and black patients, though they still had to share an exercise yard and latrines.[79] By 1907 Kingwilliamstown Lock Hospital also had separate wards for European and black patients.[80] White and black prostitutes in East London were inspected by the lock hospital doctor on different days.[81] District surgeons also requested money to build racially segregated hospitals for contagious diseases in country districts.[82] In a period when the poverty of whites was becoming a public and political issue and racial distinctions were being heightened in civil life, the different treatment accorded to white and black patients and the efforts to segregate lock hospitals helped affirm the differences between the black and white poor.

In summary, the CDPA reflected a new trend of government intervention in public health and philanthropy, reflecting widespread fears about the threat the poor represented to public health and morality.

Though the Cape Act did not differentiate according to race, in practice the way in which cases were detected and treated differed between white and black. This reflected the tendency to differentiate between the 'deserving poor' and the 'residuum' along racial lines and the growing segregation in social life and government institutions. The Act also stigmatised VD by associating poverty and disease with criminality. In the Transvaal, however, attempts to control the spread of VD gradually shifted from treating paupers to controlling the influx of diseased African workers into urban areas.

VD and pass laws in the Transvaal

The first legislation in the Transvaal aimed at controlling the spread of VD was linked to the control of labour rather than to the regulation of prostitutes and public morality. This reflected the centrality of the mining industry to the ZAR economy and laid the foundations of the government's attitude towards African health in the twentieth century. As in the Cape, the legislation arose out of a general perception that paupers, Africans and rural areas were untamed and diseased. As the legislation was refined, the government concentrated on monitoring the health of African workers and jobseekers.

By 1895, following a survey, the government had become extremely concerned about the extent of syphilis in the Transvaal.[83] The government passed the Contagious Diseases Law No. 12 of 1895, which laid down guidelines for dealing with syphilis, smallpox and tuberculosis.[84] The Act was similar to Part II of the Cape CDPA, but unlike the CDPA it explicitly provided for differential detection of and treatment for VD among whites and Africans. To detect cases in the African population, farm owners and kraal headmen were required to report the appearance of syphilis to the nearest government official. Landdrosts and mining commissioners could also instruct a district surgeon to examine townships regularly to detect cases of syphilis. No similar detection scheme was introduced for whites. The law empowered the government to establish racially segregated hospitals or wards to treat syphilis, or set aside a section of a kraal to isolate syphilitic Africans. The government planned to bear the cost of treating white paupers, but decided that Africans could finance their own treatment.[85] Thus from the start the government differentiated between blacks and poor whites in the way in which syphilis was detected, treated and financed.

The Transvaal government did not have the medical personnel or financial resources to implement the law adequately. Fewer than 30 doctors lived in the Transvaal in 1885 and the number probably had not increased substantially ten years later.[86] Several districts isolated their white syphilitics in gaol hospitals, or took the cheapest option and advised the infected individual or family to avoid contact with other people.[87] Doctors' frequent requests for lazarettos for Africans were refused. The government instructed doctors to isolate the infected kraal or send infected individuals to prison.[88] A district surgeon could order but not compel the segregation of syphilitics because patients lived such great distances from his own and police surveillance, and in some areas, such as Ermelo, the gaol authorities were unwilling to mix syphilitics with ordinary prisoners. Even farmers, faced with syphilitic workers, just had to take the precautions they saw fit, which probably meant dismissal.[89] The occasional district surgeon tried to tour his district to detect syphilitics, but this too was unsuccessful as the inhabitants ran away when they saw him coming.[90]

In the absence of an effective government treatment scheme in the Zoutpansberg and Waterberg areas, where endemic syphilis was rampant, two missionaries established hospitals to treat what they believed was venereal syphilis. Dr G. Liegme, a Swiss medical missionary, founded Elim Hospital in 1899, supported by the Swiss Mission. In Blaauwberg, Reverend Franz and his wife Helena, a trained nurse, began a hospital on their mission station in the 1890s, later renamed Bochem, catering primarily for syphilitics.

Law No. 12 was also complemented by the first attempt in South Africa to control the spread of contagious diseases among Africans through pass laws. As the mining industry moved from outcrop to predominately deep-level mining, it required ever more unskilled labour. In 1890 the gold mines employed 15 000 Africans, and the number had risen to 100 000 by 1899.[91] The mines had to battle to attract sufficient labour as many African districts still sustained viable peasant economies or Africans preferred more remunerative and less dangerous work.[92] The mining magnates began to demand assistance from the ZAR government, but until 1895 the state was reluctant to provide legislation to create a cheap, reliable black workforce as this would adversely affect the agricultural labour market.[93]

Finally, in 1895 the Volksraad enacted pass laws based on drafts drawn up by the mining industry.[94] Laws 22 and 23 introduced rudimentary efflux and influx controls in agricultural and mining districts and also prohibited the issue of a travelling or working pass to any applicant obviously suffering from an infectious disease, including syphilis.[95] This legislation tied the supply and regulation of labourers to their health status.

The 1895 laws were relatively ineffective for controlling and treating venereal and endemic syphilis, reflecting the lack of administrative expertise and personnel to enforce the laws. By the end of the 1890s, despite its close alliance with the government the mining industry's discontent had made it an enthusiastic supporter of a new British administration.[96] After the Boer War the British appointed Lord Milner as governor of the Transvaal Colony. He was keen to promote the prosperity of the mining industry. Therefore his efforts in creating and controlling the labour supply had the needs of the mining industry in mind, allowing the importation of Chinese labour and introducing minimum living and working conditions for mine workers.[97]

Over the previous few years government officials in Zoutpansberg had warned about the economic toll exacted by syphilis among Africans. The native commissioner for Zoutpansberg believed that a treatment scheme was necessary for 'restoring the people affected to the labour market, and enabling them to meet their taxation etc. which they must by necessity be exempted from during illness'.[98] The district medical officer echoed him, pointing out that the 'question of syphilis amongst Natives is undoubtedly a serious one not only for themselves but also for Whites and from an economic standpoint', as Africans returning from mining towns spread syphilis in the rural areas, affecting current and future labour supplies.[99]

In October 1906 the government decided to set up a commission to report on the extent of syphilis, especially in the Zoutpansberg district, and to submit a scheme for treating Africans.[100] The commission reported in 1907 and its recommendations were largely implemented by the new Het Volk government. The CDC had praised the Elim and Bochem missionary hospitals as examples of 'the most effectual and most economical solution' to syphilis, and suggested they should be given more government assistance.[101] The government quadrupled its annual grants. It also set aside almost £10000 from the Native Compensation Claims for War Losses account expressly to deal with contagious diseases among Africans.[102]

The government viewed missionary medicine as a cheap way to provide rudimentary health care for Africans in rural areas. The missionaries had different, though not incompatible priorities. The medical officer at Elim Hospital believed that hospitals should cater to 'the welfare of the Natives, their education, their promotion to something better than heathenism and specially to breakdown superstitions about diseases'.[103] During treatment Africans could be introduced to the notion of regular work and Christianity. Thus at Elim and Bochem, with the CDC's approval, patients were required to pay or offer labour in return for food and treatment. This was seen as part of their moral education, as well as the only way to make the institutions self-supporting.[104] In the long term, missionaries and officials hoped that their medical services would help create a civilised, Christian and healthy workforce.

In early 1909 the government decided to introduce tours by district surgeon of rural and urban areas to inspect residents for signs of syphilis and vaccinate against smallpox, under the old 1895 law. The first rural tours were disappointing. In many areas the district surgeons complained that Africans concealed cases of disease or refused to direct them to known cases.[105] The solution, Pietersburg's district surgeon believed, was to use local police to force Africans to present themselves for inspection.[106] However the government had already warned against 'the employment of harsh and exacting methods' that would lead to fear and the concealment of disease, and advised 'enlisting the sympathy and gaining the confidence of the people whom it is intended to benefit'.[107] So the following year the government instructed district surgeons to link their itineraries to magistrates' tax collecting tours to ensure they actually got to see all the local inhabitants.[108] However it was the men who paid the taxes, so in some areas the district surgeon still relied on African constables from the Native Commissioner's office to bring in women and children for inspection.[109] In the winter of 1909, 37 district surgeons examined 154965 Africans for syphilis, of whom 5120 were found to be syphilitic.[110] In 1913 the MOH for the Transvaal treated 6983 people in the Waterberg and Zoutpansberg districts alone.[111] In the most remote areas the government also issued free potassium iodide and mercurial compounds to native commissioners, missionaries and 'reliable' storekeepers to distribute to suspected syphilitics at their discretion.[112] During 1909 about 1900 Africans were treated in this way.[113] The tours came to an end in 1914.

In urban areas the tours were restricted to townships and mining settlements, especially the mines' married quarters. Driven by worsening rural conditions, women had migrated to the towns, settling in mining or informal townships and selling beer or working as prostitutes. In 1910 police estimated that 200–300 black women depended on full-time prostitution in Johannesburg, drawing most of their customers from the mining compounds.[114] These women, declared the MOH for the Transvaal, when 'brought into contact with native men living mostly lives of enforced celibacy', were 'a great power for evil'.[115]

Readily available liquor, officials believed, led to absenteeism, lower productivity and venereal disease. Mine managers were reluctant to remove the women, fearing that male workers would leave if prevented from cohabiting.[116] However by 1911 most of the irregular mining townships had been demolished and replaced by fenced, regulated married quarters for miners and their bona fide wives. All women living in the married quarters were issued with identification tickets, signed by the compound manager and attesting to their right to live there.[117]

As part of this effort to regulate the lives of African urban residents more closely, in 1909 the district surgeons in urban areas were ordered to inspect town and mining townships for VD cases, paying particular attention to women in the mines' married quarters.[118] By the end of the year the resident magistrates and district surgeons on the Rand and the director of the Government Native Labour Bureau agreed that these inspections had been unsuccessful. At several mining townships women had refused to submit to a medical examination and the district surgeon had no legal power to compel them.[119] The resident magistrate of Johannesburg warned that 'any interference with native women in the locations [townships] is likely to give rise to trouble among the natives'.[120] The only recourse seemed to be for the police to arrest women on suspicion of prostitution under the Immorality Laws, as women could be inspected and treated in gaol and then sent to Rietfontein, if necessary, at the conclusion of the sentence.[121] But the municipalities wanted a more far-reaching solution: the incorporation of women into the pass laws, which remained their regular demand over the following decades, as discussed in Chapter 6.

The CDC's recommendation to link medical examinations for syphilis and other contagious diseases to registration and passes for male jobseekers in mining and urban areas, was put into effect with the Urban Areas Native Pass Act No. 18 of 1909. The Act, which brought pass controls under central rather than municipal government control, laid down detailed regulations for medical examinations in urban areas and labour districts. Upon finding a job, a worker had to register the service contract at the pass office and undergo an examination. His contract was then endorsed 'Passed Healthy and Vaccinated'. But if a worker had syphilis, infectious tuberculosis or any other contagious disease he was not granted a pass, and if he was already employed his contract was terminated immediately. Any African who refused to submit to a medical examination was guilty of an offence and liable for a fine of £10 or imprisonment with hard labour for up to one month.[122]

The Act came into effect on 1 January 1910, but the pass offices did not have the personnel to implement the inspections effectively. The acting chief pass officer of Johannesburg reported that the 'natives are not individually examined for syphilis . . . [and] owing to the large number that pass through . . . it would be quite impossible to do this'.[123] In some areas the pass officials performed the examination themselves, relying on a government medical circular for a description of syphilis.[124] The colonial secretary also warned that 'too exact a meaning must not be attached to the term "infectious" in the case of native syphilis otherwise much disturbance of the mine labour supply will ensue without compensating benefit to public health'. He recommended that district surgeons allow 'would-be mine boys' to seek work once their lesions had healed, even though they were not fully cured.[125] The labour shortage was still sufficiently serious for the pass and examination process to 'pass the most fit of an unfit lot', commented a doctor.[126]

By the time of union on 31 May 1910 the Transvaal had developed an entirely different system from that in the Cape to detect and control VD, and this was to form the foundation of VD programmes for Africans thereafter. The government relied on missionary hospitals in rural areas to provide cheap and rudimentary health care, and most importantly it linked medical examinations to pass controls, thus introducing a framework for the systematic surveillance of the male working population.

African reaction to treatment campaigns

Africans did not passively accept the new public health measures. Biomedical explanations and treatments of diseases clashed with or ignored indigenous medical views, and public health measures were often regarded as yet another expression of aggressive colonial power.

Africans continued to rely on their own healers and remedies to treat endemic syphilitic lesions.[127] In Rustenburg and Zoutpansberg, where endemic syphilis was widespread, some communities had a longstanding practice of segregating syphilitics in a separate village or quarter, and some parents tried to prevent their healthy children from playing with children with lesions. In other areas parents were unconcerned about isolation, believing their children would recover from the disease and be immune.[128] While missionaries and district surgeons dismissed this as superstition and ignorance, it showed that, like the Dutch, some African communities had a real understanding of the course of endemic syphilis.

Endemic syphilitic lesions seemed to respond to mercurial treatment, and where the treatment was voluntary, Africans eagerly accepted it. Many visited the Elim and Bochem mission hospitals. In 1905 Elim treated 186 syphilitic inpatients (43 per cent of its total cases), and among the 1283 outpatients there was a large but unspecified proportion of syphilitics.[129] In 1912 Bochem hospital treated 3219 syphilitic outpatients (46 per cent of its outpatient load).[130] In areas remote from the hospitals, syphilitics travelled for several days to a district surgeon to receive a month's supply of ointment.

In other areas, communities resented the new attempts at government surveillance, which simply compounded their grievances about access to land and political rights. During the Boer War many Africans, especially in the Zoutpansberg and Waterberg districts, occupied white farms, believing that the white owners had been expelled and their old lands restored. At the end of the war they forcibly resisted the return of Boers to their land. Sharecroppers and rent-paying squatters were also angered by Het Volk's efforts to curtail their independence.[131] The end of the war also saw the disappointment of the black elite's political aspirations. The British administration kept the racially discriminatory legislation of the previous republics and introduced the first formal segregation of blacks in townships, an all-white municipal franchise and the first statutory industrial colour bar. Black political organisation began to grow in the Transvaal and nationally.[132]

No coordinated resistance to district surgeon tours developed, but the district surgeons of all regions reported that chiefs and commoners were refusing to cooperate with their instructions or answer their queries, and that opposition was strongest in the areas most affected by the return to the prewar *status quo*. In the northern Transvaal the MOH reported that chiefs 'often ... assume an air of ignorance' and suspicion when asked to identify cases of syphilis, and that they associated the inspections 'with the performance of acts which they resent'.[133] In Rustenburg the district surgeon similarly reported that chiefs were unwilling to identify their sick, as they 'suspect the Government of intending to segregate or deport active cases'.[134] One district surgeon complained that Chief Chigwaan of Zebedela township was 'opposed to practically any Government measure', with the result that 'his natives are very difficult to treat', while chiefs such as Matala and Malietzie of the Zoutpansberg region, who were willing to instruct their followers to present themselves for examination, had 'practically no authority over their people, with the result that they take no notice of their words and consequently will not come for examination'.[135] Justifying a tour to a hostile audience was not made any easier by the fact that many district surgeons could not speak the local languages, nor could the police.[136] Linking the medical examinations to tax collection and then pass examinations, while not overtly coercive, simply reinforced postwar resentments and fears and affirmed public health measures as a symbol of resented governmental authority.

Conclusion

By the time of union, VD detection and treatment in the Cape and the Transvaal differentiated between white and black carriers. Increasingly the focus was on Africans, especially jobseekers, rather than the poor as the origin of syphilis. Over the next decade doctors and government administrators debated the nature of national public health legislation. As will be discussed in Chapters 4 and 7, though the Public Health Act of 1919 did not differentiate on racial grounds, in practice different systems of detection and treatment of VD were evolved for whites and Africans, and the roots lay in legislation developed in the late nineteenth and early twentieth centuries.

3
VD and the 'Poor White' Problem in the 1920s and 1930s

By the time of the First World War doctors were beginning to voice concern about the effects of venereal disease on South Africa's white population. C. Louis Leipoldt, a liberal Afrikaans poet and doctor, was warned when he began work as a medical inspector of Transvaal schools in 1914 that VD 'was by no means rare' among poor Afrikaner children.[1] The *Medical Journal of South Africa* stated in July 1916 that although no accurate statistics on VD existed 'there is nevertheless, reason to believe that this prevalence is very real and alarming, and also that it is increasing, especially amongst whites'.[2] It was estimated in 1917 that 30 per cent of whites had syphilis.[3]

Doctors' fears about the hold of VD on the white population seem to have been exaggerated. After five years' practice between 1914 and 1919, and the examination of 80000 white Transvaal school children, Leipoldt discovered only 45 (0.06 per cent) with syphilis.[4] From the 1920s local authorities expanded their free VD treatment services, and on the basis of patient records the Department of Public Health (DPH) suggested in 1928 that only 5 per cent of the white population living in inland towns had VD.[5] Municipal clinics reported even lower figures: the estimated incidence of syphilis in Cape Town by 1939 was 0.09 per cent and in Johannesburg antenatal clinics it was 2 per cent.[6] No statistical survey of VD in the white population was ever undertaken.

The concern about the alleged increase in VD among whites resonated with wider political concerns about the impact of urbanisation on poor whites, and the threat that poor whites posed to the stability of white rule and the creation of a new white South African nation. The 'amateur prostitute', a woman worker who engaged in prostitution to supplement her wages, seemed to encapsulate these fears. Doctors, public health officials and philanthropists debated whether heredity or environment created poor whites and immorality. They drew on the new sciences of sociology and psychology to explore the relationship between social trends and individual deviancy. Their conclusions about the causes of and solutions to poor white immorality helped create the terms in which white, civilised identity was defined.

The poor white problem and 'South Africa First'

In 1929–30, before the effects of the international depression were felt, there were an estimated 300 000 poor whites in the Union.[7] In the rural areas of the Cape and Transvaal they were *bywoners* or labour tenants on farms, or owners of land holdings too small for subsistence. But the largest number were landless, unskilled workers who were gradually moving to the towns, a trend that had begun towards the end of the nineteenth century.[8] The rural population dropped from 52 per cent of the total population in 1920 to 39 per cent in 1931. Urban populations grew: the white population in the Witwatersrand almost doubled from 230 657 to 402 223 between 1921 and 1936.[9] The number of Afrikaans speakers doubled in Durban and Port Elizabeth and also increased in Johannesburg, making Afrikaans-speaking poor whites a far more visible presence in what were still predominately English-speaking towns.[10]

It was the daughters of *bywoners* who headed the drift to the towns. By the mid 1920s white women outnumbered white men in the largest cities and the imbalance was greater in the Afrikaans- than in the English-speaking population.[11] As mechanisation grew, skilled male craftworkers were replaced by cheaper, semi- or unskilled women workers and male unemployment rose.[12] Many of the women were drawn into the food-processing and clothing industries, and also began to replace men as shop assistants.[13]

The rapid urbanisation of whites was matched by equally rapid unionisation and frequent strikes following the end of the First World War.[14] The most prominent strike was that by the Mineworkers Union in 1922 against the Chamber of Mines' attempt to eliminate the colour bar in semiskilled work. Afrikaans speakers made up three quarters of the white mining workforce. The dispute escalated into a general strike, which was eventually quelled through martial law. The newly created Communist Party began to seek white working-class support. The First World War had also heightened tensions with Afrikaner nationalists, who were strongly republican.[15] These tensions seemed indicative of the fragility of white rule and political consensus.

By 1924 the working class had a voice in government through the alliance between the Labour Party and General J. B. M. Hertzog's Nationalist Party.[16] The Pact government's defining slogan was 'South Africa First'. This meant protecting local industry against foreign competition in the hope that increased white employment opportunities would solve the poor white problem.[17] By the 1920s local manufacturers, agricultural interests and even the mining industry were portraying local economic and industrial development as the basis for making South Africa the 'home of a white race' and 'white civilisation', a vision summed up years earlier as 'Protection, Production and a White Population'.[18]

'South Africa First' also encouraged a new national patriotism with a conciliatory attitude towards the 'racial question', then defined as the relationship between English and Afrikaans speakers. Economic independence, it was argued, could only be based on both 'races' burying their differences and cooperating.[19] Reflecting this, Hertzog's nationalism was inclusive: English and Afrikaans speakers who put South African interests before those of the Empire were regarded as Afrikaners.

The growing poor white problem seemed to put the South Africa First policy into question. One sign of the fragility of the South Africanist nation was the problem of miscegenation or racial interbreeding. In Johannesburg, despite official intervention, working-class suburbs and slums were still racially mixed in the early 1920s.[20] A visitor to Fordsburg described how 'Whites and coloured dwell together' so that 'here all shades from white to full blooded black may be seen'. In Doornfontein '[i]llegitimate children are numerous and of the most mixed description owing to the intermingling of all shades of colour with poor whites'.[21] These 'white men . . . were not ashamed to be photographed with their coloured wives and children', reported *The Star* newspaper.[22] Detective Head Constable Vowel testified that in Johannesburg, while cases of interbreeding between white women and African men were 'not . . . numerous', between white men and African women they occurred 'on a large scale'.[23] In country districts and new mining areas, where few white women lived, police reported that white men had sex with, cohabited with and sometimes paid *lobola* (bride price) for African women with whom they lived openly.[24] Poor whites' residence in mixed slums, participation in illicit liquor trafficking and their cohabitation or sexual relationships with Africans were taken as evidence of their moral degeneration. '[T]his indiscriminate herding together of white and black people under disgusting conditions', suggested a police officer in 1922, 'is slowly but surely dragging many of the Europeans down to the level of the Native'.[25]

There were also fears about the declining white birth rate and the higher fertility of poor compared with middle-class whites. John Gray, the first professor of sociology at the University of the Witwatersrand, alleged that 'it is the Poor White who breeds most prolifically and the Johannesburg bourgeois who exhibits the most sterility'.[26] Census data indicate that the white birth rate was falling. However rural whites, mainly Afrikaans speakers, tended to have larger families than urban whites.[27] And statistics from a family planning clinic in Johannesburg, whose patients were mainly poor, seem to suggest that in urban areas poor women had more children than average.[28] As infant mortality declined in the 1920s and 1930s, doctors pointed out that the high birth rate and lower death rate among unfit families resulted in perpetuating '[an] existence that is not profitable to the race and burdening the community with misfits that have to be fed and cared for'.[29] Doctors feared that the higher fertility of poor whites would lead to the number of unfit increasing rapidly. And this raised the problem not of Africans outnumbering whites, but of poor whites outnumbering the purer wealthy white stock, who were evidence of white supremacy and capable of preserving it.[30]

The fears about poor white political radicalism, degeneration and fertility reflected widespread uncertainty about the consequences of the poor white problem. Poor whites could undermine national health and virility, and bore within them seeds of the dissolution of the South African nation.[31] The fears about the extent of VD among poor whites and the role of white women in spreading such diseases reflected these anxieties.

Working women and the 'amateur prostitute'

Doctors recognised that whites 'of a fairly well educated type' did contract VD, but their greatest concern was with the poor, who were usually Afrikaans speaking, working class and relatively new immigrants to the cities.[32] Dr Simpson Wells, president of the western Cape branch of the British Medical Association and a lecturer in clinical obstetrics at the University of Cape Town, believed that syphilis was widespread among poor people.[33] The *Sunday Times* reported in 1921 that in Johannesburg VD had 'long been rampant' in 'the poorer quarters of the town'. When the new VD clinic opened in 1920, educated sufferers took advantage of the free treatment but 'the inhabitants of the slums stood aloof'.[34]

In its first six years the Johannesburg Venereal Clinic treated 5911 patients, of whom 4568 (77 per cent) were male.[35] Yet the focus of doctors' attention was on the minority of women patients (1343, or 23 per cent). It was widely accepted that prostitution was the source of VD, but by the mid 1920s, as Dr Henry Gluckman, director of the VD clinic, put it, 'the out-and-out prostitute is not the danger', but rather the 'unsatisfied female element', namely the unmarried, self-supporting woman frequently described as the 'amateur prostitute'.[36] Dr Milne, MOH for Johannesburg, similarly believed that VD was associated with 'unattached workers and not . . . the girl with a home'. The most important indicator, in his view, was that employed women – married and single – accounted for about 55 per cent of female patients, some 75–85 per cent of whom were unmarried and working.[37]

The distinction between professional prostitutes, who depended solely on soliciting for an income, and amateur prostitutes, who supplemented waged work with soliciting or accepted gifts from their sexual partners, also shaped the findings of Louis Freed's study of prostitution. Freed was a medical doctor whose sociology doctoral thesis examined white prostitution in Johannesburg in the 1930s. Freed believed that amateur prostitutes constituted 20 per cent of Johannesburg's female workforce, and on hearsay he estimated that 40 per cent of unmarried female shop assistants, 50 per cent of unmarried factory workers, 60 per cent of unmarried waitresses and 75 per cent of maidservants engaged in amateur prostitution.[38] His conclusions were based on a study of two groups: 450 streetwalkers convicted between 1932 and 1940, and 89 women discovered through contact tracing from male VD patients treated between 1934 and 1940.[39] He found that the vast majority of the streetwalkers and contacts were unmarried and all either had been or were currently unskilled workers who had taken to prostitution to supplement their incomes.[40] Among the women who had never been convicted for soliciting, Freed differentiated between 'amateur prostitutes', who solicited for the money, and 'charity girls' or 'near prostitutes', who solicited for 'a good time'. He identified the amateur prostitutes as factory workers, waitresses, maidservants, tailoresses, shorthand typists and clerks. The charity girls were office workers, nurses, newspaper reporters, school teachers, adulterous married women and society girls who were economically well off but, he alleged, used promiscuity to climb the social ladder.[41] For Freed and other writers on the subject, all employed women were potential amateur prostitutes, regardless of whether they were manual or white-collar workers or professionals, and they developed a detailed typology to account for this.[42]

Afrikaner welfare organisations also distinguished between professional and amateur prostitutes. In 1943 the Randse Armsorgraad had 172 women registered on its books, of whom 141 were defined as amateur prostitutes who worked during the day and solicited at night. The rest were defined as professionals. Most were Afrikaans speakers aged between 14 and 30 who worked in factories or cafes, or as shop assistants, domestic servants, typists or nurses.[43]

The image of the amateur prostitute – an employed woman, usually a factory worker, new to the city and living alone in the slums, struggling to survive on low wages – did not quite match the reality. Women entering industrial work in the 1930s did come from poor families, but they were urbanised rather than recent immigrants. Hansi Pollak's 1932 study of female factory workers on the Witwatersrand in 1930–31 revealed that two thirds had been born in Johannesburg or on the Reef, or had spent their childhoods in town because their families had migrated.[44] A Carnegie Commission survey produced similar findings.[45] Pollak concluded that most unmarried women lived with their parents, with just under 2 per cent living alone.[46] Even new migrants lodged with kin or friends, and only as a last resort would rent a room shared with strangers.[47] Employers frequently only employed women living with their parents or relatives to ensure their 'respectability'.[48]

Rather than all women workers being at risk of prostitution, as was widely believed, the women most likely to enter prostitution were the newest arrivals to the city and those without a family support network. These women were most likely to end up in sweatshops or in domestic work, the least desirable and most poorly paid jobs.[49] In Freed's study, most of the women tracked down because of their contact with male VD patients, and who had also been convicted for soliciting, not only had left their rural homes for Johannesburg three to 18 months before their arrest, but also lived alone because they had migrated alone, or their parents had died or divorced.[50] So it seems that women who were newer migrants and economically and socially marginal, rather than all working women, were most likely to enter prostitution.

However the image of the amateur prostitute seemed to encompass *all* working women as potential or actual prostitutes. The label 'amateur prostitute' was an attempt by social researchers to explain changing attitudes towards courting, female sexuality and premarital sex, at a time when all extramarital sex was regarded as prostitution.

Changing sexual mores

Courting customs changed as whites moved from small rural communities to large towns, where adolescents and young men and women had greater freedom to meet alone. In farming communities in the Transvaal, courting was strictly regulated through the custom of 'sitting up'. After a young man had asked permission from a young woman's parents, they would be left alone in the dining room to sit together and talk, with 'the implied and scrupulously observed understanding that the bounds of conventional courting should in no circumstances be exceeded'. If, after several such meetings the couple decided they wanted to marry, they would seek parental consent. By the late 1930s this custom had fallen into disuse in rural areas and courting was described as 'quicker' though never surreptitious.[51]

However in urban areas the uncontrolled social interaction between young male and female workers was a source of concern for doctors and social workers. It was suggested that the 'old fashioned prostitute' no longer existed as the '5/-dances provided the necessary opportunities' for young men and women to meet away from their families.[52] The Carnegie Commission noted that in the slums girls took to 'the habit of "gadding about". . . . Evenings are spent in paying visits or in the streets; immorality is only too often the result.'[53] Afrikaner welfare organisations such as the Afrikaner Christelike Vroue Vereniging (ACVV) were anxious to control young women's sexuality. One church committee and ACVV member in Mosselbay described her horror at romantic relationships unsupervised by diligent parents or employers: 'I . . . saw a pair meet their boyfriends in the shadows of trees in the evening and stand there and caress. Although I did not see anything wrong, it was not pleasant to see good Afrikaans girls, although poor, chat on the street.'[54]

Women raised in a strict Calvinist tradition may have been unwilling to discuss sex and reproduction with their daughters. One Afrikaans-speaking woman, whose 14-year-old daughter was pregnant, declared 'Sies, a person doesn't talk about such things with children'.[55] However by the 1920s more information was publically available and there were signs that sexual mores were beginning to change.

Miss Higson, an Anglican church social worker and member of the British Social Hygiene Council, which organised education about VD and sexuality in Britain, visited South Africa in 1932. After talking with students at teaching colleges, her impression was that the 'materialistic forces and the downward pull of a cheap, vulgar familiarity with sex questions is very serious'. She noted that Marie Stopes' books were best sellers in South Africa and Bertrand Russell's book, *Marriage and Morals*, was much discussed.[56] Marie Stopes' books explained human sexual and reproductive physiology, offered practical information on contraception and argued that women were capable of sexual passion.[57] Russell criticised conventional morality, which defined sexual love as sinful, and called for a new morality in keeping with the emancipation of women and the availability of contraceptives, and recognising that physical intimacy enhanced the spiritual bonds of marriage.[58] These ideas were slowly changing attitudes towards sexuality.

Dr Mary Gordon, a Johannesburg practitioner, believed that immorality was 'equally rife in all classes but . . . the better classes were able to protect themselves from the consequences'. Young, respectable, professional women with high standards of education were now asking her for contraceptives, and in some cases were cohabiting with men, even though they had no economic need to do so. She blamed the new idea in psychology that 'sex is a natural appetite and should not be restrained' for the loss of self-respect and experimentation in sex outside marriage.[59] Freed similarly remarked on the 'increasing unrest and experimentation in the realm of sex' by married and unmarried women.[60] He based his conclusion on the anecdotal views of five Johannesburg gynaecologists who in the late 1930s estimated that 95 per cent of their unmarried patients were sexually experienced. A medical officer considered that this was also true of the majority of the 600, mainly unmarried, women employed in the clothing factories he supervised.[61]

Easier access to information about sex and contraception allowed women to control their fertility, but doctors and physicians feared that it also led to promiscuity. Many of the cases described by social workers or researchers as amateur prostitution may well have been an indication of new sexual mores in the city. Rather than casual sexual relationships, young couples slept together when their intention was to marry. Pollak and Klenerman cited numerous cases of young women cohabiting with men when they could not support themselves on their low wages.[62] These cases were defined as amateur prostitution. However, fewer couples married during the depression and many men delayed marriage as they could not afford it.[63] Given an agreement to marry, it seems that some couples slept together or cohabited before marriage. Dr Gordon informed the SHC in 1926 that she knew of '[g]irls and boys of sixteen and upwards . . . living together using preventatives and waiting to marry until they have the means'.[64] Pollak cited the case of

28-year-old 'X', who 'had been friendly with the foreman, who had promised to marry her. When she became pregnant, he "cut her out" and would have nothing to do with her.'[65] In the early 1940s the Randse Armsorgraad suggested that a lack of information about marriage, as well as weak morals and low wages, led to amateur prostitution, which similarly suggests a trend in premarital sex in expectation of marriage.[66] Given public disapprobation of sexual activity outside marriage, young women workers may have found social welfare workers and researchers more sympathetic if they explained their 'illicit' relationships in terms of economic need or sexual harrassment.

It was the issue of active female sexuality that doctors, public health officials and social workers found so difficult to understand other than in terms of amateur prostitution. Active sexuality before marriage struck at the heart of the predominant perception of women as wives and mothers rearing future citizens for the *volk* (nation).

Women, work and the family

Women's economic independence, in the eyes of Afrikaner and South African nationalists, was symbolic of a far broader danger – the disintegration of the family and hence the decline of the nation or the *volk*. Middle-class philanthropists, both English and Afrikaans speaking, South Africanist and nationalist, regarded women as the embodiment of moral purity in their homes and the nation. They drew on similar themes, but harnessed them to different political projects.[67]

Afrikaner nationalists began to develop the notion of the *volksmoeder* (mother of the nation) in the late 1910s to glorify an ideal of Afrikaner womanhood and define their role in the nationalist movement. This was part of a broader cultural movement to create an Afrikaner identity by inventing Afrikaans and purifying it of its associations with poverty and 'colouredness', and by encouraging literature mythologising Afrikaner history. The *volksmoeder* nurtured her family and her *volk*, and embodied the latter's moral purity. As Willem Postma, a journalist and nationalist, put it: 'A people are what its women are. The woman is the conscience of her nation as well as the measure of its values. The moral life of a nation is controlled by the women, and by the women can we measure the moral condition of the people.'[68]

Beyond Afrikaner nationalist circles, the imperialist vision of motherhood for race and empire was replaced by the 1920s with that of mothering the white South African nation.[69] The idealised woman was the morally pure wife and mother responsible for the moral and physical health of the nation.[70] Women's 'magnificent . . . destiny' was to 'mother the nation'.[71]

Moral purity was based on the 'natural' division of responsibilities within normal families. Articles in *Die Huisgenoot* (a magazine set up as a nationalist cultural mouthpiece) presented the family as the fundamental unit of society in which the domestic world was 'God's gift to the woman' and 'a place where she feels the most at home – her sphere – her temple'.[72] Domestic work was unpaid, but part of a higher moral order and distinctively feminine.[73] In a similar way the Carnegie Commission defined the family as the basis of orderly society. A 'normal, civilised' home was one in which the 'father usually provides the supplies and the mother applies them to the needs of the family'.[74]

The incorporation of women into the workforce, and the lack of economic differentiation between men and women in the home and the workplace, brought gender roles into question. Daughters or wives were now often the major breadwinners and families relied on them for survival. Pollak found that one third of the unmarried women in her sample were responsible for supporting their families, which had no male breadwinner. The remaining women came from families with male wage earners, but they still contributed 20–40 per cent of the household income.[75] Brink suggests that women's economic leverage gave them a degree of freedom to question patriarchal authority in the family.[76] However families still tried to mask these changes. Women tried to preserve the illusion that the father was the family's sole breadwinner by sending home 'gifts' rather than money.[77] Or daughters turned over their earnings to their parents, so reinforcing the relationship of economic dependence.[78]

Factory work not only broke down the sexual division of labour in the family, it also marked women's entry into a public domain of social interaction with men unmediated by familial surveillance. Pollak and Freed reported that women workers faced a constant torrent of physical and verbal sexual abuse from their foremen and white coworkers. Factory workers told Pollack that they were 'treated like bloomin' dirt'.[79]

Racial contact in factories where white women worked alongside African or coloured men was also considered potentially polluting. In 1925 in Johannesburg laundries, white women and African men sorted and cleaned soiled linen together and were paid similarly.[80] In Cape Town, coloured foremen supervised the white and coloured female workforce, who shared cloakroom facilities.[81] The Factory Act required employers to segregate cloakrooms and toilets, so to cut costs some employers chose to employ white women and African men, or to use African foremen.[82] White and African workers cooperated in several strikes in the late 1920s in situations where the racial and gendered division of labour meant there was no competition between these groups. These strikes were seen as an ominous sign of white degradation.[83]

Waged work was also regarded as 'unnatural' for women because it disturbed 'natural' family relations and brought white women into contact with strange white and African men. Low-waged, exhausting industrial labour weakened the Afrikaner woman's physical and moral powers, leading inevitably to immorality, suggested *Die Huisgenoot*.[84] Nationalists warned that working women would abandon their role as *volksmoeders* and that 'the character of the Afrikaner *volk* will disappear if the women are lost in the factories'.[85] Freed suggested that as the differences between men and women blur, the 'differences in . . . moral behaviour . . . tend to become more and more minimized'.[86]

The abusive Afrikaans term for female factory workers was 'factory *meide*', and its layers of meaning expose the social tensions arising from the presence of women in the workforce and the changing attitude towards female sexuality. The word '*meid*' (maid) referred to an African or coloured female domestic worker, poorly paid and at the beck and call of her mistress. The implied insult was that the white female factory worker was as powerless and menial as an African servant,[87] and that industrial work, or any work for a wage, was degrading for white women. As African women were popularly perceived as prostitutes, the term also cast a slur on white women's sexual mores and suggested an affinity between working women and the African. Active sexuality resonated with the predominant view of African men and women as inherently licentious.

VD and men: unemployment and the male libido

The majority of VD clinic attendees were men, yet their sexual behaviour excited far less attention. Men were castigated for transmitting VD to their innocent wives and unborn children, but they were largely cast as victims of prostitutes and their own natural passions. While living in slums alongside Africans or working in factories was considered deeply corrupting for women, doctors and state officials sidestepped similar conclusions for men.

A health official appointed especially to draw up a VD policy for the Union suggested that VD was more prevalent 'among casual workers and loafers than among skilled artisans'.[88] It was casual workers and 'loafers' – men who were underemployed or unemployed – who were to be found in the mixed slums, while skilled artisans, who earned higher wages, could live in solidly white, working-class suburbs. And by implication, the easy social interaction with African slum inhabitants led to sexual intercourse and infection with VD. Regardless of the nature of the relationship between white men and African women – and some couples regarded themselves as married – officials tended to see African women in urban areas as nothing more than diseased prostitutes.[89]

Although social and sexual contact with Africans was considered degrading, and was believed to lead to moral and physical degeneration, this did not make white male sexuality deviant. A head constable in Johannesburg told the Stallard Commission that when adolescent white boys lived near young coloured women 'it follows as a matter of course that there is improper behaviour in many cases'.[90] In discussions preceding the enactment of the Immorality Act of 1927, which prohibited sexual relationships between men and women of different races, parliamentarians stressed that young boys were merely following their nature, and it was difficult to legislate against nature.[91] As a result, when the law was invoked white men were either discharged or given a suspended sentence, while African women received between three and nine months' imprisonment with hard labour.[92] Thus cross-racial sex did not penalise or stigmatise white men, as sex, regardless of the colour of the partner, was a natural rather than a pathological instinct.

The Carnegie Commission was quick to explain that not all poor whites would contemplate such relationships. While 'respectable whites' had a natural and 'deeply ingrained sense of superiority', it was 'poor whites of the lowest type', noted for their 'absence or loss of self respect', who were to blame.[93] This resonated, firstly, with the fear that poor whites might be a degenerate white race mid-way on the racial continuum between pure African and pure white, and that as a hybrid race they were capable of gross immorality. Secondly, the distinction between the respectable and immoral poor was an older, late-nineteenth-century, definition related to attitudes about work. In the early 1920s state officials and police still distinguished between poor people who were 'very respectful and respectable' and despite their living conditions still 'endeavour to make an honest living', and poor people who were 'moral criminals and irreclaimably vicious'. The latter lived off the illicit liquor trade or criminal activities, or cohabited with Africans and earned their living 'by other methods than real honest hard work'.[94] Work was a duty owed by a man to himself and to his community and defined the difference between the 'respectable' and the 'vicious' poor.

The source of male immorality and deviancy thus lay in the refusal to work. The solution was relief work programmes, privileging white job seekers over African, and for the most intransigent 'won't works', compulsory labour colonies were set up to teach them the ethical value of labour.[95] The Work Colonies Act of 1927 provided for work colonies to detain and train unemployed men. The colonies, explained the minister of labour, aimed to deal with people 'who have become indifferent to discipline, to habits of industry and . . . to their own self respect and who have been sliding down the social scale'. The colonies would 'rehabilitate them', and through 'industry and discipline . . . make them once more useful citizens and members of the community'.[96] There were also calls for white paupers and 'won't works' to be deprived of their parliamentary and municipal vote.[97] This suggests that for men, refusal to work was considered a betrayal of citizenship and of the responsibilities of being white.

By the late 1930s male VD cases were associated with poor family lives rather than aversion to work, possibly reflecting the increasing number of men drawn into the labour market after the depression and the decline in male unemployment.[98] Freed's study of 770 male VD patients showed that some unmarried men blamed their infections on their fiancees or 'charity girls', thus construing female sexuality outside marriage as contaminating. Others explained that they had visited prostitutes because their fiancees refused to sleep with them before marriage, or they could not afford to marry. For married men, neglect by their working wives had driven them into the arms of prostitutes. These cases Freed attributed to the expression of male libidinous instincts, rather than deviant sexuality.[99]

For men, VD did not signify corrupt sexuality and similarity with the African in the way it did for women. Male sexuality was natural and normal. Even interracial relationships, while believed to be the source of VD infection, were not considered a sign of pathological behaviour. Men with VD were always seen as the victims of women – whether prostitutes, fiancees or working wives – rather than being stigmatised as deviant. It was the absence of a work ethic rather than deviant sexuality that marked men as suspect.

Heredity versus environment? Poor whites and the 'quality' of the population

Poor whites' poverty and residence in racially mixed slums, female industrial labour and male unemployment seemed to be the antithesis of qualities that were deemed respectable, civilised and white. Fears about miscegenation, criminality, feeble-mindedness and racial degeneration were widespread in official and intellectual circles and among the public. As medical and social researchers investigated the cause of the poor white problem they increasingly saw the poor white as an identifiable social type, different from ordinary whites, and they drew on eugenic language when debating the relative importance of heredity and the environment in creating social problems.[100]

The eugenic movement, which began to emerge in Britain in the 1880s and gained currency in the 1910s and 1920s, directly challenged the optimism of environmentalism. Environmentalism had shaped Victorian public health reforms with the idea that individual progress and morality were shaped by the environment, and hence were malleable. Eugenicists, drawing on new theories of genetics and heredity, concluded that heredity determined character and tinkering with the social environment would have little effect.[101] Modern medicine, public housing, public health services and philanthropic welfare, eugenicists argued, had destroyed the effects of natural selection. As a result the worst racial stock – the unfit, diseased and degenerate – was increasing while the best was dying out, leading to national deterioration.[102] The high VD rates in Britain's civilian population during the Boer and First World Wars were seen as a sign of this physical and moral degeneration, and as a threat to stability, family and empire.[103]

In South Africa these ideas were reinterpreted in light of local problems, particularly the poor white problem and the threat it seemed to pose to the forging of a new South African nation. The most outspoken 'hard' eugenicists, who regularly contributed articles to local journals, were educated professionals, prominent in medical, scientific or intellectual circles. They saw themselves as modernisers, applying scientific principles for the improvement of society.[104]

The alleged high incidence of VD among poor whites – doctors and other professionals believed – reflected the general physical degeneration that was evident among poor whites 'compared with the magnificent physique of the older generations'.[105] Evidence of mental deterioration was also cited. The first intelligence tests, conducted in

South Africa in the late 1910s, tried to compare the relative abilities of whites and Africans. The poorer performance of African school students was taken as proof of Africans' innately inferior mental abilities and lower level of civilisation.[106] However poor whites also fared badly in IQ tests and their average IQ was lower than the average for the white population.[107] This seemed to suggest that poor whites had an affinity with Africans in terms of mental ability.

Some doctors and politicians blamed mental deficiency and the resulting moral degeneration on inbreeding. They argued that the subdivision of land had led to sexual intimacy in families. The result, claimed a district surgeon in Bethal, was that 'the younger generations' brainpower seems to have shrunk at the same rate' as 'the shrinking of their farms'.[108] Isidore Frack, for many years a doctor in the rural Transvaal, maintained that '[c]onstant intermarriage between cousins has perpetuated the breed, the defective strains have multiplied. . . . Insanity in adults, feeblemindedness in children have caused illegitimacy, prostitution and homosexuality in both sexes. . . . They are a drain on the country and irreclaimable.'[109]

Poor white deterioration was also popularly blamed on racial interbreeding and the decline of pure white stock. Hard eugenicists believed that continued racial mixing would lower the physical, psychological and mental fitness levels of whites. Harold Benjamin Fantham, a professor of zoology and comparative anatomy and president of the South African Association of Science in 1926–27, and his wife, Dr Annie Porter, a parasitologist, believed that with racial mixture 'the white man loses', since their research showed that intermarriage led to physical abnormalities, and mental and moral problems such as sexual instability.[110] Popular literature, such as the books of Gertrude Millin, also explored the dangers of miscegenation in defiling pure racial stock and laying the seeds of the eventual dissolution of the white race.[111] Africans and poor whites who had sexual relations would 'run loose and breed disease, vice and betray the black races and white alike into a common welter', warned one parliamentarian.[112]

VD, miscegenation, feeble-mindedness and the decline of the white 'race' seemed inextricably connected. Many doctors believed that not only did VD lead to mental disorders, but that feeble-minded women were most likely to spread the disease. 'It is now generally recognised that a very great percentage of prostitutes are imbeciles and feebleminded persons', declared the Pretoria branch of the Medical Association in 1916.[113] C. Hugh Bidwell, in his presidential address to the medical congress twelve years later, suggested that 'the unfit', a category that included people defined as subnormal, defective or feeble-minded, were carriers of VD.[114] Biological unfitness, he went on, inevitably led to moral degeneration. The unfit could not compete with their more efficient brethren since 'stupidity leads to dismissal from employment, low wages, poverty and consequent temptation to theft', and gradually the unfit 'drift into dependence, prostitution and crime'.[115]

For the hard eugenicists, who believed that 'poor whiteism' was biologically determined and attributable to inbreeding or miscegenation, the solution was sterilisation or contraception for the mentally unfit, criminals and the racially unfit.[116] 'Eliminating the feeble-minded', suggested another writer, was the only way to diminish the rate of miscegenation and avoid 'the danger of South Africa becoming a coloured country'.[117] The Race Welfare Society (RWS) was formed in 1930 by a group of prominent natural scientists, headed by Fantham, to lobby public and government support for the eugenic application of birth control as a solution to the poor white problem.[118] It regarded as 'comparatively ineffective' the attempts by civilised labour policy and 'charitable, slum-clearing and rehabilitation efforts' to ameliorate the poor white problem. Instead, birth control would be of the 'greatest assistance in solving the Poor White problem' and would 'lessen the stream of recruits to the poor-white class'.[119] Doctors voiced similar opinions in the *South African Medical Journal*, declaring that birth control would lead to the development of better racial types and strengthen the nation.[120]

However the Department of Health discouraged close association with the RWS, and the strict eugenicists never successfully influenced central or local government health policy. Heredity and eugenics could explain the poor white problem in objective, physiological and scientific terms, but they posed intellectual difficulties in respect of differentiating inferior white from African racial stock, and called into question white supremacy. This was untenable in a period in which segregationist social legislation was being strengthened.

A 'softer' eugenics shaped the language of some public health professionals and criminologists, who looked for environmental or psychological explanations of degeneration, that allowed the possibility of social and individual improvement. When officials resorted to judgements about white heredity they stressed the elite European heritage that all whites possessed as the basis for a new white South African nation. For example, Dorothy Tonkin, a factory inspector, praised 'the soundness of the British, Dutch and the French stocks from which these girls originally sprang', which would come to the fore in a new, white environment.[121]

Public health officials claimed that the experience of work, low wages and contact with Africans in the slums created amateur prostitutes, and that poverty, poor health and slum living created the poor white problem. MOH for Johannesburg maintained that 'the Wages question bore a very definite relationship to Venereal Disease and . . . [that] bad trade conditions were frequently reflected in increased immorality'.[122] Louise Scandrett, president of the SHC and philanthropic welfare and rescue worker, and Fanny Klenerman, a unionist, similarly argued that low wages forced young women to supplement their incomes through immoral means.[123] *Die Huisgenoot* also suggested that 'the moral circumstances which affect the girls stand in direct relation to their economic circumstances'.[124] The solution, suggested Klenerman, was to raise wages so that men could support their families on their pay-packets and women could leave the labour force.[125]

Klenerman also pointed out that 'miserable quarters and lack of suitable accommodation could be held responsible for much of the immorality in this town'.[126] Living in a city slum or any other 'area thickly populated with natives', in addition to 'a non-living wage', forced 'girls . . . in positions where they are unprotected from their weaknesses'.[127] The idea that slums were detrimental to the physical and moral health of the people was widely espoused by local and central government public health departments.[128] For T. Shadick Higgins, the MOH for Cape Town and professor of public health at the University of Cape Town medical school, slums 'represent disease and premature death, economic inefficiency, degradation and vice, and political instability and revolt'.[129] The crux of slum degradation was that poor homes made poor families – the poor physical environment mirrored poor marital and moral relationships. If a family did not have proper housing the wife did not become a 'decent housekeeper' but 'the very opposite', causing 'considerable trouble'.[130] Married women required a decent home and the economic support of their husbands, and single women required the careful supervision offered in a family or a hostel to preserve their moral status. In their natural environment – a civilised home and family – white women would show evidence of their essential healthy stock, attend to their familial duties and avoid vice.

The implication was that poor whites were not genetically inferior and irreclaimable, but that in the appropriate environment and with adequate state intervention to create good 'habits', poor whites would rise above their poverty and tendency towards immorality – the conditions that gave rise to similarity with Africans. The belief that a new environment would make the race or nation strong and create 'virile' citizens shows that public health officials were not immune to the language of race and degeneration. But their focus was on intervening in the urban physical and personal environment as a way of strengthening the white population – a notion quite in keeping with South Africanist ideology.[131]

Social welfare workers and criminologists offered a different perspective on the causes of amateur prostitution and poor whiteism that stressed the heredity of individuals, rather than of poor whites as a group. In the opinion of H. E. Norman, the first probation officer in South Africa, low wages were not the sole cause of immorality, as not all poorly paid women resorted to prostitution. He suggested that 'low intelligence was generally the accompaniment if not the cause of a low standard of Morality', thus implying that immorality was innate, and perhaps hereditary.[132]

Investigations by the Johannesburg Social Services Department into the background of convicted streetwalkers illustrate similar premises. Prostitution among juveniles was attributed not only to low wages, growing up in a broken home and lack of parental discipline,[133] but also to inferior heredity and degeneration. Some of the women were described as coming from 'bad stock'. Many were also defined as 'mentally retarded', 'abnormal but not certifiable', having the 'appearance of a defective', of 'low intelligence' or 'not . . . very bright mentally'.[134] Women who appeared mentally normal from IQ tests were defined as 'psychopathic', 'moral imbeciles' or 'psycho-neurotic' to account for their refusal to work and their engagement in prostitution.[135] The concern with the mental capabilities of women implied that sexual promiscuity was due to feeble-mindedness that was innate and perhaps the result of heredity.

British social hygienists and American sociologists believed that sexual precocity and promiscuity in women was a sign of an underdeveloped and feeble mind. Sexual promiscuity and the inability to control bodily desires and instincts were associated with animal or primitive behaviour, or in other words a lower level of social development than that which characterised the 'normal' white population.[136] The conclusion that the delinquent was a primitive form of human found currency in South Africa. For example E. Clarry, a probation officer, suggested that the young delinquent was 'little more than a wild barbarian at play. His emotions and instincts are too strong for his intelligence or his intelligence is too weak for his instincts and emotions. In either case he remains uncivilised and uncontrolled.'[137] The image of the normal child developing from a primitive, instinctual stage to the zenith of self-control resonated with a Social Darwinist view that lower races were promiscuous, but with ascendancy up the scale of civilisation they became sexually restrained and modest.[138] The white amateur prostitutes' lack of rational control over their sexual instincts and apparent primitive development – signs of abnormality – were regarded as typical of the normal African population. Thus the amateur prostitute's abnormal behaviour classified her as the same as or at least similar to the African.

However feeble-mindedness and immorality were seen as faults in particular individuals rather than as characteristic of a social group.[139] By defining the amateur prostitute as a deviation from the norm, assumptions about normal white behaviour and morality were thrown into relief. And although abnormality was associated with similarity to the African, the causes were sought not in heredity but in social influences and the environment. Probation officers such as Norman and Clarry suggested that the causes of immorality were to be found in early childhood experiences and poor home discipline, which in Clarry's view 'often retards the development of the real self'.[140] This poor social environment could be remedied.

Public health officials, social welfare officers and criminologists believed that whatever the cause of degeneration and immorality, an improved environment would improve the quality of the poor white population. In both the public health and the criminological explanations of amateur prostitution, the apparent similarity with Africans in terms of licentious behaviour was recognised, but the fundamental difference of whites was affirmed. And by highlighting what was objectionable behaviour for white women, the criteria of civilised womanhood were clarified. In a decent home away from the slums, and supported by a husband, a woman could satisfy her duties as mother and wife, and fulfil her obligation to build the nation or *volk*.

Urbanism and the poor white problem

At the root of the concern that poor whites were degenerating was a broader question about the possibility of constructing a new South African nation made up of English and Afrikaans speakers. If VD was associated with the incorporation of women into the workforce, male unemployment and the intermingling of whites and Africans in the slums, was urban living appropriate for poor whites?

The Carnegie Commission's five reports were the definitive work on the poor white problem and its solutions in the 1930s. The commissioners were influenced by American sociology, which from the turn of the century had focused on social reform and slum improvement, and saw itself as the new science of society.[141] It also built upon the indigenous environmental approach espoused in public health and municipal circles.

The Commission regarded the poor white problem as larger than the issue of heredity. It placed the problem in the broader process of urbanisation and proletarianisation and sought to discover social causes for the particular psychological, familial and mental failings of poor whites. This approach was influential in Freed's study of white prostitution in the late 1930s. He tried to establish general social laws to explain prostitution. He defined the prostitute as 'a bye-product of the problem of societal disequilibrium'[142] and a symptom of 'social pathology',[143] and he established 'functional interrelationships' between migration, family and morality that he encapsulated in universal social laws – the sign of sociology's status as a new science. He explicitly criticised the hereditarian argument that morality was related to IQ and considered that most white prostitutes were normal.[144] He argued that poverty was a more important cause of prostitution than excessive sexual desire, and that prostitution reflected the impact of overarching socioeconomic trends and familial conditions on an individual's psyche.[145]

The Carnegie Commission suggested that poor whites were ill-equipped to deal with modern society. The transition of 'simple and inexperienced people' from a rural life to the 'nervous haste and competition' of a modern industrial town, left them 'subject to the demoralising influences of life in the city all the more easily because of the uprooting effect of leaving their old environment with its sanctions and customs'.[146] On the surface this seems similar to the segregationist argument that Africans were innately tribal and rural, and when transplanted into an urban environment they lost their culture, leading to 'detribalisation' and moral collapse. This justified a policy of preventing African urbanisation. However the Commission did not draw a similar conclusion for poor whites. Rather it considered them capable of adapting to urban life.

The Commission suggested that it was poor whites' isolated, pioneer lifestyle and nomadic existence that had caused 'certain psychological traits to develop among the people, by which ... they were handicapped in the adjustment ... to the new demand of modern conditions'.[147] This life had undermined poor white women's natural maternal role and abilities, and encouraged in men an unwillingness to work and lack of habits of industry'.[148]

The idea that whites seemed to degenerate in the colonies and that the colonial seemed to be a distinct social, psychological and physical type with particular psychotic disorders was widely accepted in metropolitan and colonial medical circles in the 1920s and 1930s.[149] Mental disorders, which in the metropole were blamed on modern civilisation, were in the colonies attributed to prolonged distance from civilisation and the European community, and proximity to the indigenous people. The cure was a return to civilisation, regimented regular work, sexual moderation and family life.[150] From the viewpoint of the Carnegie commissioners, poor whites had for too long been out in the wild, the natural home of the African, and too isolated from European civilisation. Even the city slums were in a sense the wild part of the city, where the 'lack of . . . civilised . . . conditions, easily lowers the standard of living to that of the natives, or even worse'.[151] Through state intervention poor whites could be made at home in an urban terrain and rehabilitated into white standards of living and behaviour.

This view of poor whites as properly urban is evident in relief and welfare policies. During the 1910s state relief policies had encouraged the agricultural resettlement of poor whites as aspirant landowners or *bywoners*, rather than the provision of industrial training. But in the 1920s and 1930s the focus was urban and industrial.[152] Along with artisan training, the Wage Act of 1925 protected unskilled white workers by introducing minimum wage rates that allowed a 'civilised' standard of living, while the 1926 Colour Bar Act legalised the job colour bar to safeguard the jobs of semiskilled and skilled white workers. The government funded white relief works, and the new parastatals, such as ISCOR (the Iron and Steel Corporation), created in 1927, were aimed at white employment. The Customs Tariff Act of 1925 made tariff protection conditional on employment of white labour.

To channel women out of the labour force, labour legislation defined the 'civilised wage'. This, declared the Wage Board in 1929, 'should be taken to mean . . . a wage on which a person . . . can maintain himself . . . and . . . his wife and family, with a reasonable degree of comfort according to European standards'.[153] Women's wage levels should be lower, recommended the Industrial Legislation Commission (1935), to ensure they sought a husband for support.[154] Married women were also excluded from paid employment in certain fields, on the assumption that once married they could rely on their husbands.[155] Thus the intention of wage legislation was to create 'civilised' white families where husbands worked, and wives reared children at home, and the moral problems resulting from low wages for women supposedly would not arise.

The strong environmentalist approach also encouraged the building of subeconomic, segregated housing for whites in urban areas. In

Johannesburg in the 1920s, MOH Charles Porter defined the city's housing problem as one of racial mixing, rather than a shortage of working-class dwellings. The remedy was to remove Africans from the inner city, demolish the inner-city slums and relocate whites to segregated, subeconomic housing project areas.[156] English and Afrikaner charitable and church groups also built hostels for single women workers.[157] Although limited in size, the housing programmes were hailed as successful examples of the moral rehabilitation of poor whites in new, supervised environments. Modelled on the British Octavia Hill management scheme, the housing programmes were based on the assumption that 'it was not enough to improve the dwellings, . . . it was even more important to improve the tenants'.[158] Rehousing not only removed whites from the racially mixed slums, but through careful supervision of tenants' home lives it converted slum inhabitants into 'reliable citizens who would be assets to the community',[159] 'preserve family life and build up ideal homes'.[160]

English-speaking church leaders, social workers and public health officials also advocated supervised leisure activities for young adults to ensure that young men and women socialised in a moral atmosphere.[161] The Johannesburg social welfare department ran several boys' and girls' clubs during the 1930s.[162] The public health department issued a sex and moral education booklet in English and Afrikaans, instructing adolescents in the appropriate social etiquette between whites and Africans.[163] Clubs established by Afrikaner nationalists for female factory workers also offered supervised socialising but inculcated pride in *kerk, taal en volk* (church, language and nation) as well.[164]

A Johannesburg Councillor reviewing the slum clearance and welfare programme in 1938 concluded that 'South Africans . . . were not hereditary slum dwellers. From the so-called "poor whites" could be built a race of which the nation and the whole world would be proud.' The housing schemes 'had brought to the individual undreamed of happiness and content; to the city they had given regenerated and virile human beings'.[165] According to other sources the rehousing programme was 'essential to a healthy life' and made 'the race' strong,[166] and 'the quality of a nation's home life is one of the determining factors of a nation's strength'.[167]

This new environmentalism shaped government policy throughout the 1930s, but by the end of the decade Afrikaner nationalist intellectuals had begun to develop their own theories about urbanisation and criminality that drew heavily on eugenic ideas and German anticapitalist and racist criminology.[168] While the Carnegie Commission emphasised rural–urban migration as the cause of social disorder, Afrikaner nationalists regarded the social interaction between different races and the corrupt values of the city as the source of criminality and immorality. The problems of urbanism were contrasted with a mythological view of the unity and moral well-being of the *volk* in its precapitalist rural past.[169] The nationalist intellectuals' focus on urban vices, eugenics and blood purity justified more rigid racial separation, moral conservatism and sexual purity to strengthen the Afrikaner home and soul.

Conclusion

From the late 1910s doctors became increasingly anxious about the prevalence of VD among whites, particularly poor whites. Eugenic fears about racial degeneration threatened the solidity of white political supremacy and the possibility of building a white South African nation.

Doctors and social welfare workers focused on working women as the source of VD among whites. Their economic independence seemed to threaten the family and the state, as it was feared women would neglect their duties as wives and mothers. At the same time as urbanisation and poverty were leading to changes in courting and attitudes towards premarital sex, there was growing professional and public awareness of active female sexuality and wider access to contraception. This too fed the anxiety that the amateur prostitute was threatening the stability of the family and the nation.

Promiscuity among white women also suggested a similarity to what was considered to be the naturally licentious state of Africans. Although doctors and researchers realised that poor white men also contracted VD, this was never seen as a similar threat. Even when VD was associated with interracial relationships, the men were excused since male sexuality was taken to be naturally promiscuous.

Public health and welfare officials emphasised the role of adverse socioeconomic factors rather than heredity in shaping immorality in individuals, thus implying that poor whites were not racially degenerate as a group, and that unlike Africans they were not innately immoral. Immorality was shaped by outside factors – low wages, slum housing, careless family discipline, ingrained habits of rural life, all of which could be remedied. Housing, education, strengthening the family and affirming women's maternal and domestic roles were solutions to the problems of the amateur prostitute and the poor white.

4
VD Treatment and Educational Propaganda for Whites, 1910–1930s

The Public Health Act of 1919 led to the establishment of free municipal VD clinics for whites, and marked a shift from a moralist to a scientific approach to VD. The *Rand Daily Mail*, reporting on a newly
opened clinic in Johannesburg, dismissed as outdated the 'old attitude
of regarding venereal disease as a well-served punishment'. The modern
approach was to recognise VD as a 'nation-destroying' evil that had to
'be tackled on national lines and from the standpoint of national health
alone'.[1] VD and promiscuous sexuality were public and national matters
now because they affected the health, virility and future of the new
South African nation. And this perception required a more interventionist role by the state. The state was now obliged to provide accessible medical services and educational propaganda, so that citizens could
honour their national obligation to avoid VD and if necessary seek treatment without fear of judicial sanction.

The concern with white health and the creation of a health service
specifically for whites complemented a more general attempt to
improve the socioeconomic circumstances of poor whites and institutionalise racial segregation. As important was the attempt to create
models of white femininity and masculinity. VD propaganda affirmed
racial identity by helping define the boundaries of 'normal' white sexuality and differentiating it from African sexuality.

VD and the Public Health Act of 1919

The Union Act of 1910 had overlooked the field of public health. As a
result the control and treatment of people with VD continued to be
regulated by different pre-union legislation in each province.[2] In the
discussions on VD legislation and services preceding the Public Health

Bill, a debate developed over the appropriate way to deal with VD patients.

Some doctors, especially William Darley-Hartley, the editor of the *South African Medical Record* and an outspoken eugenicist, continued to view prostitution as the source of VD, and VD as a just retribution for sin. They favoured maintaining the Contagious Diseases Prevention Act (CDPA).[3] Darley-Hartley believed that legislation should be targeted at women only, as 'a woman . . . is, in the nature of things . . . a commercial purveyor of disease'.[4] The CDPA would at least ensure that prostitutes were healthy, and would allow diseased women to be detained in lock hospitals to prevent them from contaminating the rest of the community, both morally and with disease.[5]

The anti-CDPA lobby was an alliance of doctors, and of philanthropic and suffragette organisations. The latter consisted of the International Federation for the Abolition of State Regulation of Vice, established in the Cape in 1912, and later the National Committee for Combating Venereal Disease (NCCVD) which set up a Cape and Transvaal branch in 1917.

In the Cape, religious, philanthropic, temperance and suffragette organisations had fought for the repeal of the CDPA since the 1890s.[6] The International Federation and the NCCVD followed in that tradition, arguing that the CDPA tacitly condoned prostitution. The aim of the CDPA, the NCCVD suggested, was 'to empower the Government to secure at public expense healthy women in order that men may gratify their passions without fear or risk of disease to themselves'. Yet the CDPA was ineffective as the examination of prostitutes proved only that they were free of infection at that moment, and this 'false sense of security' was 'a direct inducement to thousands to contract disease'.[7] Also, instead of reducing the incidence of VD the CDPA 'did much harm by identifying disease with crime, which led to the concealment and spread of disease',[8] The solution was to treat men and women similarly.[9]

In England the social purity alliance was strongly influenced by the feminist stance of 'Votes for Women and Chastity for Men', which linked an equal moral standard with equal political rights. The Cape branch of the NCCVD similarly linked its anti-CDPA stance with the demand for suffrage. Extending the franchise to women, it believed, would spread moral purity from the private to the public domain. However female suffrage was not a popular issue and did not attract the sympathy of parliament.[10] The NCCVD may well have realised that if it was to have any gainsay with the medical profession and the Public

Health Department, it had to drop the demand for franchise. The call for moral equality and personal chastity for men and women could stand without the request for franchise.

What drew the anti-CDPA alliance together was the new scientific understanding of syphilis as a bacterial disease and new treatments that offered the possibility of a total cure. In 1905 Fritz Shaudinn and Erich Hoffman identified the spirochaete. The following year August von Wasserman announced his discovery of a sensitive serodiagnostic test. These developments meant that the efficacy of treatments could be proven. In 1905 Ilya Metchnikoff and Pierre Roux discovered that if sub-chloride of mercury (or calomel) in ointment form was applied within a few hours of infection, the spirochaetes were destroyed. This treatment was adopted by the German army in 1907 and the American and British Forces in the First World War and drastically reduced the rate of infection.[11] Then in 1910 Paul Ehrlich announced the synthesis of salvarsan, also known as '606', a drug specific for syphilis. The drug was an arsenic compound that homed in on and destroyed the spirochaete and assisted the body's natural immunological responses to disease.[12] Later Ehrlich developed neosalvarsan, or '914', which though less effective was also less toxic. Ehrlich's products ushered in the age of modern drug treatment, and also earned him, along with Metchnikoff and Roux, a Nobel prize.

These developments made syphilis a treatable disease, like any other. For sufferers to seek treatment, however, the disease had to be relieved of its moral stigma. The NCCVD, for example, called for 'the treatment of Venereal Diseases as maladies not crimes . . . in the same category as other contagious and infectious diseases' – a position supported by the 1914 Medical Congress.[13] The alliance called for the provision of ample, free diagnostic and treatment services.[14]

The anti-CDPA alliance was also drawn together by an undercurrent of eugenic assumptions that tied the health of individuals to the strength of the nation, and justified state intervention to ensure public health. The alliance regarded VD as 'a national danger'. Men with VD infected their innocent wives, who then bore diseased children, thus putting the survival of whites into jeopardy, explained Dr Ernest Hill, chairman of the public health section at the 1914 Congress. As Chapter 3 showed, the health of the nation was seen as crucial to forging the new South African national identity. Making VD a public health and national issue meant not only that the state had a responsibility for the health of its citizens, but also that leading a healthy life was a citizen's duty to the state. A person with VD had to realise, explained Hill, that by seeking treatment he was 'doing not only good service to the State, but most of all to himself, to those in his own immediate circle, and to his own possible descendants'.[15]

The new view that VD was a contagious disease and not a moral crime did not mean that moral questions were unimportant, but the way they were defined was new. 'People cannot be made moral by Act of Parliament', suggested Hill. 'The real cure must come from within, from the people themselves. They must be educated and taught what the dangers are . . . and how they can be avoided.'[16] Dr W. E. de Korte, chairman of the Cape branch of the NCCVD, felt that 'a sense of individual responsibility must be awakened' in the general populace.[17] Education about normal sexuality and the symptoms and consequences of VD was the way to do this. This was antithetical to the stance of the pro-CDPA lobby, which opposed public health education, arguing that explicit knowledge about sex would excite the layperson's imagination and simply lead to more disease. What was more appropriate was a 'policy of silence' and 'a resolute avoidance of thinking about sexuality'.[18]

The views of the anti-CDPA alliance were given added grist by the findings of the 1916 English Royal Commission on Venereal Disease, which recommended that free treatment be complemented by moral education.[19] Charles Porter drew up a VD scheme for Johannesburg modelled directly on these recommendations. Porter, the MOH for Johannesburg since 1901, was an extremely influential figure in public health and urban planning circles at both local and national level, and continually sought inspiration for his plans from trends in Britain and throughout the Empire.[20] So it is not surprising that his proposal was duplicated by several other large municipalities, publicised in the medical journal and presented before the public health conference that debated the Public Health Bill in 1918.[21] Porter argued that 'scientific measures against venereal disease' were the way of the future, and that providing adequate treatment facilities did not condone the 'sin', as some doctors suggested.[22] The new schemes were 'for the protection of the public health and the production of a healthy race', by which he meant, of course, the white population.[23]

The new view of VD as a contagious disease deserving of modern, voluntary treatment in general hospitals shaped the Public Health Act of 1919. The Act made the government responsible for the provision of free laboratory diagnosis, for funding two thirds of the costs of local authorities' VD treatment schemes and for partially funding public health education.[24]

The new public health ethos implied a move away from coercive, overt control of sexuality to a more subtle surveillance that relied on people policing their own sexual behaviour and following social norms. Instead of using the legal system to define people with VD as criminals and controlling their behaviour with the threat of legal penalties, the Public Health Department advocated preventive health measures: free treatment so that people with VD would not infect others, and education so that people would take advantage of the new facilities and act morally to avoid VD in the first place. People were defined as individuals with rights in the polity, and thus bound by responsibility to themselves and the community.

This new approach to VD thus revolved around the central government intervening in public health matters in a way it had not done before. Chastened by their experience of the paucity and poor coordination of local health services during the flu epidemic of 1918, medical practitioners and government medical officers now showed greater tolerance for the idea of state responsibility for public health. The new ethos of state intervention was summed up by a 1919 government housing commission, which declared that there was 'an undeniable duty upon the State to ensure that all members of the community are healthy and useful citizens, and that no section of the community is allowed to sink to such depths of discontent, depravity, or disease, as to become a menace to the well-being of the rest'.[25]

Central and local government officials and doctors involved in public health sometimes used the rhetoric of race and degeneration to explain the deterioration of poor whites, but tended to emphasise the influence of their social and physical environment. Their conviction that immorality was largely environmentally determined meant that it was possible to change the lifestyle and mores of poor whites and create respectable citizens by placing them in a carefully supervised, healthy and racially segregated environment. The new approach to VD outlined in the Public Health Act was one aspect of a broader programme of state intervention in the 1920s and 1930s in health, housing, education, employment and social welfare aimed at alleviating the effects of urbanisation, improving the social and economic circumstances of poor whites and incorporating them into the 'respectable' white body politic. The 'civilised labour policy', which introduced minimum wage rates and the job colour bar, together with segregated subeconomic housing projects, relief employment schemes and the broader provision of state education and social welfare helped segregate whites from Africans and prevent social interaction, and affirmed the notion of white difference and superiority. The state was now seen as responsible for creating the conditions for ensuring the health and virility of the white nation.

From lock hospitals to VD clinics

The impact of the Public Health Act on VD health services for whites can be illustrated by comparing the conditions at a private clinic and at the Rietfontein lazaretto before the Act was implemented with those at a government-sponsored VD clinic that opened in Johannesburg in 1920 after the passage of the Act. This comparison demonstrates how perceptions about VD and its treatment changed and how, in line, with segregationist policy, white patients began to be treated differently from Africans, so reinforcing white racial difference and superiority.

Wealthier whites who could afford private treatment could escape the moral stigma of being treated in a lock hospital or lazaretto and the 'indignity' of close association with Africans and white paupers. These patients could consult their personal doctors, or go further afield to specialist venereologists. The key to the popularity of a private practice specialising in treating VD in Umzinto, Natal, was the secrecy the doctor promised his patients. He met them at the station, housed them in a private room alongside his clinic, and returned them to the station for their departure. 'The patients see only the doctor and the nurse, and all unnecessary gossip, staring of frightened hotel-keepers, awkward questions, and possible damage to reputation are avoided.'[26] These luxuries of secrecy and privacy were, of course, beyond the means of poorer whites and paupers, who had to rely on public institutions for treatment.

Rietfontein had opened as a smallpox lazaretto in 1895, and then become a home for African and white pauper patients with incurable diseases. After the Boer War it again became an isolation hospital for smallpox, scarlet fever and measles – and increasingly for VD. The hospital was situated seven miles north-east of Johannesburg to distance contaminating people from healthy and respectable society.

The intention of lock hospitals was to provide treatment, but the conditions were appalling. A select committee investigating hospital conditions in 1914 described Rietfontein as 'the most dirty, disgraceful and dilapidated premises that ever pretended to the name of a hospital'. Patients were housed in tents and 'temporary wood and iron erections which have long since served their time and . . . should be forthwith burnt'.[27] Security was lax. At the entrance to the hospital was a board warning the public away, but there was no guard and one reporter was able to slip in unchallenged and tour the buildings in 1915.[28] The medical superintendent and police frequently complained that white and African patients with infectious syphilis absconded from the hospital, either to avoid treatment or to visit a nearby poor white settlement or Alexandra Township near Johannesburg to buy illicit liquor. In 1918 the superintendent described desertion as a daily occurrence, and often 60 patients were absent at a time.[29]

As discussed in Chapter 2, from the 1890s the Cape Colony had begun to segregate patients and prisoners in state asylums, hospitals and prisons along racial lines, as well as according to gender and class. At Rietfontein, by 1915 African and white men were being housed separately but white women and juveniles were housed with African female patients and in sight of African male patients. The medical examination of African men, who were required to strip, was easily watched by white patients.[30] In 1914 this was viewed as 'nothing short of a scandal and an abomination'.[31] A select committee recommended that Rietfontein be rebuilt to cater for Africans, and that whites be transferred to special wards at a general hospital.[32] The Transvaal Provincial Council passed an ordinance in 1915 to this effect, but it was rescinded by the government. The government noted that while accommodating white syphilitics 'within sight of native syphilitics is obviously undesirable', there were no finances to build a new hospital.[33] By 1922 white patients still had to meet at the Pass Office and travel with African patients in the mule-drawn ambulance to Rietfontein – a situation the medical superintendent regarded as 'undesirable'.[34]

Accommodating white and African women together in Rietfontein, as in reformatories, symbolically cast these delinquents from white society and affirmed their similarity to African women.[35] VD among white women was associated with active sexuality and promiscuity, which were regarded as signs of primitive, inherently African behaviour, and so indicative of poor white degeneracy.

As the state began to shape a more segregated society, notions of white racial degeneracy became untenable. Stoler suggests that in the colonial context, European power was associated with good health, virility and strength. Thus aged, ill, insane or poor whites were not admitted to the colonies or were shipped home.[36] As the Public Health Act took effect, the government began to segregate VD patients, removing white patients from the gaze of African eyes and providing whites with confidential and superior outpatient treatment. This not only emphasised the difference between white and African but also, perhaps, served to protect the mystique of white supremacy.

Only the most severely infected white patients continued to be admitted to Rietfontein in the 1920s. In 1927–28 the hospital treated an average of 27 white patients and 425 African patients a day.[37] The hospital was now strictly racially segregated. A new white female VD ward was completed in 1927 and the fence around the African male quarters was raised from seven feet to ten feet and a serrated top added.[38] Two years later the hospital planted a hedge of quick-growing evergreens along the fence to block out the view between the African male and white female wards.[39] In a period in which segregationist ideas were being consolidated, this physical division between the white female and African male wards emphasised racial difference. The fence prevented social interaction, and by hiding white women from African men's eyes, it prevented African men from assuming equality. But VD was still a sign that a woman might be promiscuous, so the fence also prevented African men from viewing white women who were morally degraded and an insult to white womanhood.

By 1928 the government was supporting 26 local authority VD clinics for whites.[40] A description of the development of treatment services in Johannesburg illustrates the impact of the Act. The Special Treatment Clinic opened in 1920. It was set up in the General Hospital to stress the new view that VD was a disease like any other, rather than having to be treated in a separate and isolated unit. It offered sessions for men and women on separate days and promised 'treatment . . . free from unwelcome and embarrassing conditions of discrimination or publicity'.[41] To allay fears that 'some friend or relative . . . [would] find out his [the patient's] plight', the clinic entrance was inconspicuous. Patients entered through the main hospital and followed signboards so they could avoid the embarrassment of asking directions.[42]

In contrast to the white experience, the treatment of VD among the African population became far more coercive. The pass laws were used to exclude infected men from urban areas while urban women who were regarded as prostitutes, but were exempt from the pass laws, were arrested on suspicion of being infected with VD. Africans with VD were treated in gaols or, on the Witwatersrand, detained in Rietfontein, where patients were treated *en masse* in public. Urban local authorities established limited outpatient clinics for Africans only in the 1930s, but without the same effort to ensure patient confidentiality.

Thus the government used the Public Health Act to provide accessible and affordable treatment to the white population. This complemented a general shift in government policy towards a modern, interventionist, welfarist state for whites that tried to ensure social segregation, institutionalise the privileges of being white and uplift the poor white population.

The professionalisation of welfare and VD education

The emergence of a welfarist state ran parallel with a shift from philanthropic to professionalised social work to deal with the problems of the poor white population. This shift was reflected in the changing composition of the NCCVD, the South African Social Hygiene Council (SHC) and the Red Cross Social Hygiene Committee (RCSHC), which were all partially funded by the central and local government health departments.

The Transvaal NCCVD members included the bishop of Pretoria and dean of Johannesburg, the Johannesburg MOH, Dr Porter, the assistant MOH, Dr Milne, and members of the National Council of Women. The president was J. D. Rheinallt Jones, a prominent segregationist liberal who was particularly active in promoting African social welfare. The vice presidents were Dr Henry Gluckman, director of the Johannesburg VD clinic and lecturer in venereology at the University of the Witwatersrand, and Mrs Charlotte Louise Scandrett, who had a long history of participation in welfare work in the areas of health, education and indigency, and was a founder and president of the non-suffragettist National Council of Women of South Africa.[43] The Cape Town branch of the NCCVD similarly included several doctors, the archbishop of Cape Town, several churchmen, and liberals concerned with philanthropy. For example Emily Solomon and Julia Solly were prominent in the Women's Enfranchisement Association of the Union, as was Lady Rose Innes, wife of the president of the Cape NCCVD, Sir James Rose Innes. Solly and Mrs John Brown had been involved in campaigns against the CDPA for many years and had been officeholders in the International Federation for the Abolition of State Regulation of Vice.[44] The NCCVD was thus an assembly of individuals whose interest in VD was motivated by liberal opposition to coercive and unfair legislation, and promotion of philanthropic and religious welfare rescue work, Christian salvation and rescue from sin. It arose out of the earlier Victorian tradition of private, voluntary philanthropic organisations dominated by middle-class reformers imbued with a strong sense of Christian duty and moral propriety and belief in women's superior moral outlook.

In 1926 the NCCVD changed its name to the Social Hygiene Council (SHC), following the lead of its British parent body. While retaining its links with philanthropic groups such as the National Council of

Women, the South African Temperance Alliance and the Women's Reform Club, it also drew on a wide range of professional social welfare organisations and individuals. These included the District Nursing Association, the South African Trained Nurses Association, the Central Rand Teachers Association, the Children's Aid Society, the Mental Hygiene Society, representatives from the Municipal Health Department, the British Medical Association, and H. E. Norman, the first probation officer to be appointed in the union (1916).[45] Scandrett was the president, and while she may have been a symbol of the older moral philanthropy, the vice presidents, Dr Porter, Dr Orenstein, the chief medical advisor to the Rand Mines, and Dr Peirson, were all active in public health activities in Johannesburg and represented the SHC's new medical and professional character. In 1927 Norman took over as president, followed by Gluckman, so consolidating the gradual professional approach of the organisation.[46] Despite the more professional personnel, the SHC still maintained contact with its parent body, which sent out lecturers and trainers. The secretary of public health described these as being 'neither medical women nor nurses' who addressed VD 'mainly from the religious point of view', which he wanted to discourage.[47]

The SHC was absorbed by the Red Cross in 1927 and by the late 1930s doctors dominated its membership. There were medical officers of health from all the Reef municipalities, in addition to representatives from professional welfare and educational organisations. Representatives from women's organisations and the church were no longer evident (except where churchmen were also experts in 'native affairs').

The shift from religious to professionalised social work was mirrored in the emergence of a new moral language couched in terms of scientific health laws rather than sin and moral purity of the soul.[48] The NCCVD, building on the platform of a single moral standard for men and women, had aimed to provide 'accurate and enlightened information' about VD and its treatment 'to raise the standard both of health and conduct'.[49] The Red Cross, however, provided educational material on a range of diseases, including VD, from a resolutely scientific point of view. It urged citizens' obedience to 'proven laws of health' as 'a vital part in the development of a vigorous nation'.[50] The 'law' of sex was that it was a positive instinct when it was associated with reproduction in marriage, but led to disease and suffering in all other situations.[51] The new language was shaped by the growing acceptance of sociology and psychology, which identified the 'scientific' laws governing social life, health and the psyche.

The NCCVD, SHC and RCSHC also had close links with the local municipal departments of health, which together with the central municipal health departments tended to emphasise the need to redress the social conditions in which people lived: rehousing in a new environment, education and solving the problem of poverty were heralded as solutions to poor white immorality.[52]

Professionalisation gave precedence to the rationality of the state-sponsored expert and this reflected a shift to a new form of social control. Criminal laws could still regulate public morals as in the past, but now education and social rehabilitation were considered a preferable way to channel sexual instincts towards socially approved goals.

Foucault's term 'normalisation' describes the process of creating conformity in moral behaviour; an individual was surveyed by professionals and measured his or her own behaviour against the definitions of 'normal' and 'abnormal' behaviour developed by social scientists. VD propaganda focused on defining the contours of 'normal' white sexuality and morality. The propaganda emphasised the differences between whites and Africans, but also defined different meanings of sexuality and morality for white men and women.

Education, race and morality

The propaganda of the NCCVD, SHC and RCSHC was distributed through pamphlets, posters, lectures and films. The CNA, a major newsagent, refused to stock educational literature,[53] but when the NCCVD placed advertisements in daily papers it received a deluge of requests.[54] The RCSHC distributed VD posters for whites to all municipalities and distributed pamphlets in rural and urban areas.[55]

Much of the work for whites involved the holding of 'film lectures'. There are no figures on the number of people reached in this way, but isolated examples do give a sense of the activities. Early in 1926 Gluckman and Milne gave a lecture to 400–500 people in the Parys Town Hall, to 600 people, including education students and nurses, in Potchefstroom, and to 600 people in the Vereeniging Town Hall. Each lecture was followed by a screening of a film entitled *Waste*.[56] Over 20 000 people were estimated to have seen *Whatsoever a Man Soweth*.[57] Other films screened in the 1920s included *The End of the Road*, *The Shadow*, *The Flaw* and *Memories*.[58] In 1934 the SHC screened *The Irresponsible* and *Any Evening After Work* in 21 towns to 20 000 people.[59] In the Transvaal in the late 1930s, the RCSHC organised hundreds of lectures to trade unions, schools and societies, and organised health days and health weeks in small towns. The committee felt its lectures and displays were 'very enthusiastically received' and estimated that, especially in the smaller towns, sometimes 75 per cent of the population attended.[60] To prevent embarrassment, the films were screened separately to white male and female audiences. Only occasionally were the films screened before a mixed white audience, and these publicly advertised showings were intended for married couples.[61]

The NCCVD, SHC and RCSHC believed that these films were unsuitable for Africans and recommended developing 'African' materials (see Chapter 7). Despite the differences between the mostly middle-class and English-speaking educationists and their poorer, Afrikaans-speaking, white audience, the organisations did not think that poor whites needed separate educational propaganda. Lectures and pamphlets in English were translated into Afrikaans. The emergence of national patriotism – the call for 'South Africa First' – emphasised the common norms of English and Afrikaans speakers as whites, while differentiating white civilisation from African tribalism.

The pamphlets and films were aimed at an adult audience, but local authorities, the NCCVD and its successors viewed school-going adolescents with particular concern. The Johannesburg Public Health Department and the RCSHC published *Facts About Ourselves for Growing Boys and Girls* in the early 1930s, and reprinted it in 1939 in English and Afrikaans.[62] The aim was to provide professional guidance and information for adolescents, in the belief that the 'natural educators' – the parents – were failing in their role. The level of immorality, commented Gluckman, indicated that 'the parent of to-day, both male and female, . . . has abundantly proved his or her instability, and we must look for something in the way of education more dependable than the parent'.[63] Since parents were not performing their roles adequately, the nation's health could be safeguarded only if state-sponsored experts – public health officials or the SHC – took on the responsibility of educating the adult public and instructing school-going adolescents in moral hygiene. This endeavour, Milne noted, was important to 'the future welfare of the country' and had 'a very direct bearing on the solution of our Poor White problem'.[64]

Many doctors were concerned that the larger families of poor whites would swamp middle-class whites, as well as about the illegitimacy, prostitution and more casual attitude towards sex that they believed was rife among poor whites. By educating white adolescents and adults, the DPH and educational bodies believed they could redress the neglect of moral issues in poor families, perhaps prevent moral failure, and instil the values of a morality appropriate to whites and reflecting the different social roles of men and women. Treatment was simply the first step in dealing with VD, and had to complemented by what Fraser called 'a programme for moral and mental sanitation'.[65] Educational propaganda prescribed the terms of moral behaviour, and where the direct or implicit contrast was with African morality, it defined the norms of white behaviour too. VD propaganda constructed its audience not only as moral subjects but also as racial subjects.

By the 1930s the prescriptions for morality and sexuality provided in VD propaganda and adolescent sex education aimed at white audiences were explicitly contrasted with an image of promiscuous, uncontrolled African sexuality. During VD lectures, householders were warned of the perils of venereal infection from promiscuous house servants. During a Transvaal lecture trip, Dr J. H. Rauch 'stressed the fact that in South Africa we were living in the midst of a large native and coloured population which held very primitive ideas on matters of hygiene and sanitation as judged by civilised standards'. The 'native', already a 'reservoir' for endemic diseases, was 'now being gradually invaded with . . . venereal diseases'. Since Africans made up all the labour force, this constituted a 'danger to the health of the European population'. Rauch assumed that Africans would inevitably contract VD once working in town, and then 'innocently' transmit the disease to their white employers.[66] His ideas were in line with segregationist conceptions of African sexuality (see Chapter 6). Africans were depicted as naturally promiscuous in their tribal environment, but in an urban environment, free from their tribal sanctions and customs, this promiscuity became dangerous and led to VD.

Facts About Ourselves suggested that all humans had the same animal sexual instinct, but that evolutionary development had resulted in racial differentiation. Europeans had the 'advantage of two thousand years of civilisation . . . with all that it means in knowledge, self-control and care for others'. Africans were less developed mentally and morally, and thus incapable of rationally mastering their baser instincts. 'Their instincts are exactly the same as ours, but it is not reasonable or just to expect that they will have the same control over the working of them.'[67] The evolutionary advancement of whites had led to greater intelligence and the ability to judge whether an act was moral or not.[68] Civilisation meant rational control of mind over body; promiscuity was primitive and implicitly African.

These racial moral differences meant that whites had to observe appropriate etiquette when dealing with Africans. *Facts About Ourselves* warned girls that they should dress 'sensibly, nicely and comfortably without exposing too much of the body' to avoid attracting the attention of African men. It instructed boys to avoid vulgar jokes and conversation with African men, and instead to talk 'sensibly and to remember they [white boys] have a higher standard of civilisation to uphold'. The intention of these rules was to make clear that Africans were easily sexually aroused, and to break down the camaraderie or sense of social equality that officials feared existed among poor whites and Africans in the slums. 'If the natives have a real respect for our boys, they will be the more likely to have a genuine respect for our girls', the booklet concluded.[69]

VD education also clarified 'normal' and 'abnormal' sexuality for white men and women. Normal sexuality was associated with marriage and parenthood, rather than with personal gratification. 'The sex instinct demands satisfaction, but it is wrong to imagine that real satisfaction can come by indulging in the sex act. Sexual intercourse ... must take place only under the proper conditions, and for civilised people the only suitable conditions are provided by marriage.'[70] The result of sex outside marriage was VD.[71] Active sexuality was animalistic outside the confines of marriage. Thus white promiscuity and VD were signs of backward and primitive behaviour and were 'uncivilised'.

VD films contrasted images of the wholesome mother and the diseased good-time girl or amateur prostitute. Motherhood was portrayed as the focus of women's sexuality and the basis of her membership of the political community, her claim to being a citizen. The NCCVD claimed that having children was a national duty, 'the best work we can do for our country'.[72] A slide show entitled 'Love–Marriage–Parenthood' depicted women as the moral saviours of their families and the educators of their children into purity and chastity.[73] Sex for pleasure denied a woman's natural destiny as a mother and was abnormal. The message of The End of the Road, a popular VD film screened nationally, was that sex, love, marriage and motherhood were women's proper destiny. Excessive flirting and sexual experience before marriage led to VD and personal destruction. The sex instinct was only human when it was guided by love and the desire for children in a marital relationship; sex for pleasure had no meaning other than prostitution.[74]

The messages about normal male sexuality were more contradictory. The theme of British VD films, many of which were screened in South Africa, was that male sexuality was naturally promiscuous and led to VD, but this was not immoral as long as the infected man sought treatment.[75] For example the film *The Shadow* depicted a young man who visited a prostitute when drunk and contracted VD. He later passed on the infection to his innocent, newly wedded wife. But both went for medical treatment and ended up a cured, happy family. Medical treatment absolved the man of his moral failing.[76] Chastity and marital fidelity were held up as the ideal behaviour for men, but the natural force of the male libido meant that promiscuity was not a sign of inherent immorality, as it was for women.

This acceptance of a strong male libido did not mean that boys and men escaped the message of chastity. The legacy of the anti-CDPA lobby's association with suffragette and Christian organisations was the belief that men could learn to be as moral as women, and that society should insist on an equal moral standard.[77] The NCCVD stressed that male self-restraint was 'compatible with perfect health' and 'led to no loss of strength and virility in mind or body'.[78] The association between self-control and purity as the basis of masculinity continued into the 1930s. VD propaganda continually stressed that self-restraint was compatible with good health for men. Sexuality was a primitive instinct, and the mark of civilisation was disciplining the body with the mind. Sports could dissipate the sexual urge and at the same time promote greater physical prowess and self-control. A strong mind meant a healthy body. *Facts About Ourselves* urged boys to 'Keep your purity . . . it belongs to the girl you will marry'.[79] If sexual instinct linked men to animals, self-control separated them. The highest freedom 'is a freedom from our own bodies', . . . 'conscience and reason . . . should . . . dictate what our bodies are to do'.[80] For men, civilisation was a contradictory state of being: promiscuity was natural, and not deviant, yet its rational control was the acme of perfection.

During the 1920s and 1930s VD among poor whites was attributed to miscegenation, inbreeding, loss of racial self-respect and the difficulty of adjusting to a new urban environment. Constructing a South African nation of English- and Afrikaans-speaking whites involved specifying their difference from Africans and a uniform, 'civilised' moral and sexual code. Throughout this period VD propaganda was characterised by consistent themes explicitly contrasting white and African morality and behaviour, and defining the norms of white sexuality: chastity and the rational control of sexual instincts led to white moral and physical prowess; the undifferentiated promiscuity of the African contrasted with the individualised sexual identities of white men and women, bound by their whiteness but separated by their gender. In South Africa the message that continence preserved the health of the family and the nation, and that sex was healthy and a national duty within the confines of marriage, had the added resonance that moral behaviour was also civilised and white.

Conclusion

This chapter has shown how the Public Health Act marked a new direction in the treatment and prevention of VD and also helped affirm white racial identity and privilege. Until the 1920s, poor people with VD (usually women) were subject to criminal legislation and forcibly rounded up and confined to lock hospitals. When the provisions of the Public Health Act of 1919 were implemented the government set up free VD clinics for outpatient treatment. Now the dominant medical view was that VD was a disease like any other, rather than a crime or moral illness.

The Public Health Act also reflected the new welfarist approach to white health and well-being that was evident in the new housing, education, social welfare and employment schemes. These helped to segregate whites from Africans and affirmed the idea of white superiority. Free treatment, far from being a sign of pauperism, was the right of every white citizen and it was the duty of the state to ensure the healthy virility of its citizens. Treatment was complemented by educational propaganda. VD propaganda prescribed the boundaries of normal sexuality and morality, and was part of a process of moralising the white population and making individuals, rather than just the police and judiciary, responsible for regulating their own behaviour. While professional experts assumed the role of monitoring and 'uplifting' almost every aspect of white social life, citizens were expected to take responsibility for seeking treatment to ensure their own and the national health, and for conforming to the norms of white moral behaviour.

5
Migrancy, Prostitution and VD, 1920–50

In 1937 General Jan Smuts warned: 'The natives of this country are becoming rotten with disease and a menace to civilisation, instead of a first class nation.'[1] His fears were echoed by Dr O. P. Theron of the union's Public Health Council, who reported that VD and tuberculosis had spread to such 'alarming proportions' that in some areas 'colonies of Natives were almost living *en masse* in a putrescent state'.[2] In Nongoma district in Zululand in 1939, Regent Mshiyeni voiced his disquiet about 'a dreadful town disease which is threatening to destroy the whole country'.[3] The Transkeian Territories General Council expressed similar concerns.[4] These sentiments reflected the recognition that venereal syphilis had become a serious urban health problem and had spread to rural areas, which had been relatively unaffected at the turn of the century. Syphilis seemed to have an especial hold on the African population, and although doctors would occasionally report cases of gonorrhoea the focus of the medical literature was on syphilis. This reflected the continuing presence of endemic syphilis in parts of the country, resulting in inflated estimates of the extent of venereal syphilis in the African population.

The extent of VD in urban and rural African populations was a reflection of the general decline in African health by the interwar years. Government commissions during the 1930s and 1940s drew attention to the appalling health conditions in urban and rural areas: high infant mortality rates, widespread malnutrition and alarming morbidity rates for diseases associated with poverty, lack of sanitation and poor nutrition.[5] High morbidity rates of preventable diseases, including VD, were a sign not simply of decades of neglect of African health and medical services in urban and rural areas, but also of the toll exacted as the precapitalist, rural and agricultural society was transformed into a capitalist, industrial economy dependent largely on migrant labour.[6]

This chapter assesses the relationship between the increase in VD and the socioeconomic transformation of South Africa from the 1920s to the end of the 1940s, when rural living standards gradually declined and increasing numbers of men and women were drawn into a migratory life or settled permanently in the growing urban slums.

A statistical portrait

Lack of proper statistical surveys did not prevent doctors and laymen from making wild estimates of the extent of VD in the African popula- tion. Press reports in the early 1920s alleged that 50–60 per cent or even 80–90 per cent of Africans had syphilis. These estimates were rejected by the Department of Public Health (DPH), which believed that 10 per cent was a more likely figure.[7] The issue arose again in 1930 when the Native Economic Commission (NEC), which was investigating the socioeconomic circumstances of Africans as a basis for policy proposals to regulate urbanisation, questioned witnesses about the health of and the extent of VD in the African population. A Roman Catholic priest in Flagstaff, Transkei, told the NEC that 80 per cent of Africans had VD, but a district surgeon in the area considered that only 7–10 per cent were affected, while an Umtata African practitioner believed that only 1–2 per cent of rural Africans had syphilis.[8] In the face of such con- flicting reports the NEC called for a country-wide survey to establish the extent of VD in the African population, but the government and medical authorities never acted on this suggestion.[9] Even into the 1940s doctors continued to make wild estimates.[10]

The confusion over the extent of syphilis among Africans, and their unique symptoms, was, as in the late nineteenth century, probably due to the lack of recognition of endemic syphilis. As explained in Chapter 1, endemic syphilis is transmitted by non-sexual contact, primarily affects young children and is an indicator of poor personal and com- munity hygiene, rather than sexual promiscuity. Doctors first defined endemic syphilis in the 1930s, a decade after they had begun to accept the separate existence of yaws, a similar disease but confined to more humid areas.[11] However in South Africa, doctors still resisted explanations that did not point to sexually transmitted syphilis, pre- ferring to argue that the African symptoms of venereal syphilis were unique. In particular Africans were supposed to suffer destructive bone and joint lesions, rather than tabes and general paralysis, the more common sequelae of tertiary syphilis typical in the white population. The secretary for public health, for example, pointed out in the early 1920s that in Africans 'syphilis takes a milder form than in Europeans', with skin lesions being particularly common. Tertiary syphilis was not very common and had little impact on fertility.[12] A district surgeon in Vryburg also reported this to the NEC in 1931, noting that 'in spite of the fact that syphilis is rife amongst them [native women], they are most prolific – which is contrary to European standards'.[13] Even in the 1950s, many doctors remained blind to the possibility that the extent and characteristics of syphilis in Africans were unique because they were not the result of venereal syphilis, but of a related but different disease.[14]

As discussed in Chapter 6, doctors sought an explanation for the strange characteristics of syphilis in Africans' inherent racial difference, rather than in the aetiology of disease. However the absence of congenital and tertiary syphilis in the presence of other apparently syphilitic symptoms is suggestive of endemic syphilis. In addition the regional distribution of endemic syphilis in the 1920s and 1930s resembled the distribution patterns of the late nineteenth century. In the 1920s and 1930s the DPH reported that syphilis was still widespread in districts in the north-western Cape, Bechuanaland (Botswana) and the western and northern Transvaal.[15] However the disease seemed to be declining, a trend the DPH attributed to widespread treatment.[16] In 1920, for example, 600–700 cases were treated in hospital, 9895 cases by district surgeons and 15 336 cases at Rietfontein and the mission hospitals of Elim and Bochem, which were situated at the heart of the endemic syphilis areas.[17] Mercurial treatment did not result in a complete cure, but the infectious lesions usually disappeared and cases became latent. As the pool of active endemic syphilitic infection decreased, the incidence of cases would gradually decline.[18]

The uneven regional distribution of syphilis is illustrated by the results of a survey of African mine recruits conducted by the Witwatersrand Native Labour Association (WNLA) in 1930 (Table 5.1). The incidence of syphilis did not necessarily correspond to the number of migrant labourers in these particular areas. In 1938, in the high prevalence zone of southern Bechuanaland, only 40 per cent of economically active males were migrants,[19] but 70 per cent of males in the Transkei and 66 per cent in the Ciskei were absent from their homes in 1936, and these were both low prevalence areas.[20] Only among British Basotho (Lesotho) workers did the high prevalence rate seem to match the relatively high migration rate of 50 per cent,[21] but in the late nineteenth

Table 5.1   Syphilis incidence among African mine recruits, examined by the Witwatersrand Native Labour Association in 1930

Group examined	Number tested	Positive Wasserman reaction (%)
Transvaal Basuto	200	29.5
British Basuto	200	25.5
Bechuana	100	22.0
Mpondo	200	8.5
Mozambique	300	7.0
Xhosa	200	2.0

Source: Kark (1949), p. 78.

century some doctors had suggested that the Basuto suffered from endemic rather than venereal syphilis.[22] As exposure to endemic and venereal syphilis result in a seropositive reading on the Wasserman test, it is possible that the high prevalence among the Basuto and Bechuana recruits reflected their earlier infection with endemic syphilis, rather than venereal syphilis.

In groups with a low prevalence of syphilis such as the Mpondo and Xhosa, and in urban areas, the clinical descriptions of primary, tertiary and congenital syphilis seemed to indicate sexually transmitted venereal syphilis. One doctor, describing symptoms of syphilis in the Transkei in the 1940s, noted that the primary stage was often evident, particularly amongst men, and it was seldom extragenital. He had also seen tertiary symptoms such as cardiovascular disease and neurosyphilis. Tertiary symptoms also appeared among mental asylum inmates – 7 per cent of African inmates in 1936–40 suffered from cerebral syphilis.[23] Autopsies on African hospital patients between 1924 and 1938 showed that 5.9 per cent had died from undetected syphilitic heart disease.[24] Another six-month study of postmortems conducted after natural deaths revealed that 12 per cent had been due to syphilitic aortitis.[25]

Congenital syphilis occurred in both urban and rural populations. A breakdown of the admission records of the East London Location Dispensary between 1932 and 1936 showed that of a total 137 syphilis cases, 58 (42.3 per cent) were due to congenital syphilis.[26] In Alexandra, a freehold township near Johannesburg, among 506 infants who had died in 1940 during their first year, 19 (3.8 per cent) of the deaths were attributable to congenital syphilis.[27] Records from King Edward VIII Hospital in Durban in 1941 showed that 22 per cent of infantile deaths were due directly to syphilis.[28] Figures were also high in rural areas. Between 1941 and 1946 in Polela, Zululand, 20.6 per cent of newly born infants had congenital syphilis.[29]

Sexually transmitted diseases are also associated with sterility and miscarriages among women. The assistant health officer for the union noted in 1922 that among Mpondo women 'a history of miscarriage suddenly appearing and remaining, formerly most uncommmon, is now most common'.[30] In the early 1930s Mpondo informants told Monica Hunter, an anthropologist, that women did not bear as many children as had their mothers and grandmothers, and many women were sterile.[31] There were also reports about an increase in sterility and stillbirths in Natal.[32]

The emergence of venereal syphilis in Pondoland and the eastern Transvaal[33] was regarded as a new trend by doctors, who associated the disease with migrancy. The assistant health officer of the union commented in 1922 that '[s]yphilis was practically non-existent in Pondoland thirty or even twenty years ago, and has only become so terribly prevalent since the Mpondo went to Durban, Johannesburg and Kimberley'.[34] In Sibasa in the eastern Transvaal, VD cases were still comparatively rare in 1936, and the district surgeon reported that in 'nearly every case it was possible to trace the infection to an individual who had recently returned from town'.[35] The pattern was similar in Natal, where syphilis appeared to be increasing and related to migrancy. A study tracing the sources of venereal infection in rural Polela (Natal) in the 1940s showed that most married and single women patients had been infected in their rural homes by husbands or lovers who had recently returned from working in a town or on a farm. Only two out of 20 male patients had been infected by their wives, who were assumed to have been adulterous.[36] Tables A2.3 and A2.4 (Appendix 2) suggest that during the interwar years the incidence of venereal syphilis in the rural population was still relatively lower than in the urban population, and that the disease was usually contracted in urban areas and then transmitted to rural areas when migrants returned home.

Migration, prostitution and VD

Transient sexual relationships in urban and rural areas, and the constant traffic of men between rural and urban areas probably contributed to the high rate of VD in the African population.

At every small country rail station channelling migrant men to the mines or larger cities, or marking their return home, were groups of women who depended on these migrants for their livelihood, offering them food, sex and companionship before they continued on their journeys. The routes between Basotholand and Johannesburg, and from Mpondoland to major railheads at Umtata, MacLear and Port Shepstone, where men entrained for Johannesburg or Durban, were dotted with 'rest camps' where prostitutes gathered, reported state and mine administrators in the 1920s and 1930s.[37] Officials in Umtata, the central station in the Transkei for migrants departing for and returning from work at the mines and in the towns, warned in 1929 that 'this area is the focus for the disease for the whole country served by this railhead'. A detective sergeant reported that women living in the nearby slum township 'are meeting Join boys going and coming from Johannesburg and giving this disease to them. These Join boys carry the disease all over the Union and Umtata.'[38] There were similar complaints by administrators and chiefs in Basutoland about the activities of women in the border towns,[39] and from administrators in Zebedelia in the northeastern Transvaal when the extension of the railway opened the area for migration to the Rand.[40] Throughout the 1930s the mining industry also complained that its recruits were contracting VD on their way to or from the mines by consorting with prostitutes.[41]

Administrators considered that women living in the urban slums or in squatter settlements on farms surrounding the mines were the source of VD. 'The large majority of cases are contracted in locations adjacent to compounds, over which, of course, the Mining Companies have no jurisdiction', the Chamber of Mines complained to the Director of Native Labour in 1922.[42] During the 1930s the mining industry continued to blame the women in urban townships for spreading VD, and noted that outlying mines, far from townships, had fewer cases of VD.[43]

Likewise, in the eastern Transvaal in the mid 1920s and Natal by 1930 the collieries regarded the uncontrolled settlement of women in and around the collieries as responsible for VD among their male workforce.[44] In 1925 a local magistrate in the Breyten area described the married quarters as 'a refuge for all kinds of loose characters' and the cause of 'the liquor traffic . . . and the spread of disease'.[45] The squatter settlements of wives and single women in the surrounding farms were 'a hotbed of the disease and drunkenness. . . . Most . . . if not all' of these women 'were probably infected with syphilis' and were 'spread[ing it] through the district'.[46] In the late 1930s several government commissions continued to blame women from Basotholand and Mozambique for 'indulging in immorality and spreading disease' at the coalfields and on the Witwatersrand.[47] By 1930 the collieries of northern Natal and nearby towns such as Dundee, Newcastle and Dannhauser were facing a similarly huge female influx from the reserves, and especially the farms, which they too linked directly to the spiralling VD rate.[48]

Migrant travel clearly helped to spread VD from urban to rural areas. The impact of migration and proletarianisation on social relationships in rural and urban areas also encouraged casual sexual relationships. Longer periods of migration and infrequent contact with their rural homes made men more likely to seek relationships with women in towns. Young men's access to an independent income gradually diminished the social relationships and obligations that bound traditional marriages. Abandoned wives and single women who migrated to towns had few economic opportunities, and relationships with migrants offered a degree of financial and social security.

The impact of migrancy on social relationships

The institutionalisation of the migrant labour system and urbanisation reflected the gradual collapse of the rural agricultural economy. The Land Act of 1913 had defined the restricted boundaries of African reserves and, together with antisquatting legislation, facilitated the demise of the independent African peasantry.[49] Increasing population density and land degradation meant that by the 1920s the reserves were producing less than half the subsistence needs of their population and some homesteads no longer had access to land or owned cattle, though the pattern varied between areas.[50] As conditions worsened, dependence on migrancy began to dominate rural economies. Older men and women as well as the usual complement of young men entered the migrant labour market. In relatively conservative areas such as Pondoland, the proportion of economically active men aged 15–45 working away from home increased from 24 per cent in 1911 to 34 per cent in 1921, and to 43 per cent by 1936. Other districts were more heavily involved in migrancy, and the overall proportion for the Transkeian Territories steadily rose from 41 per cent in 1911 to 57 per cent in 1936.[51] In Basutoland the number of men absent from home rose steadily from 10 per cent of the total male population in 1911 to 15 per cent in 1921 and 25 per cent in 1936, levelling out at 28 per cent by 1946.[52] This exodus from the reserves was accompanied by emigration from white farms. Labour tenancy was also in decline by the late 1920s and white landowners began to evict their labour tenants to put more land into intensive use with the help of waged labourers.[53] By the 1940s the exodus from farming areas was greater than that from the reserves.[54]

As migrant men became increasingly dependent on their income from work at the mines or in white towns, they spent longer periods under contract and shorter periods at home, gradually losing contact with their rural homes. In 1931 the average time worked at the mines was 10.88 months, and an average of 8.1 months were spent at home. Within six months, 40 per cent of miners returned to work, and 44 per cent after a year. By 1942 on average migrant mine workers were spending 13.6 months at the mines and 7.6 months at home. Within six months 44 per cent returned to work, 36 per cent after a year, but 20 per cent returned to work 'after what may be regarded as no more than a holiday visit to the Reserve', according to the Lansdown commission investigating conditions at the mines. It noted that 'a considerable percentage of the Reserve natives have to work here almost continuously with relatively short breaks to earn a living'.[55] Isaac Schapera, an anthropologist, studied several migrant labour source regions in the Bechuanaland Protectorate (Botswana) in 1932–34 and 1943. He found that younger migrants spent longer periods away on contract and had longer migrant careers than older men, and that visits home had shortened.[56]

The long absence of men from their homes, wives' dependence on inadequate remittances and fear of abandonment imposed a great strain on marital relationships, as reflected in increasing male accusations of adultery. Wives living in their husbands' homesteads became the *de facto* heads of their households, but without the equivalent social or financial authority. When a husband failed to remit sufficient funds or abandoned his wife, she had to seek additional support. In some cases kin might take her in, but such relationships were beginning to break down.[57] Some women, facing economic and social marginalisation, chose to return to their parents' home and become *amadikazi*: women living temporarily or permanently in their father's or brother's homestead, including abandoned or divorced wives, unmarried women with children and married women visiting their parental homes for a while. *Amadikazi* had far greater social freedom than wives living in their husbands' homesteads, who had a heavier workload, were required to observe *hlonipa* (respect and avoidance) restrictions in their relations with senior male agnates, and whose social activities were restricted. *Amadikazi* could go to *itimiti* (formalised meetings at which beer was sold and men and women danced, modelled on the 'tea meetings' of the school people) and enter and drink inside the hut with the men, rather than drinking outside with other wives; and they could accept lovers at 'beer drinks', although if the woman was married the relationship was still defined as adulterous.[58]

In her study of the Mpondo in the early 1930s, Monica Hunter reported that African men thought that although *amadikazi* had always existed, their numbers had increased by the 1930s and that adultery by wives was on the increase. At one time the Native Recruiting Corporation gave a coloured kerchief to men upon their enlistment for a work contract, which many gave to their wives. The kerchiefs became unpopular, she reported, because husbands felt that when donned by their wives they indicated to other men that their husbands were away and they could be seduced safely.[59] Several anthropologists reported that men relied on protective medicines to prevent adultery by their wives in their absence and to harm prospective lovers.[60] In the early 1930s missionaries reported that when a wife contracted VD, either from her husband or through close cohabitation with infected women, she was accused of adultery and witchcraft.[61]

For women abandoned by their husbands or lovers, brewing and selling beer, and sexual relationships with returned migrants were a means of survival. Becoming an *idikazi* was also a way for a woman to reject the privations and dependence of marriage. Their new independence was symbolically captured in *famo* dances and songs, often performed at beer drinks or shebeens in urban areas, in which women offered moral commentary on their experience of poverty and abandonment while provocatively soliciting male company and rejecting their authority.[62]

By the mid 1930s these social changes were beginning to have an impact on the spread of syphilis. Missionaries who ran the Raleigh Fitkin Memorial Hospital in Bremersdorp, Swaziland commented in 1936 that while '[p]reviously the majority of our cases could be traced to the townships', now the 'congregation of natives of both sexes at beer drinks is becoming increasingly the source of spread of this disease'.[63] Ten years later the Umtata Native Welfare Society tendered similar evidence to the Fagan Commission in respect of conditions in rural Transkei. 'The women at home tend to lead an uncontrolled life and become . . . "Amatshawekazi", which means prostitutes who spend nights, often for several days, at beer drinks in the company of men other than their husbands, especially men who have returned from the mines and can spend a lot of money on these women, buying them Kaffir beer and giving them a good time in all possible ways.'[64] While men despaired of curbing the immorality of their wives, for women, taking lovers was a way to procure some emotional and economic support during the long, uncertain and possibly permanent absence of their husbands.

Other young women chose to leave the rural areas for the towns. From the early twentieth century first Mozambican and then Basotho women constituted a disproportionate number of female migrants to the Rand, while Mpondo women remained traditionalist even in the 1930s. This reflected the earlier and more severe impact of migrancy on Mozambican and Basotho society.[65] The estimated number of Mozambican women in the Rand and at the coalfields in the early 1920s was about 2000, and in 1930s in the Rand it was around 6500.[66] The number of women absent from Basutoland increased from 1.3 per cent of the total female population in 1911 to 3.3 per cent in 1921, levelling out at 9.3 per cent in 1936–46.[67] Those most likely to migrate, suggests Philip Bonner in his study of Basotho women, were those who, under the strain of rural pauperisation and the migrant labour system, had become socially and economically marginalised in rural society.[68] For women whose access to and investment in rural resources was often minimal, the move to town was permanent.

A few of the women were from polygynous households and were probably cowives or junior wives, or the divorced wives of men who had accepted Christianity and monogamy. Their prominence declined as the number of polygynous marriages in Basutoland decreased from 18.7 per cent in 1911 to 8.4 per cent in 1946 due to poverty and shortage of land. In other areas, such as Ngqeleni, a conservative district in Pondoland where land was still plentiful by the 1930s, 15 per cent of men were polygamists in 1932, but this had declined to 4–5 per cent by 1950.[69] Other migrants were widows who faced either a levirate marriage to male kinsmen of their husband or were perpetually vulnerable to men. They also lacked protection against chiefs' demands for fines and labour, and were often arbitrarily deprived of their land, which was reallocated to young male taxpayers.

Another category of Basotho migrants were women who had not been properly married and had subsequently been abandoned. *Bohali* or bride-wealth payments had escalated in the late nineteenth century as a way of entrenching the chiefly lineage in Basotholand, but this had made marriage extremely difficult for commoners. By 1910 abduction, seduction and elopement had become a common way of marrying on the cheap as the compensation (*chobale*) paid to the woman's family acted as the first payment of *bohali*. Similarly, in the Keiskammahoek district of the Ciskei marriages by abduction (*twala*) increased from 5 per cent before 1890 to 36.6 per cent in 1940–50.[70] Without the transfer of significant bridewealth the men had only limited rights over their children, weaker bonds with their wives, and were more likely to disappear to South Africa and never return. These abandoned wives, with few claims on their husband's kin, were likely to migrate to town.

However the largest number of migrants were women who had been properly married, owned cattle and lived with their children in monogamous homes. Within a few months of marriage their husbands had returned to an urban-based job and remained away for long periods, returned infrequently, sent home remittances intermittently and sometimes abandoned their families. Wives had to deal not only with insecurity and poverty, but as new wives they lived in their in-laws' homesteads and had to cope with conflict over the allocation and distribution of their husband's remittances, *hlonipa* restrictions and conflicts over the allocation of work.[71] Women who went in search of their husbands often found that their men had disappeared without trace or refused to renew contact, so they had to establish themselves independently in town.

For a newcomer to the city, whether married or not, finding a way to support herself and her children was not easy. Women were excluded from formal employment by a rigid sexual and racial division of labour. Domestic work was dominated by men in the Rand and in Durban, though women did take in washing and ironing from white families. Men's wages were extremely low, pegged at the level migrants had to accept, which was insufficient for an urban family and meant that even married women living with their husbands had to work. For many women informal sector activities – hawking and beer brewing – were the only way to supplement their husband's income or establish an independent livelihood and look after their children.[72]

Beer brewing was often associated by administrators and anthropologists with 'prostitution', though a range of different relationships were recognised. These ranged along a continuum from a straight cash-for-sex exchange, preferred by some men because it implied no responsibilities, to becoming an *intombi*, or girlfriend whom a man could seduce and ensure her fidelity by giving her gifts, to entering into a relationship with an *ishweshwe* or *nyatsi*, undertaking domestic services in return for regular support from one or more male partners.[73] Ellen Hellman, an urban anthropologist studying an inner-city slum in Johannesburg, noted that '[m]any women [beer brewers], hardpressed to balance expenditure and revenue . . . must be expected to succumb to prostitution as an additional means of supplementing their incomes'. This was true not just of unmarried women, but also of married women. Sometimes a married woman 'unbeknown to her husband succeeds in earning part of her alleged beer money by having one or more *nyatsi*

who pays her for the favours she extends them'.[74] Several commenta-
tors also noted that domestic workers often depended on one or several
lovers to make ends meet. Mabel Palmer, a member of the Durban Joint
Council, noted that '[w]hat appears to develop is not so much organised commercial prostitution, . . . as a system of free love whereby young
women earning a partial wage from European employment change
lovers frequently'.[75] A relationship might last until a male migrant
returned home, but until then, in exchange for home cooking, companionship and sex, 'the men . . . pay their share of housekeeping and
. . . such household equipment as a primus stove'.[76] This suggests that
domestic workers and migrants cohabited, accepting the obligations of
marriage without formalising the relationship. Municipal housing was
only available to married couples, so women also sought a partner to
gain access to housing.[77] Marriage also protected a woman from being
deported from urban areas, as married women were not defined as
'habitually unemployed'.

Administrators, missionaries and philanthropists commented widely
on the trend towards informal relationships. In half of marriages in
Orlando in 1939, according the township superintendent, 'the couples
are not married but just live together', and similar situations were
reported in other townships. Some of these informal relationships lasted
for six to eight years, and in one case 16 years, but on average they
lasted two years.[78]

In many cases the informal unions were entered into for economic
reasons. Traditionally a son depended on his father and male relatives
to collect *lobola* for him, and even migrants frequently turned over their
earnings to their fathers to use as they saw fit. But by the 1930s many
young men were keeping their wages and paying their own *lobola*.
According to Krige, even if the father was still considered responsible
for *lobola*, 'there is a masked tendency for men to pay *lobola* out of their
own earnings'.[79] A couple might cohabit while the marriage negotiations were taking place and the man was saving for *lobola*.[80] But if a man
could not afford gradual marriage negotiations, or the feasting and
display associated with a wedding ceremony, he might postpone the
marriage indefinitely.[81] Some men refused to register a civil marriage as
the marriage officer was often the pass officer and poll tax collector and
might discover that his tax had not been paid.[82] Other men found it
impossible to pay for their marriages and provide for their own children
as they were already responsible for the 'illegitimate' children of their
sisters.[83] Eventually some couples legitimated their informal relationships through *lobola* or Christian marriage.[84]

The commoditisation of bridewealth also undermined the social and legal rights it had once implied, making the marriage tie more tenuous and women more vulnerable to abandonment. Formerly bridewealth was a settlement in cattle passed from the groom to the bride's family, which guaranteed the wife protection if she was maltreated by her husband or his kin and established the legitimacy of her children. Anthropologists and administrators noted that bridewealth was increasingly being paid as an exact cash settlement and was seen as a 'purchase and sale' rather than a sign of mutual conjugal responsibilities and respect. Janisch reported that marriages were more stable when *lobola* was paid in cattle: 'where *lobola* is paid in money, the protection of the marriage by both the bride and groom's clans is being broken down. Not only are heavy cash debts involved, but as the Africans say: "Money has no calves", and once it is spent the beneficiaries cease to feel responsible for the marriage from which they have received advantages.'[85] Failure to pay *lobola*, or payment of only part of the sum, made it easier for a man to abandon his wife when she became pregnant as he had no rights over the child. Without the security of *lobola*, a deserted wife had no kin to turn to, and had to fend for herself. She then might seek another partner to ensure economic support.[86]

With the decline of the social and legal protection offered by *lobola*, women turned to the courts to enforce their rights, though men resented even these limited legal powers, which challenged their own domestic authority. Some women insisted on a civil as well as a Christian or customary marriage as protection against desertion or being usurped by a second wife, and as a way of making their husbands legally responsible for household maintenance.[87]

The apparent acceptance by urban and rural African communities of premarital pregnancy and illegitimacy reflected not only changes in customary marriage, but also the decline in customary sanctions over adolescent sexuality. In traditional society girls had received explicit sex education not from their mothers, but from their female peers. Initiation schools and coming of age songs had been commonplace throughout South Africa and had instructed girls on their rights and duties as women, and etiquette in marriage. Some groups had practiced premarital intracrural sex, but this had been strictly regulated by the peer group and girls were examined to ensure their virginity. If a girl fell pregnant, her lover was fined and both were publically disgraced. Anthropologists such as Hunter concluded that this public recognition and control meant that it had been 'unusual for a girl to have a child before marriage'.[88]

By the early twentieth century missionaries had banned puberty rituals and intercrural sex among adolescents as they associated these customs with promiscuity and lack of respect for women. Even in non-Christian communities, with ever increasing numbers of young men becoming migrants, it was difficult to impose sanctions or hold young men responsible for their illegitimate children. The absence of fathers from their homes also left discipline to the mothers, who were customarily expected to be more indulgent.[89] By the 1930s among the Mpondo and Xhosa, for example, girls often refused to submit to an examination by older women, and though boys might be fined for seduction and pregnancy, the stigma had declined.[90] By the 1930s older Christian women who had seen initiation songs and teaching being condemned as obscene, and had accepted reticence and the use of euphemisms about sex as Christian, were unwilling to speak candidly to their daughters about sex and reproduction, as missionaries urged. Thus explicit advice on how to avoid pregnancy became less available to girls from Christian homes, just as premarital sex became easier to experience, since girls led less supervised school lives and adopted ideas of romantic love.[91]

Parents found it difficult to control adolescent children who socialised with migrants free of the discipline of their peers or relatives. In rural areas, girls were often pressurised by returning migrants to submit to sexual intercourse during their brief period at home, though if a girl fell pregnant the young man might abscond.[92] In urban areas adolescents were freer of parental and community discipline, and parents blamed premarital pregnancies on the 'loose' sexual ethos of *marabi* dances, and on the shebeens where their daughters met and were seduced by young urban and migrant men.[93]

The changes in marriage practices and the controls over sexual behaviour, together with widespread migrancy helped to create an environment in which VD could spread. Longer periods of migrancy and infrequent contact with their rural homes made men more likely to seek relationships with women in towns. Women in rural areas who had been abandoned by their husbands, or those who migrated independently to town, had few economic opportunities and relationships with migrants offered a degree of financial and social security. In an environment where formalised marriage and informal relationships were unstable, and where economic pressures made sexual relationships a source of income, sexually transmitted diseases were bound to spread.

Contesting sexual behaviour

Yet to assume that migrancy inevitably led to VD is too simplistic and implies that Africans were inevitably promiscuous. The possibility of migrants abandoning their rural families, or seeking transient relationships in urban or rural areas that might result in VD, did not go unchallenged by male and female migrants, their families and rural communities.

From the early twentieth century migrant associations attempted to control migrants' sexual activities in towns. These associations not only provided protection and comfort in an alien urban environment, but also reasserted rural ties and values. Among the Pedi, urban areas were termed *makgoweng* ('place of the whites') and young migrants were warned that townships and urban women were dangerous and disease-ridden. In urban areas Pedi often lived with men from their home village and districts, and the ethos of these migrant networks was that men's prime responsibility was to their parents and later to their own households. Men who became involved with urban women were shunned and punished. A similar rejection of urban lifestyle and association with urban women occurred among *amalaitas*: groups of uneducated, non-Christian youths from the northern and eastern Transvaal who mainly engaged in domestic work.[94] If a migrant was suspected of infidelity by his wife, her mother-in-law would often side with her in pressuring the man to remember his responsibilities to his rural home.[95]

Homosexual relationships in mining compounds and municipal barracks were also a way of preventing migrants from meeting urban women. Older men, who were often in positions of authority at the mines, took novice male recruits as 'wives' and expected sexual and domestic services in exchange for gifts of money, material goods or a transfer to a better job. The men practiced *metsha* (intracrural sex), which meant that the risk of contracting VD was minimised. For a young man a 'mine marriage' was a way of avoiding entanglements with town women, increasing his wages, reducing his number of contracts, paying bridewealth and establishing his own homestead more quickly. It was a means of strengthening his commitment to his rural home.[96] Rural wives were aware of and not necessarily opposed to migrants' homosexual relationships, believing that this meant men were less likely to form permanent relationships in town and less likely to contract VD.[97] Migrants themselves saw homosexual relationships as a way of avoiding VD. An anonymous memo to the NEC about migrant worker barracks in Durban reported that

> Those who practice Homosexualism give the following explanation for it. Nowadays here in Durban good, healthy and moral girls are hard to find because they are so few; the majority of single females are possessed of venereal diseases. . . . Bitter experience has therefore taught these people that Native town women are to be shunned altogether. . . . If you have sexual union with males you get an outlet for your carnal desires and at the same time escape getting diseased.[98]

Abstinence was also a way to avoid infection. Among the Pedi, some homosexuality occurred in compounds, but young men were usually encouraged by the elders to go home to Sekhukhuneland, which was relatively near the Rand, if they could no longer cope with compound isolation and wanted the companionship of their wives or girlfriends.[99] Reverend H. P. Junod reported to the Fagan Commission in 1946 that migrants in Gazaland (Mozambique) had a 'more seasonal, less permanent' libido. He went on to explain that a migrant had told him that 'sexual abstinence had been almost automatic . . . and that, as soon as the sexual urge re-appeared, after about eighteen months he went home'.[100] This 'automatic' abstinence may have had its origins in a taboo on sex observed during hunting trips lasting several months by hunters and their wives at home. The taboo was supposed to prevent mishaps, death or injury to the hunters.[101] The Chamber of Mines also suggested that a married man's customary abstention from intercourse while his wife was pregnant or lactating, coincided with many migrants' contracts and resulted in celibacy at the mines.[102] Certainly, gold mine morbidity rates from the mid 1930s to the mid 1940s remained at about 0.6 per cent for syphilis and 0.2 per cent for gonorrhoea (though the rates at coal mines were occasionally higher), which was far lower than the rates in urban and rural areas (Appendix 2, Table A2.5). This may reflect the impact of homosexual relationships and abstinence as ways of controlling migrant sexuality and preventing VD.

In rural areas too, young men tried to regulate their relationships with young women. In Pondoland in the 1930s the *indlavini* youth groups emerged just as migration to the Rand began to escalate. They attempted to regulate their own social behaviour towards women through a set of formal rules governing courtship and *metsha*, and prohibiting members from initiating relationships with girlfriends of other members. They saw themselves as more disciplined in sexual relationships than youth described as *amanene*, who had more education and longer urban experience, and showed less restraint about impregnation. Although the *indlavini* were less respectful to their elders, reflecting the erosion of homestead and parental control and their economic independence, they still paid bridewealth, married and sought to establish their own homesteads.[103]

Migrant men also tried to control the sexual behaviour of women in rural and urban areas. In Mozambique in the late nineteenth century, to protect his wife against her own sexuality and procreativity, for a fee, a migrant usually left his wife and family in the care of his father, brother or heir – a protective role known as *basopa*, from the Afrikaans or Fanagalo expression 'to watch out'.[104] In the eastern Cape in the inter-war years, some men appointed a male substitute to offer intercrural sex to their wives during their absence, thus gratifying and safely channelling their wives' sexual desires and controlling their fertility.[105] Of equal concern to men was women's rejection of *hlonipa*, the levirate and marriage, and their economic and sexual independence in urban areas, which undermined male authority and was regarded by men as evidence of female promiscuity, insubordination and financial greed. On the Witwatersrand some men responded to this new independence individually through assault, or collectively through gangs such as the MaRashea, made up of Basotho migrants. A woman living with a MaRashea member had to submit to a code of male authority and fidelity, or else risk being seized, assaulted and raped.[106] Similarly in eastern Cape rural townships in the late 1940s, magistrates noted an increase in the number of cases of sexual violence, as men tried to control women who had 'got out of hand'.[107] This violence was an attempt to regulate women's sexual activities, and to ensure their fidelity and acceptance of male authority.

Christian communities also tried to regulate the sexuality of youths and migrants. *Manyanos* (uniformed prayer associations) tried to instil Christian norms for marriage, domesticity and courtship among mothers and their daughters, especially emphasising the significance of premarital chastity.[108] The Bantu Purity League, established in Natal in 1919, also formalised a puritan, Christian etiquette for courtship, betrothal and marriage as a way of forging a respectable, progressive identity among the young Christian elite.[109] The Zulu Cultural Society, established in the 1930s, tried to reconcile the 'traditional' values of wifely submission and obedience with Christian values.[110]

Migrant women similarly tried to regulate their relationships with men in the towns. Bozzoli's study of mostly Christian women migrants from Phokeng in the western Transvaal documents how these women saw migrancy as a rite of passage into adulthood, which allowed them to bring a dowry into their future marriages. Eminently respectable, these women defended themselves from unwanted advances by walking in groups at night, sharing sleeping accommodation and writing letters to shame a less educated suitor, or to initiate social pressure from a man's parents.[111]

Migration certainly disrupted social relations and encouraged transient sexual relationships, but rural, urban and migrant communities also tried to regulate the sexual behaviour of men and women to reinforce traditional or Christian norms and alleviate the disruptive impact of the migrant labour system, and sometimes explicitly to prevent VD.

Conclusion

The rich supply of documents on syphilis in the African population, despite their limitations by modern statistical standards, allow one to construct a portrait of the incidence and causes of syphilis between the 1920s and 1940s. I have suggested that the reportedly high prevalence of venereal syphilis in the African population must be tempered by recognition of the presence of endemic syphilis in certain rural areas, though in contrast to the late nineteenth century, sexually transmitted syphilis was increasingly evident in urban and rural areas.

The extent of VD in the African population seems to reflect the consequences of the migrant labour system on African social life by the interwar years. Rural immiseration, increasing dependence on migrant labour by men and women, longer periods of migration, inducing some men to seek transient relationships with urban women, urban women's economic dependence on sexual relationships for survival, and migrant workers carrying disease from urban to rural areas, all led to the spread of VD. However this was tempered by African communities' attempts to control the sexual behaviour of migrants, and informal relationships did not necessarily imply prostitution.

What remains unanswered is why doctors believed that VD was so pervasive among Africans and failed to recognise endemic syphilis, and why it was widely assumed that Africans in urban areas became rampantly immoral and spread VD. In other words, one has to analyse how the fears and perceptions of VD were socially constructed.

6
Moral Tribes and Corrupting Cities: VD and the 'Native Question', 1920–50

In the early 1930s the Department of Public Health (DPH) blamed the 'increased prevalence [of VD] especially amongst the urbanised and detribalised class of natives' on 'the slackening or absence of moral restrictions amongst them'.[1] Administrators and liberal and missionary philanthropists linked the extent of VD in the general African population to widespread cohabitation, illegitimacy, prostitution and beer brewing, which they attributed to the presence of African women in the towns. The belief that urban life was corrupting and town women were diseased prostitutes was also shared by Africans in urban and rural areas. By the late 1920s, among rural and urban communities the terms 'Basuto woman' and 'town woman' were euphemisms for a prostitute.[2] A genre of African literature also emerged around the themes of the provocatively sexual 'loose town woman', who was promiscuous and enticed by money, and the evils of city life luring young men and women from the country to disease and personal destruction.[3]

The influx of women into the towns hit at the central problem of segregationist policy: how to control the pace of African urbanisation, shore up rural society and regulate the lives and activities of Africans in urban areas to establish a stable social order. The presence of African women in the towns reflected the decline of African men's authority over the sexuality and mobility of their wives and daughters, the decline of tribalism and the fragility of white power. In the eyes of administrators, VD seemed to be the result of the influx of women into towns and their release from tribal controls. They associated VD with prostitution and cohabitation, which symbolised the dangers of urbanisation for Africans. However, as I explore in this chapter, their efforts to control the flow of women into towns continually met with failure.

Doctors' interpretations of the causes of VD in the African population were filtered through the distinctive language of segregation, which drew on anthropology to construct 'the African' as rural and tribal. Medical discourse helped affirm notions of racial difference in cultural terms, objectifying the African as part of a homogeneous tribal group and defining the process of urbanisation as pathological for 'normal' tribal society. This approach differed from explanations of VD in the white population, which associated VD with the 'abnormal' sexual character of individual men or women and with racial degeneration due to environmental conditions. Only in the late 1940s did some doctors and liberals begin to suggest that VD in Africans, like whites, could be attributed to the social disruption wrought by the impact of migration and urbanisation and begin to see Africans as individuals reacting to changes around them and making moral choices.

Social crisis

During the interwar years, white rural impoverishment, proletarianisation and urban militancy was matched by a similar process in the African population. The most visible aspect of the social crisis was the growing number of African men and women who became migrants or settled permanently in urban slums. The African male population resident or working in urban areas expanded most dramatically during the early 1920s to the mid 1930s, and continued to increase, but at a slower rate, into the 1940s (Table 6.1).

This influx reflected the gradual disintegration of the reserve economies (due to land shortage, population pressure, soil erosion and overstocking), as well as the decline in labour tenancy on white farms and the emergence of capitalist agriculture. In the early 1930s the Native Economic Commission, set up to investigate the social and economic conditions of Africans in urban areas, warned that the deterioration of the reserves could lead to a 'poor black problem' on a larger scale than the already existing 'poor white problem', and that this would pose a social and political threat to white supremacy.[4] 'The real racial danger in South Africa today', proclaimed the secretary of public health, was 'that the Europeans may be elbowed out or swamped and absorbed by the natives'.[5]

Another sign of the depth of the social crisis in rural areas was the presence of women in the cities. In 1924, local authorities drew the government's attention to the 'growing tendency amongst Native women

Table 6.1   African male and female urban population, 1911–46

Census year	Total urban population	Number of Men	Average increase (%)	Number of women	Average increase (%)
1911	508 142	410 161	–	97 981	–
1921	587 000	439 707	7	147 293	50
1936	1 141 642	784 359	78	357 283	143
1946	1 794 212	1 152 022	47	642 190	80

Sources: UG 22-32, p. 61; Herbst Report (1937–39), p. 77, para. 436; UG 28-48, p. 6, para. 7, p. 10, para. 13.

to abandon their mode of kraal life and migrat[e] to the towns, whether accompanied by their men-folk or not', and this refrain continued throughout the interwar years.[6] Although the male population in urban areas still outnumbered the female, the percentage increase of women far exceeded that of men (Table 6.1). Some of the women accompanied their husbands,[7] but many arrived in town on their own.

Vaughan suggests in her study of VD in east and central Africa that in the shared discourse of African men and administrators, African women represented tradition and order in a period of rapid social and economic change, and when they stepped outside this role they came to be seen as the source and reflection of social disintegration.[8] This seems to be true in the South African case too. For government administrators, the influx of women into the towns seemed to embody a range of problems resulting from uncontrolled urbanisation. It was African women who were blamed for the physical and moral decline of the African population, and – through miscegenation – for the potential downfall of the white population as well. It was African women who brewed liquor illegally and engaged in prostitution, creating a culture of lawlessness. And it was they whose uncontrolled urbanisation signified the potential fragility of white political and administrative power.

Administrators' concerns were matched by the concern of rural and urban African men about the fragility of their own power. The flight of women from their rural homes, the number of young men settling down with urban women and the changes in customary marriage directly undermined the basis of rural society and male authority. The authority of older men in African society depended on their control of marriage, and the ties of dependence between younger and older men. Young men's economic independence and their tendency to pay their own bridewealth, rather than rely on their male elders, undercut this directly. Without economic ties and social obligations to his father, not only could a young man abandon his rural homestead, but he could also marry whom he wished, and if he wanted to dissolve the marriage he had fewer family obligations to consider.[9] Young men were unlikely to return home to establish their own homesteads or send home remittances if they settled permanently in urban areas with their wives, sought relationships with other urban women or were deserted by their wives. If a young wife left her in-laws' homestead to return home or migrate to a town, the parents-in-law lost the rights to the young woman's labour and the seasonal labour of her husband. The perception that adultery and the number of *amadikazi* were increasing was another reflection of males' concern about their declining authority.[10]

These views were reflected in the findings of the Native Affairs Commission, a body of 'experts' who were regarded as 'friends of the Natives', advised on native affairs and considered African views. During the early 1920s the Native Affairs Commission consistently attributed the physical and moral decline of Africans to the disintegration of the traditional tribal system and the decline of chiefly authority, leading to an absence of discipline, the loss of parental control over adolescents and young adults, and uncontrolled mobility and immorality on the part of women.[11]

The 'new African elite' also viewed with dismay the activities of town women and whites' perceptions of African women. The term 'new African' referred to men who were educated, urbanised and Christian, and tended to be small entrepreneurs or landowners, professionals, court interpreters, teachers or priests. From the 1920s their economic independence was undercut as the government reserved certain jobs for whites or refused to grant trading licences, so that despite their aspirations they experienced similar hardships and poverty to the urban working class.[12] They saw themselves as civilised, respectable and progressive in their espousal of values such as temperance, hard work, self-improvement and the assimilation of Western norms.[13] Eales suggests that they sought acceptance by white society, but realised that this could not be on the basis of individual merit, but required the upliftment of the race, symbolically represented by the status and behaviour of African women. The stereotype of African women as immoral prostitutes and liquor sellers was an affront to the elites's aspirations.[14]

Another sign of white fears about the fragility of the social system was the ongoing refrain that VD would decimate the labour supply. In 1921 Dr Reith Fraser, the newly appointed medical officer for the union, warned that syphilis was 'steadily depleting the labour market'.[15] A rural district surgeon warned that infected migrants returning home undermined the region's prospects as a labour supply area, for which it was 'necessary to have the native clean and fit as far as possible'.[16] Fears about the impact of VD on the birth rate, the quality of labour and the future of the country's economic development continued throughout the 1930s.[17] Industry also depicted African women as a danger to efficiency and profitability. Burnside colliery in Natal, for example, complained that women placed 'the continued operation of the industries ... in danger ... owing to the inefficiency of the labourers due to diseases communicated by these undesirables'.[18] Between 1927 and 1930, on average the colliery lost over 1000 shifts per year due to workers being incapacitated by syphilis.[19] And the Smit Report of 1942 regarded VD as a 'threat ... to urban industry itself'.[20]

Another sign of the impending calamity was the politicisation of the African urban and rural population. The South African Native National Congress (eventually renamed the African National Congress, ANC) sponsored a passive resistance campaign against the pass laws in the Rand and a spate of strikes between 1917 and 1924, galvanising a more aggressive militancy among workers and the elite.[21] The Industrial and Commercial Workers' Union (ICU) began as a trade union in 1919 but grew into a successful mass movement in the Transvaal and Natal countryside in 1927 and 1928, appealing to rural workers' grievances over their lack of access to land and increasing obligations as labour tenants. At its peak the ICU claimed a membership of 250000, before its decline in 1933.[22] The South African Communist Party, formed in 1921, initially focused on white workers, but by 1928 had allied itself with the ANC and the ICU, and involved itself in the unionisation of white and African workers.[23] Responding to the political volatility of the 1920s and 1930s, government officials and philanthropists continually drew attention to the 'awakening of race consciousness' among Africans, the spectre of cross-racial class alliances and the threat of 'Bolshevism and chaos'.[24]

Saul Dubow suggests that the emergence of a coherent policy of segregation during the 1920s and 1930s was an attempt by the state to preserve the social structure during a period of rapid industrial growth, contain African political radicalisation in urban and rural areas, and legitimise white rule.[25] The issue of African women and the control of

VD struck at the heart of the debate on the position and rights of Africans in urban areas.

During the 1910s and early 1920s there was as yet no consensus on the exact meaning of segregation. Pass laws for men, job discrimination and territorial separation were inscribed in legislation, but still not seen as a coherent package.[26] During the 1920s and 1930s politicians and administrators' views on urban problems and policy were filtered through Smuts-like inclusionist and Hertzogist exclusionist visions of segregation.[27]

The inclusionist vision grew out of the old Cape liberal tradition. Inclusionists accepted territorial segregation and did not wish to encourage urbanisation, but recognised that a segment of the African population was permanently urbanised. By stemming the influx of unskilled, casual labour, supporting an urban labour preference policy and improving the living conditions for urbanised Africans, inclusionists hoped to create a small, stable urban African community as a bulwark against labour and political unrest. The inclusionist vision was represented by the Godley Report, the Native Economic Commission and the Young-Barrett Committee.

The exclusionist vision, as described by Hertzog, Colonel Stallard and Heaton Nicholls, was stridently racist and highlighted the danger that racial assimilation, political equality and a politicised African proletariat posed to white supremacy. It was premised on limiting the number of Africans in town and developing the reserves so that Africans could 'evolve' in their own areas, under their own tribal laws and leaders. Exclusionists recommended strict influx controls to regulate the size of the urban population until the reserves were developed sufficiently, and providing minimal facilities in towns to reduce the attractiveness of urban areas.

The key legislation controlling African urbanisation was the Native Urban Areas Act (NUAA) of 1923 and its subsequent amendments. The terms of the Act were based on the continuation of the migrant labour system and limiting the influx of Africans into cities to 'protect' them from the dangers of urban life. It aimed to tailor the influx of African male jobseekers to the labour needs of white urban areas by tying the right to employment to the availability of housing. The intentions of the legislation on influx control proved easier to commit to paper than to implement. A key hindrance was administrators' inability to control the influx of women into town, and their activities once there.

The NUAA and 'redundant women'

In the discussions preceding the enactment of the NUAA, the Godley Report and the Stallard Commission examined the role of women in urban areas. Their perceptions were shaped by the Victorian notion, discussed in Chapter 2, that legitimate work determined an individual's moral status, and they drew on a Christian and assimilationist discourse in which work was the basis of salvation and the key to differentiating between the 'respectable' and 'vicious' poor, regardless of race.[28] It was the absence of legitimate employment for men and women that threatened health and morality. The Godley Report identified unemployed 'native undesirables and loafers' as 'a fruitful source of danger to the community and a malevolent influence contaminating impressionable and innocent natives'. It suggested that as soon as an African became unemployed or had no legitimate reason for remaining in town, he became 'a ready victim' of corruption.[29] The Stallard Commission noted that the 'masterless native in urban areas' was 'a source of danger and a cause of degradation of both white and black'.[30] African women who were not legitimately employed by whites or legitimate wives were 'masterless' – that is, outside the control of an employer, the administration and an African husband or father – and were considered likely to become concubines or prostitutes.[31]

Local authorities saw African women as a threat to the health and morality of male migrants.[32] African women were represented as predators, and migrant men as the victims of their wiles and diseases. Thus Kimberley officals described how miners were 'preyed upon by loose coloured women',[33] while in Johannesburg the commissioner of police warned that 'boys are being debauched' in the slums.[34] And at the collieries a medical officer argued that it was not the men who had VD but the women who preyed on them.[35] In a political climate where African urban influx was tailored to white labour needs, women had no place. And local authorities and the DPH regarded women as 'redundant' to the needs of white towns.[36]

One way to control urbanisation was to introduce passes for women. Male jobseekers in urban areas were already subject to pass controls and a medical examination upon entering a city, but women were excluded from these provisions. The Godley Report opposed the introduction of influx control for women, but the Stallard Commission favoured it.[37] Beyond this difference, both commissions advocated similar measures for expelling from urban areas 'idle', 'dissolute' or 'undesirable natives', categories that included women who were neither legitimately employed nor married. They would be repatriated to their rural homes and placed under the control of a chief, or sent to labour colonies or indentured to farmers.[38] In this way the women most likely to spread VD would either be subject to control at the point of entry to towns, as the Stallard Commission suggested, or be deported, as both reports advocated.

The Native Affairs Department (NAD) seems to have accepted the caution of the Godley Report on the issue of passes and medical examinations for women. The secretary for native affairs explained to the secretary for public health in 1921 that the benefits of examining women were outweighed by the possible discontent such action might engender: 'having regard to the present state of native feeling, it would be extremely impolitic to require native women to submit to a medical examination . . . [the] comparatively little advantage [gained] . . . would be wholly outweighed by the irritation caused'.[39]

Wells suggests that in the 1920s the state was reluctant to introduce passes for women because its previous efforts had provoked strong resistance.[40] However Eales suggests that it was the views of African men that influenced the state. One senior Transkeian magistrate and NAD official gave evidence to the Native Pass Law Commission in 1920, and on being asked whether African women should carry a pass he replied: 'The government should have nothing to do with the regulation of women. . . . *They* [native men] should look after *their* women and I see no reason why we should accept the responsibility.'[41] Both white administrators and African men regarded African women as the wards of African men and felt that the state should not interfere in the African domestic sphere. African men were as concerned as administrators about the uncontrolled mobility of women and their activities in urban areas, and were not averse to stricter controls.

Rural and urban African men believed, as did the state administration, that the solution to immorality was greater control over women's mobility and the restoration of tradition and propriety to women's behaviour. At the Native Conference in 1924 African attendants recommended that young women should not be allowed to leave rural areas without parental consent, and should be repatriated from urban areas by the government. Also recommended was a strengthening of chiefly and (male) parental powers to regulate young men and women's behaviour.[42] Similar views were expressed to the Godley and Stallard commissioners.[43] The urban elite also called for greater controls to keep women at home, off the streets and with their husbands.[44] The African male urban and rural elite thus called for controls over women's mobility, where these enhanced parental or chiefly power and shored up traditional male authority.[45] However they rejected passes and medical examinations for women as these were imposed by the government and overrode their own domestic and chiefly authority.

The state and the white public seem to have recognised this. When the possibility of compulsory VD examinations for African women was discussed again before the Public Health Act was passed, church representatives warned that 'tampering with their land or their womenfolk would lead to trouble', implying that women were the property of men, and instead proposed public education and voluntary treatment of VD.[46] At issue was not whether controls should be introduced, but their imposition by government officials rather than African men. The government chose not to introduce passes and medical examinations for women, instead it hoped to control their migration and monitor their economic and social lives once they were resident in urban areas in an indirect way – namely through slum clearance.

Doctors and administrators continually portrayed black women and the urban slums in which they lived as the source of VD infection for the entire country. Government officials described Kimberley's municipal townships as 'disseminating centres of venereal disease amongst natives throughout South Africa'.[47] The Stallard Commission described Johannesburg's slums as 'plague spots in the social and moral life of the community' that 'ought to be extirpated'.[48] *The Star* newspaper similarly described Johannesburg's slums as the place where '[v]enereal disease is being propagated'.[49]

The NUAA empowered local authorities to *proclaim* parts of their cities, most importantly urban slums where poor whites and Africans might cohabit or live alongside each other, and where African women could maintain an independent existence. The local authority could then compel Africans with the right to live and reside in the city to move to newly built hostels or family accommodation in segregated African townships.

Following the suggestions of the Godley and Stallard Commissions, the NUAA chose to deport what it deemed as the surplus population, redundant to the needs of the town and a potential cause of immorality. Section 17 of the Act allowed municipalities to send to labour colonies or repatriate to rural areas men and women deemed 'habitually unemployed', 'without honest livelihood' and 'leading an idle or dissolute life'.[50] The secretary for public health promised optimistically that the NUAA 'will prove a valuable adjunct in safeguarding the natives in the towns against venereal infection', as Section 17 meant that 'the diseased native prostitute' could now be controlled.[51]

The government hoped that through the dual measures of tying employment to approved housing and expelling the surplus population it could limit the size of the urban population, and thus reduce the number of Africans exposed to urban life or tempted into potentially illegal or immoral activities. By implementing the Act a local authority could cleanse its inner-city or peri-urban slums morally, physically and racially. It could condemn slums and control overcrowding and racial integration by sifting Africans out of white residential areas and into approved housing in areas of their own. It could house legitimately married and permanently resident couples in family locations and genuinely employed, single men and women in single-sex hostels. The detritus, consisting of unmarried cohabiting couples, 'dissolute' women dependent on brewing beer and prostitution, and other 'idle' and 'dissolute' Africans who were regarded as the source of VD and criminal and immoral behaviour, would be sifted out and expelled. The NUAA thus had a clear moral dimension.

Implementing the NUAA in the 1920s

Large cities such as Johannesburg, small towns such as Umtata, and the eastern Transvaal and Natal collieries all tried to use the provisions of the NUAA or similar regulations to control the size of the urban population and exclude 'undesirables', with the sometimes explicit intention of controlling the spread of VD. Administrators found that their inability to restrict the influx of women and control their conduct in town immediately threw into disarray their plan to cleanse the city through slum clearance.[52]

Section 17 offered some controls over women's conduct after arrival, but it was difficult to prove that a woman was 'without honest livelihood' and 'leading an idle and dissolute life'. She might provide evidence that she was a washerwoman, but actually live off the proceeds of prostitution and liquor selling; and a married woman could not be considered habitually unemployed or lacking means of honest livelihood. No farm colonies existed for women, and if the administration could not ascertain the rural origin of a woman who was declared undesirable it could do little more than send her to gaol for a few days and release her back into town.[53]

The Natal collieries complained that the police refused to prosecute women living on nearby farms who were suspected of prostitution or of cohabiting with mineworkers and blamed for spreading VD. If these women ever appeared in court they were simply cautioned and told to return to their kraals. As they no longer had a rural home, they just moved to a nearby town or mine to evade detection, and continued to spread VD.[54] The secretary for native affairs was unwilling to recommend repatriating these women as he feared that without proper treatment facilities in rural areas the women would simply 'aggravate the situation' and also spread VD in these areas.[55]

The absence of control over the influx of women into urban areas and their activities once there had direct implications for slum clearance and housing programmes. The Johannesburg council tried to monitor applications for official housing, but many slum residents facing eviction simply moved to another inner-city slum. Officials found that, when selecting residents for the housing programme, it was difficult to determine whether a woman was 'reasonably necessary to the community' and whether she was genuinely married, an issue discussed in further detail below. By the late 1920s the council was losing rent on empty properties and was forced to let houses to unattached women, the very people the Act was meant to discharge from the city.[56]

In Umtata the magistrate regarded the municipality's plan to destroy the slum settlement, move Africans to a municipal township and repatriate single women as a direct solution to urban women infecting migrants with VD at the railhead. In 1929 he instigated a police raid on slum and municipal townships to serve notice on all women who were over 13 years old, unmarried, widowed or beer brewers to submit to a VD examination. The police arrested 94 women and subjected them to an examination.[57] However two years later the magistrate complained that these efforts had come to nought as the municipality had failed to 'provide sufficient location accommodation to enable it to enforce an order for the removal of all natives to the urban location where undesirables could be culled'.[58]

The collieries also began a dual policy of evicting 'dissolute' women and restricting the right to residence. Mozambican women were the largest group of female immigrants during the 1920s, and from 1926 native affairs officials began a concerted programme throughout the eastern Transvaal and on the Witwatersrand to arrest and deport them as illegal immigrants. The selection criteria were more overt than the provisions of Section 17 of the NUAA. In order of priority, the local police were to select women convicted under the liquor laws for illegal brewing, 'unattached women', women of 'known loose character', women living with labourers known to be discharged, women who were known to have transferred their allegiance to men other than their husbands, and women found in mine locations without permits. Married women were excluded from these provisions on the assumption that they were supported by their husbands and their sexual activities were bounded within a conjugal relationship. The government planned to repatriate 25 women a week, but by September 1927 it had only deported 160 women. Again officials found it difficult to establish which relationships were legitimate.[59] The Mozambique Convention of 1928, which reduced the number of male recruits to the mines, solved this problem by endorsing the repatriation of all women, regardless of their relationship to male migrants.[60] By January 1929 at least 1000 women had been deported from the Transvaal.[61]

Under pressure from the government, the collieries had to restrict the number of married quarters so that the proportion of married to single labourers did not exceed 15 per cent, and limit the 'privilege' of residence to labourers with three or more years of service in the district who could provide proof of marriage.[62] Thus only workers who already seemed permanently settled and legally married – though this was hard to prove – were eligible for family housing. Residence in townships was now dependent on medical proof of freedom from VD.[63] If a woman refused to be examined she could be prosecuted under the Public Health Act, and might be denied residence.[64]

As the 1920s progressed it became evident that the NUAA did not offer officials the legal powers and administrative machinery to deal with the influx of women into urban areas, or their activities once resident, and in fact only 11 municipalities ever tried to implement it.[65] In 1928 the DPH admitted that its hope that the NUAA might 'exercise a measure of control and supervision over Native females and . . . exclude from urban areas undesirable and redundant Natives of both sexes . . . has not been realised'.[66] The shortcomings of the NUAA meant that by the end of the decade local authorities were blaming the uncontrolled influx and settlement of women for their inability to limit the permanently urbanised population and control the spread of VD, crime and alcohol.

'Civilisation means syphilisation': VD and medical discourse in the 1920s and 1930s

As liberal analysts and government officials tried to understand the causes of the economic and social decline of Africans in rural and urban areas, they began to develop a new understanding of race. Segregation-ist thought, suggests Dubow, drew on two intellectual traditions – assimilationism and scientific racism (see Chapter 1) – and thus appealed to a wide range of political and economic interests in the white political community and among the African elite.[67] Dubow argues that English-speaking liberals were influential in developing and refin-ing segregationist ideas and new perceptions of race in the interwar years. Many liberals were actively involved in the anthropology or Bantu studies departments established at all four teaching universities during the 1920s, which offered courses tailored to the needs of native administrators. They viewed anthropology as a source of 'applied knowledge' that could help find a solution to the native question. Their efforts had little direct effect on state policy, suggests Dubow, but they were influential in shaping the development of the ideology of segregation.[68]

These 'new' liberals were uncomfortable with the pessimism of sci-entific racism, but also felt that assimilation was incapable of arresting the physical and moral decay of Africans that resulted from their contact with urban and industrial life. Their anthropological notions of culture and society meant they could begin to view Africans and African society not as a less developed version of themselves, but as intrinsically dif-ferent on cultural rather than biological grounds.[69] The African, in their view, was primarily a rural and tribal being, regulated by tribal law and needing protection from contact with urban life. The intention of seg-regationist policy was to recreate a stable society by limiting the extent and impact of proletarianisation and European ideas on Africans, strengthening traditional structures of authority and customs in the reserves, and making rural tribal life the focus of African economic and social development.

The language and concerns of medical discourse during the 1920s and 1930s was shaped by this broader socioeconomic and intellectual context of segregation. In the early 1930s many doctors commented that urban Africans seemed less hardy and virile, and their physique less impressive than the rural Africans of bygone times – a phenomenon that was blamed on the effects of exposure to civilisation and racial sus-ceptibility to disease rather than dire poverty.[70] A significant body of medical opinion accepted that Africans reacted to a range of European diseases differently from whites and hence required different treatment. Randall Packard shows that doctors associated with the mining houses in the 1920s and 1930s believed that Africans were 'virgin soil' and would gradually acquire immunity to tuberculosis if they experienced industrial life for limited periods, separated by rest and recreation in the open air of the reserves, so justifying the industry's preference for migrant labour.[71]

Doctors drew on a similar theory for syphilis, suggesting that Africans were culturally unsuited to urban life to explain why syphilis was so widespread and displayed unique symptoms in the African population. G. J. M. Melle, a district surgeon in Potgietersrus, believed that syphilis had spread rapidly among Africans because it 'showed a peculiar malignancy when it attacked a virgin soil'.[72] 'It is common knowledge', he reported, 'that . . . as natives come in contact with civilisation they adopt our mode of living and acquire or develop our diseases'.[73] With longer exposure to syphilis, he believed, Africans would perhaps develop similar symptoms to whites. The DPH attributed the gradual decline in the peculiar symptoms of syphilis in customarily high prevalence areas not only to treatment but also to the progressive immunisation or salting of Africans.[74] Melle described syphilis as a tribal disease, and the DPH's theory of 'salting' also implied that Africans were inherently syphilitic. Doctors' focus on racial difference, described in cultural terms, meant they were blind to the possibility that unique syphilitic symptoms might indicate a different disease.

The assumption that civilisation had a deleterious effect on African health threw into question the advisability of urbanisation for Africans. Urban life seemed to lead to moral degeneration and susceptibility to what were termed European diseases. For example a Natal practitioner, though he admitted he did not keep statistics, confidently informed the Native Economic Commission (NEC) that 25–50 per cent of Africans employed at the mines or living in towns were probably syphilitic while only 5 per cent of 'raw natives' were diseased.[75] Doctors drew on anthropological views of 'the African' to suggest that the loss of tribal customs in urban areas was to blame for the high incidence of VD in the African population. A pathologist for the Pretoria Hospital and Mental Hospital suggested in 1921 that the lower incidence of syphilis in rural areas was due to the possibility that 'the standard of morality is still slightly higher among the less "civilized" natives and irregular sexual intercourse, therefore, less frequent among them'.[76] Thus he seemed to imply that Africans were simultaneously naturally promiscuous and yet more moral in tribal surroundings, but outside their tribal terrain their promiscuity took rein. A health officer for the union suggested in 1922 that VD in Pondoland was 'due to . . . indirect interference with tribal control' arising from migration, 'which has separated them . . . from the control and discipline of their tribal chiefs, laws and customs'. This 'special tribal control', particularly of women, he maintained, 'possesses many and peculiar methods for maintaining their freedom from infection and its detection when found to be present'.[77] Thus he too suggested that tribal customs and authority kept African nature in check. Very similar assumptions predominated in the 1930s. Durban's MOH concluded that 'civilisation means syphilisation'.[78]

The consensus among medical practitioners was that Africans were predisposed to VD because under the pressures of urban industrial life they lost the tribal customs that had kept their natural promiscuity in check. Implicit in the notion of the corrupt urban and more moral tribal African was the idea that Africans were inherently unsuited to urban life, that urban life was corrupting and tribal life, even if 'backward', was morally purer. This ambivalence about African morality and sexuality in rural areas implied that all Africans were different from whites and diseased and potentially contaminating, but pathologised the urbanised African in particular. The urbanised African blurred the margins of difference between civilised and uncivilised society, and seemed out of place in both urban and rural environments, leading to moral chaos and collapse. The 'normal' African, though suspect, was healthy and unthreatening in the rural areas where he belonged, but became diseased and contaminating in an urban environment.

Detribalisation and the urbanised African

The onset of the Great Depression in late 1929, with the consequent rise in unemployment until 1933, increased the influx of migrants from rural areas. In addition to single men and women settling in urban areas, many men were now bringing their families with them. The proportion of Africans continually resident with their families in urban areas reached 30 per cent by 1936 and had risen to 38 per cent ten years later. As the urban population stabilised, the proportion of men to women gradually declined from 3:1 in 1921 to 2.2:1 in 1936, reaching 1.8:1 by 1946.[79] Another indication of permanent settlement was that, nationally, the number of urbanised Africans completely dependent on a wage increased from 75000 in 1925 to 85000 in 1930 and 155000 in 1936, an increase of 2.5 per cent per year up to 1930 and 10.5 per cent from 1930 to 1936.[80] Far from indicating greater stability, urbanised Africans seemed to epitomise the moral dangers of detribalisation and urban life for Africans.

The most striking illustration of the dangers of urbanisation lay in the apparent disappearance of marriage among urban Africans. A Johannesburg magistrate declared to the NEC that traditional marriages in the Witwatersrand 'are seldom heard of' and that '[c]ohabitation without marriage is unfortunately greatly on the increase especially in urban areas. Emergence from native life into the changed conditions in or near the towns is undoubtedly productive of moral laxity.'[81] Ellen Hellman, an urban anthropologist who conducted a study of an inner-city slum in Johannesburg, concluded that 'adultery, illegitimacy and prostitution even if not completely condoned, are accepted as social norms'.[82] In 1942 the Smit Commission spoke anxiously of a 'moral vaccuum' in towns and the utter lack of 'any moral standards, either Native or European' where cohabitation was the norm.[83] Likewise African and white missionaries believed that most urban marriages were irregular and that this was 'responsible for . . . the wholesale moral depravity of urban Africans'.[84]

The cause of this moral degeneration was widely agreed to be detribalisation, an argument now clearly based on anthropological conceptions of African life and on the significance of tribal life and the family in promoting stability. The NEC of 1932, which systematically outlined segregationist ideas and policy, painted a picture of a rural tribal idyll as the natural abode of the African, in which tribal laws preserved social stability by governing family life and clearly delineating social roles and obligations between chiefs and their subjects, and between men and their women and children. It depicted customary marriage, or *lobola*, as the root of the social structure, which had 'a far reaching wholesome effect on the morality and character of the society, the tribe, family and of individuals'.[85] Morality in traditional tribal life was sustained by customs and punishment for transgressions. In urban areas, however, 'there are no sanctions . . . to secure the observance of tribal morality' and this led to loose morals. The uncontrolled influx into the towns was thus the cause of detribalisation and 'a great deal of immorality'.[86]

Without the protective patina of tribalism Africans' innate hypersexuality came to the fore – a sign of their fundamentally different nature and lower level of development compared with whites. For an American Board missionary actively involved in African social welfare, the informal relationships were a 'hangover of the polygamous outlook', a result of the transition from the controlled promiscuity of tribal society to the collapse of tribal sanctions in urban areas, with the resultant absence of sexual restraint.[87] Some local government officials similarly saw cohabitation as a sign that Africans were in an evolutionary phase leading to civilisation.[88]

Women were considered a central cause of this moral chaos. Local authorities were well aware that once male migrants settled with urban women they neglected their own families, with the result that their deserted wives might also decide to migrate to town, establish new relationships and bear children. The migration of women to towns seemed to undermine the rural social life upon which the migrant labour system and segregation depended, and contributed to an expanding population of urban families cut off from their rural roots, as well as a rise in VD.

Even when men and women were formally married, urbanised women appeared to be unsuitable wives and mothers. The 'present illicit-liquor-selling mother' and the 'absent labouring mother'[89] were further indications of the absence of moral and social order in African urban life. The root of the problem seemed to be that wages for urbanised African men were too low, with the result that women had to work and this undermined the stability of the family. In the eyes of missionaries such as Clara Bridgman, the ideal, happy family was one where 'the man earns the money and his wife keeps the home and really tries to bring up the children'.[90] Womens' bread-winning activities, while economically necessary, disrupted what were regarded as appropriate family roles for men and women, undermined male authority and led to the decline of family life – an argument similar to that about white amateur prostitutes.

The African urban male elite, influenced by Christian ideals of the family, similarly voiced their concern about the assertiveness of women, the decline of male authority and the consequent demoralisation of all Africans. As one African correspondent to *The Bantu World* put it:

> Our women of today ... just marry out of curiousity to divorce tomorrow. ... They have lost their respect, discipline and manners to the opposite sex. ... Other nations look at us disgustedly through our women ... who have substituted foreign customs, which have been detrimental to them. ... Let us wake up and destroy this immorality from our womenfolk which retards our marching forward.[91]

Where prostitution, cohabitation and illegitimacy flourished, VD was a natural consequence, concluded doctors, officials and philanthropists. An American Board missionary doctor working in Natal pinpointed urban Africans' apparent preference for informal cohabitation rather than *lobola* or Christian marriage as the cause of VD: 'The lower the type of matrimonial alliance the greater the prevalence of disease. . . . [I]llegitimacy is a fair basis for judging of the increase of venereal disease in towns.'[92] A member of the Durban Joint Council similarly believed that 'irregular sexual intercourse' meant that illegitimacy, '[v]enereal disease and general degeneracy spread'.[93] The prevalence of informal relationships and VD were proof of the pathology of urban life and urbanisation for Africans, and the unassimilable, cultural distinctiveness of Africans.

In the early 1920s African women were regarded largely as prostitutes, but now administrators began to recognise that some women were wives and mothers or respectable workers. It was women who depended on brewing beer, cohabitation or prostitution, rather than all African women in towns, whom officials now blamed for spreading VD. The Durban MOH concluded: 'From the VD point of view, Native women in Durban may be said to belong to one of two categories – firstly, those in regular employment in the City many of whom are married women; and secondly, those who are unemployed and for the most part unmarried.' It was this latter group that was 'probably responsible for at least 75% of the infections'.[94]

These women were also regarded as subversive. In Durban, women spearheaded protests against the municipal monopoly on the sale of beer, and beerhalls were boycotted between 1928 and 1930. The boycott directly undermined Durban's slum clearance plan as it had intended to use beerhall profits to subsidise the housing programme.[95] Similar efforts to clamp down on home brewing in the Pretoria–Witwatersrand–Vereeniging area in the late 1930s also resulted in violent clashes with police as women defended their livelihoods.[96]

Thus by the 1930s health officers had begun to draw a distinction between women whose sexuality was confined safely to a marital relationship and whose behaviour was monitored by an employer or a husband, and single women living in the slums and relying on prostitution or cohabiting, who seemed beyond the reach of any authority and were now regarded as the 'real reservoir of infection in the City'.[97]

Moralising the urban African

Legislation passed during the 1930s intended to allow local authorities to differentiate between migrant and urbanised women, and between married or working and 'dissolute' women. The legislation tried to evaluate women's moral status on the basis of their relationship with men in urban areas. The intention was to limit the immorality associated with the uncontrolled influx of women into urban areas and to stabilise family life in urban areas. The local authority programmes were three-pronged: medical examinations and influx control to limit the number and control the type of women entering and residing in towns; housing and welfare programmes to encourage marriage and moral stability; and, despite the fears about the consequences that work would have on their families, encouraging women to enter the domestic labour market.[98]

Influx control and medical examinations

Local authorities had never abandoned the idea of introducing medical examinations for women after the measure was explicitly excluded from the 1923 NUAA. Every year the minister of native affairs received endless resolutions from municipalities, citizens' associations and medical officers urging its introduction, especially among domestic workers. The lobbying was particularly fierce in the periods leading up to the 1930 NUAA amendment and the Native Laws Amendment Act of 1937. The government remained unsympathetic. This was partly due to miserliness about funding African welfare services (especially during the depression), but also to the concern about the political fracas that might result and its reluctance to intervene in the African domestic sphere. As in the early 1920s, African men still supported the introduction of greater controls on women's mobility where this reinforced their own authority, but not passes. And they still opposed compulsory state medical examinations of women on the grounds that they were racially discriminatory and undignified.[99]

Legislators thus returned to influx control measures as a way to control the entry of women into urban areas, differentiate between married, job-seeking and undesirable women and strengthen African male authority. The amendment to the NUAA, passed in 1930, was aimed at restricting the influx of women into urban areas by sifting out respectable from dissolute women on the basis of their legal relationship to a male guardian. Section 12 required all women entering an urban area to provide a certificate of approval from the urban local authority that accommodation was available. The certificate could not be issued to a minor without the consent of her guardian, nor could it be issued to a wife joining her husband or a daughter joining her father unless she had proof that the man had been resident and continuously employed in the urban area for not less than two years. This document had to be produced on demand.[100] The amendment was significant for two reasons. Firstly, it tied the legitimacy of a woman's presence in an urban area to her relationship to a man – either father or husband – and thus strengthened male authority in the family. Secondly, it implicitly recognised the controlled urbanisation of respectable women in a family relationship. Independent women who flaunted African male authority and their obligations in rural areas by migrating to the towns, where they seemed to contribute to immorality and the breakdown of social order through prostitution and cohabitation, were deemed undesirable and subject to the deportation provisions of the NUAA.

The promise that the 1930 NUAA, by differentiating between respectable and dissolute women, would control the type of women living in cities proved impossible to uphold. A woman either had to enter the city so that she could apply for a certificate, which contradicted the intention of the Act that she should possess a certificate upon entry; or she had to apply in advance in writing for a certificate, which was difficult given that most Africans were illiterate.[101] Johannesburg abandoned its efforts in 1932, and Durban in 1936.[102]

A similar measure to the NUAA amendment was applied in Basutoland, where from 1931 all African women were to be prevented from leaving unless they had a certificate of permission from their parents or husbands. This measure too was impossible to enforce. The secretary of native affairs also appealed to the railway authorities not to issue tickets to Basotho women leaving for the Rand, which the railways refused to do, arguing that they had no basis upon which to distinguish a legitimate from an illegitimate purpose for visiting the Rand. So officials were reliant on rounding up suspected illegal aliens and deporting them across the border, often with the support of Basotho men.[103]

Local authorities had to fall back on the provisions of Section 17 to expel undesirable women from the city. In 1936 Durban's administration received eight applications a day for the deportation of 'immoral' women.[104] At the eastern Transvaal collieries, the government continued to deport Mozambican women as illegal immigrants. It repatriated 133 women in 1935, 122 in 1936 and 67 in 1937.[105] In Umtata the local authority 'culled' undesirables by raiding the slum township in 1931, 1933 and 1935 and subjecting women to VD examinations.[106] Deporting women was still no solution as the authorities in their home areas often refused to have them back for fear that they would contaminate local people, and even if banished they could still return to an urban area under a new name and continue their activities as before.[107]

The government tried to redress the failure of the NUAA amendment with the Native Laws Amendment Act (NLAA) of 1937. In order to enter an urban area, women now required a certificate of approval from the urban local authority and the magistrate or native commissioner in their rural district of origin. Thus the Act was aimed at controlling the mobility of women at both the rural and the urban end, rather than just the latter, as had been the case with the 1930 NUAA amendment. The Act also tightened up Section 17, for example by making it applicable to persons arrested for the first time for supplying or being in possession of liquor. Police were given the power to arrest offenders without a warrant. Women could also now be sent to the Leeuwkop farm colony, which had opened a section for women.[108]

In September 1937, at a meeting of municipalities it was agreed that these new provisions were as impractical as the previous ones as there was no procedure for coordinating rural and urban administration.[109] Local authorities found it so difficult to get convictions against so-called undesirable women that in the 1940s Leeuwkop Prison never had more than 14 female inmates at a time – often there were just two, and occasionally none.[110] Local authorities never implemented the stricter controls on men and women prescribed in the NLAA. On the Rand on the eve of the Second World War, surplus male labour had already been quickly absorbed by rapid industrial development before Smuts relaxed the pass regulations for black men. Thus there was no need to control their influx, and women continued to flood into towns without impediment.[111]

Stabilising the family – housing and recreation

Local authorities continued their programmes of slum clearance and the creation of segregated African townships they had begun in the 1920s, with their moral intent becoming ever clearer. The slogan 'one man, one wife, one house', adopted by officials of the Johannesburg council, summed up the hope that by limiting access to housing to married couples and encouraging Africans to formalise their relationships, the council could perhaps limit the number of casual relationships exploited by single women to gain access to municipal housing, and thereby stabilise African family and moral life.[112] Durban's officials similarly regarded their housing programme as a way to restrict 'indiscriminate sexual intercourse'.[113]

However local authorities found that housing policy seemed to contribute to detribalisation, rather than limit it. The failure of the regulations to control the influx and settlement of women in 1930 and 1937 meant that local authorities still were unable to identify whether women were legitimately resident in urban areas as jobseekers or wives, and this hindered the selection process for family accommodation. Eligibility for family housing was based on two factors. Firstly, municipal family housing was restricted to permanent residents: prospective tenants had to provide evidence that the male head had been in legitimate employment for at least two years, so that only respectable Africans without rural ties would be eligible. This was in line with policy to restrict the size of the permanent urban population. Secondly, couples had to provide evidence that they were legitimately married.[114] This was intended to prevent cohabitation and encourage marital stability, and thereby minimise the effects of detribalisation on family life and morality associated with VD.

However it was difficult for local authorities to establish proof of marriage. Until 1927 customary marriage, because of its association with polygamy, had been defined as 'repugnant to the laws of civilisation'. It was only recognised as a legal contract in Natal. The Native Administration Act of 1927 recognised tribal authority and customary law and thus implicitly accepted the validity of customary marriage.[115] This was in line with the segregationist view that Africans could best be protected from the dangers of urbanisation by strengthening traditional laws and customs.[116] However the Act made no provision for registering customary marriages. Officials were worried that by recognising informal marriages, especially where there were children, and admitting such couples to housing projects they were contributing to immorality, resulting from detribalisation, and to the destruction of rural families.[117] Housing policy thus seemed to contribute to rather than alleviate the effects of detribalisation on marriage and morality.

When Durban was proclaimed in 1937 the city took a more authoritarian approach to sifting out married and working women from what it regarded as the unwanted detritus. From March that year the police began to raid African homes in the early hours of the morning and to stop women on the street, demanding that they produce their marriage certificates or a 'special' as proof of their right to reside in the city (a special was a 'complimentary' service card issued by the Durban Native Affairs Department to women workers. It required women to register their work contracts and was a surreptitious attempt to introduce passes for women.) Under section 162 of the Natal Native Code, illicit intercourse was an offence. So the purpose of a police demand for a marriage certificate was to assess whether a couple were legitimately married or were cohabiting, and thus guilty of an offence. Women involved in informal relationships were immediately under suspicion of being prostitutes and spreading VD.[118] Protests forced the council to withdraw the specials, but the raids to determine whether couples were married continued into the 1940s.[119] Clearly the administration was attempting to restrict Durban's female population to married or legally working women, and expel any women who fell outside these categories.

Efforts to use housing to control the single working female population were also unsuccessful. Durban had introduced women's hostels as early as 1911, and in 1936 and 1939 built two new hostels.[120] Johannesburg built its first hostel in 1929, but so few single women opted to live there that the council had to reduce its tariffs to attract residents. Even so it was only in the mid 1930s, when extensive slum clearance had restricted the possibility of moving to another inner-city slum, that women reluctantly began to turn to the hostel.[121] Both cities introduced medical examinations for women residents if the matron felt it was in the interest of the institution and public health.

To complement the housing programme in Durban, the Native Administration Committee suggested to the NEC that planned leisure activities would 'have the effect of deviating superfluous energy from an immoral standard of living and consequent degeneration'.[122] If sexual desires were not dissipated, warned the MOH, 'a bottled up state' might develop, and explode into rioting, sexual gratification with prostitutes and wild drinking bouts.[123]

Organised recreational schemes were introduced first in Johannesburg in the 1920s by Ray Phillips and F. B. Bridgman of the American Board Mission with the support of the mining industry and the municipality.[124] Durban appointed a Native Welfare Officer in 1930, and his activities had the support of the Joint Council, the American Board of Foreign Missions and the Christian, urbanised African elite.[125] These groups set up different sports and social activities for urbanised workers or migrants, and for elite Africans. The intention was to draw African men away from radical political activities and to promote their efficiency as workers by creating outlets other than shebeens for relaxation.

These efforts were complemented by an attempt to reach out to respectable women and encourage a Christian view of family life that was particularly appealing to elite Africans, affirming the dominant authority of men in their families and elevating the role of women as moral guardians of the family and the nation. From 1937, with the creation of a municipal welfare department, Johannesburg's welfare officers made a special effort to contact women living in the new townships, setting up mother and housecraft clubs. The aim of these activities was to make women more competent household managers, and to help them live on meagre incomes while avoiding liquor brewing. Similar women's associations were set up in Durban.[126]

Domestic work for women

As the economy recovered after the depression the shift from male to female domestic labour in the Transvaal and Natal quickened as men moved into the newly expanding and better-paying manufacturing industry. In Johannesburg in the early 1930s, about 5000 African women and 21 000 men worked as domestic servants.[127] The drop in wages due to the depression reinforced the trend of women moving into domestic work since, with fewer options in the job market, women were more willing than men to accept lower wage rates. By 1945 women outnumbered men and of the 60 000 full-time domestic servants, 32 000 were women.[128] In Durban, it was only when the city's sluggish manufacturing industry expanded with the outbreak of the Second World War, attracting male workers, that women began to replace male domestic workers in greater numbers.[129] In 1921 white households employed 1345 women, constituting 15 per cent of the domestic labour market of 8944. By 1936 this had increased to 5508 women and 14 432 men, a rise to 28 per cent. Ten years later women made up 36–41 per cent of the domestic workforce (11 750 women) and between 16 776 and 21 295 men were still employed in domestic service.[130] The growth in the number of female domestic workers was accompanied by a fear that African women's promiscuity, disease and acculturation might be brought into white homes.

Urban employers were reluctant to employ female servants, believing that men were 'more amenable to discipline' and 'give more service' while women were 'most unreliable'.[131] This was partly true as the pass laws, medical examinations and registration for service contracts and tax applied only to men, and these gave employers greater control over the conditions of employment and dismissal. Householders frequently complained that female servants stole property or left their jobs after a few days, and were impossible to trace because no form of registration existed.[132] Employers' also complained about their inability to control their female servants' sexual relationships, and thus their contact with the wider urban African population. A Johannesburg magistrate commented to the NEC that '[e]mployers prefer not to have them as owing to moral laxity they are a source of anxiety'. He himself had dismissed five women when they became pregnant and complained that it was impossible to prevent female domestic servants from being visited by male friends.[133] The active sexuality of women was taken as a sign of their intrinsic African nature, the dangers of the absence of tribal sanctions and the decline of male authority.

Most often it was the threat of contagion from a servant to sexually innocent children that aroused alarm. In a parliamentary debate in 1935 on medical examinations for domestic servants, a member of parliament warned that children could contract VD from domestic servants in the 'negligent family' where the mother 'who does not look after her child ... is the parent who will be punished for her neglect'.[134] In Durban in the 1940s, the MOH reported that many employers and their servants were ignorant of how to care for children. The scarcity and cost of mothercraft nurses and home visiting meant that many white households went unsupervised.[135] As discussed in Chapter 3, motherhood was believed to be the basis of a healthy home and virile white race and nation. White women's willingness to entrust their children's upbringing to African women was thus a potential threat to white civilisation. If African women cared for white children, they might be acculturated into tribal or African rather than white, 'civilised' norms. 'Going native' was a constant threat to the morality and sanity of white men living in isolated areas away from white communities, and African nursemaids carried this threat into white homes. The fear that African nursemaids might contaminate white children with VD thus symbolically represented a fear about the fragility of white identity and the consequences of intimacy between whites and Africans.

Concern about female servants' promiscuity shaped calls for the introduction of contract registration and medical examinations for VD among female jobseekers. The Durban council, the police, the public health department and local citizens' associations were particularly vocal about the issue. The Durban City Council also began to discuss a scheme for a nursemaid panel to complement contract registration and a medical examination with health and domestic education.[136] Trained women – employers, missionaries and municipal officials believed – made better servants and better wives. Training would also safeguard the health of white families by ensuring that servants were acculturated into white norms of child care and lifestyle.[137] The scheme was never implemented but it does illustrate the fears associated with the employ-ment of African women.

The attempt to draw domestic servants from the urbanised popula-tion was linked to broader debates on native policy. An urban labour preference policy, it was hoped, would improve wages and employment opportunities for urbanised women, and prevent new migrants from gaining a foothold in urban areas. It was also another way to ensure morality. With a permanent urban population, it was suggested in the early 1930s, whites could employ 'respectable native girls, the daughters of native families living in the neighbourhood'.[138] In Western Native Township in Johannesburg, the wife of the superintendent set up an employment agency for domestic workers from permanently urbanised families. The agency interviewed applicants in their own homes so that employers could be informed about their personal back-grounds, and if problems arose, could contact the servant's family.[139] The Native Welfare Committee of Rotary in Durban also recommended that domestic servants should be drawn from the villages and town-ships around Durban.[140] For employers the choice seemed to be between a single migrant workforce subject to detribalisation and immorality and an urbanised population living in families and thus moral. The increasing settlement of families during the 1930s meant that white households could often employ urbanised, settled workers,[141] though the stricter controls they demanded were only implemented in the mid 1950s when the government was finally able to introduce passes, influx control and labour bureaux to control the influx of women migrants into the city.[142]

VD as 'social pathology': the emergence of a universalist discourse in the 1940s

In the 1940s the government was still facing problems with rural im-miseration, uncontrolled urbanisation and mushrooming squatter slum settlements, despite all its legislative attempts to rehabilitate the reserves and control the influx of Africans into urban areas. VD was still regarded as a serious health problem among Africans, but the debate on its causes had broadened. Some doctors continued to attribute VD to the cor-rupting effects of urban life on tribal Africans, while others focused on socioeconomic, rather than cultural factors as the cause of VD in the African *and* the white population, thus implying that Africans were not inherently different from whites, and not fundamentally unsuited to urban life. This debate reflected the ongoing, wider discussion on the place of Africans in urban areas, which was brought to a head by the appointment of the Fagan Commission in 1946 to examine the problems of urbanisation.[143]

During the 1940s many doctors, particularly those associated with the mining industry, continued to hold to the notion that Africans were essentially part of nature and unsuited to urban life, and that migration was good for their health and morality. In its evidence to the Fagan Commission, the Chamber of Mines portrayed rural areas as an idyllic utopia of orderly social relations, obedience to authority and restrained sexuality. It explained that 'the very strict moral code of his society' 'served to restrict the excessive physical impulses of the Native of the reserves'.[144] The reckless sexual abandon that took place in cities, and the consequent high VD rates, illegitimacy and unstable marriages, so often blamed on the migrant labour system, were, it believed, an indictment of detribalisation and urbanisation. 'Moral standards are generally lower in detribalised communities than in the territories', the Chamber argued in justification of the benefits of migrant labour.[145] The mining industry thus stressed the advantages of the migrant labour system for African health and social stability in rural and urban areas, basing its argument on the notion that Africans were fundamentally rural, tribal and custom bound.

A small but vocal group of doctors began to develop a different approach to explaining the causes of disease. Based on their experience in municipal clinics and rural areas, they began to examine the impact of social dislocation and poverty on African and white health profiles. In previous decades there had been a virtual consensus among doctors that Africans experienced 'African' forms of disease, but doctors were now beginning to attribute disease to the adverse social and economic conditions in the industrial economy, thus following the wider reformist thought of the time and accepting the permanence of African urban settlement and the necessity for socioeconomic development. By the 1940s some doctors were offering a socioeconomic explanation of widespread tuberculosis in the African population[146] and an environmental and nutritional explanation of physiological growth,[147] and they began to examine the part played by the migrant labour system in the spread of VD. In emphasising the socioeconomic determinants of health, they offered a universalist rather than a cultural explanation of African ill-health. This was in line with attempts from the mid 1930s by liberals working in the universities to refute racial science. Influenced by new ideas from Europe, I. D. MacCrone, a psychologist, and Hilda Kuper, an anthropologist, for example, argued that Africans and whites were part of the same human species and that there was no evidence that physical differences affected culture.[148]

George Gale, the secretary for public health emphasised that whites and Africans suffered similar diseases when living in similar slum and poverty-stricken environments. Even in 1950 he felt it necessary to stress to a medical audience that 'it is environment and not race *per se* which determines the incidence of disease. . . . [T]here is no evidence to show that there are any fundamental differences between the physiology and psychology of the European and those of the Bantu, nor between the pathological processes . . . of ill-health among Europeans and those among the Bantu.'[149] Doctors began to suggest that universally valid sociological laws determined the incidence of disease in any population, regardless of race. Louis Franklin Freed, for example, sought to apply to Africans the same 'laws' of social life he had derived from his study of VD and prostitution among whites.[150] He concluded that the incidence of VD could be expected to be proportionately higher among Africans compared with whites since Africans had a higher rate of urbanisation.

An examination of the socioeconomic determinants of health led these doctors to focus on the structural consequences of migrant labour for family life, rather than the effects of detribalisation on urbanised Africans. Under Gale's influence, in 1947 the DPH declared that the 'most important single contributory factor in the production of a high incidence of venereal disease among the Natives is the system of migratory labour'.[151] Migration not only caused men to contract VD in urban areas by encouraging prostitution, but also facilitated its transmission to rural areas when migrants returned home. Debilitating diseases such as syphilis, Gale concluded, were 'symptoms of a disordered socio-economic system'.[152] Similarly Kark argued that VD was a sign of 'social pathology' manifest in individual psychological maladjustment to the immediate environment, and indicative on a broader scale of a society that 'does not allow for the healthy development of the individual' and where 'society itself is pathological'.[153] Migration had 'led to instability and pathology in family relationships' in urban and rural areas, and was 'not conducive to the development of a moral social code, which might influence behaviour as it would be in the case of a stable community'.[154] These medical arguments were repeated by those liberals who, in the 1940s, were critical of segregation and condemned migrant labour as an economically inefficient system that encouraged transient sexual relationships in urban and rural areas, leading to the breakdown of family life and the spread of VD.[155]

The recognition that Africans were individuals, with individual psychological responses to unstable social lives, was different from the segregationist perception of Africans as possessing a collective tribal identity.[156] Segregationist discourse had defined Africans as tribal and fundamentally different from whites, and had pathologised African society and urbanisation. The new belief that disease in the African and white communities had similar causes and effects, and that the incidence of VD was influenced by socioeconomic forces rather than cultural difference, implied that Africans too could lead healthy lives in an urban environment. This implied that urban social welfare provisions – higher wages, better housing, health education and services – and stable family lives were the solution to VD and not the limiting of Africans' contact with urban areas and the strengthening of tribal traditions. This understanding informed a proposal for the establishment of a preventive rather than a curative medical service, as discussed in the next chapter.

Conclusion

The inability of the administration and African men to prevent women from migrating to and settling in urban areas symbolised the disintegration of the social order in rural areas and the difficulty of establishing a moral order in urban areas. Although all Africans were considered potentially diseased, African women were blamed for the spread of VD. From the 1920s to the 1940s, women who escaped the authority of their fathers, husbands or employers were depicted as prostitutes and purveyors of VD.

However administrators' perception of African women changed as they began to recognise that a permanent urban population existed. During the 1920s immorality among African urban women was linked to their being superfluous to urban needs and their release from tribal roles. By the 1930s, as administrators were forced to recognise that the permanent settlement of some Africans was irreversible, they began to differentiate between married, working and 'dissolute' women and attributed immorality primarily to detribalisation and poverty, which affected migrant and urbanised women in different ways.

Doctors' explanations that VD was attributable to detribalisation, and later to socioeconomic destabilisation, were shaped by particular historical contexts, implied particular medical and political solutions, and were a way of symbolically representing white fears about the fragility of the social order in a period of massive social change. Medical discourse also helped construct ideas about racial difference, drawing on anthropology or sociology for legitimacy.

The state hoped to preserve the social order by reinforcing traditional male authority to shore up tribal society, and limiting the pace of urbanisation by linking housing to employment and slum clearance. This dual strategy helped shape the state's VD treatment and education programmes for Africans, as discussed in the following chapter.

7
VD Treatment and Educational Propaganda for Africans, 1910–50

In his evidence to the Native Economic Commission (NEC) of 1932, Dr Alfred Bitini Xuma, a Rand medical practioner, criticised government inaction in respect of VD programmes for Africans. VD was 'common to both communities of European and Bantu', he pointed out, 'but our method of approach to them in the way of treatment and treatment facilities has been more racial in its point of view than being dictated by public health principles'.[1] Several other African witnesses to the NEC complained that the government spent more money on the much resented cattle dipping than on African health, and if the government could afford supervisors to examine cattle it could invest in doctors to look after people.[2] Their observations were apt: VD treatment facilities for Africans were meagre and mostly concentrated in urban areas, and the ethos of these VD detection and treatment schemes was very different from that underpinning the programmes aimed at whites.

VD policy for the white population, as discussed in Chapter 4, was based on a new ethos of welfarist state intervention to monitor and improve white health in the national interest. This involved the establishment of accessible, segregated treatment centres and initiating a programme of public health education to clarify the terms of civilised, 'normal' morality and sexuality for white men and women. In the African population, health services in the 1920s and early 1930s were underpinned by repressive state regulation of migrant labour, and a conviction that the African was a different cultural type, an object rather than a person, predisposed to VD and requiring authoritarian supervision. In the 1940s the government expanded the VD treatment and education services for urban African populations, reflecting official recognition of the permanence of these populations. This new welfarism was founded on authoritarian state surveillance of urban populations, and an ambiguous and grudging recognition that Africans were individuals who made choices about their moral behaviour. The shift in health policy reflected a gradual acceptance by the state, as discussed in Chapter 6, that the African population in urban areas was not simply migrant, but permanently settled, and that the health – and by implication morality – of both migrant and urbanised Africans had to be carefully monitored to control the spread of VD. The shift in health policy was shaped by new medical ideas about the benefits of welfarist over simply repressive controls, and changing perceptions of racial difference, the nature of 'the African' and his predisposition to VD.

The 1919 Public Health Act and 1923 Native Urban Areas Act

Government proposals to deal with VD in the African population in the 1920s were shaped by late-nineteenth-century legislation in the Transvaal, which had tied medical examinations for African men to the system of pass laws and marked the beginning of a differentiated policy towards the treatment of syphilis in the white and African populations. If the late-nineteenth-century attempts to control VD in the African population had been vigilante-like, the size and complexity of the state now allowed it to approach the problem more in terms of a military campaign, as occurred in other colonies.[3] The proposals were also influenced by the widespread assumption since the turn of the century that Africans were potentially dangerous and diseased, which justified racial and residential segregation.[4]

After the First World War the government began to consider measures for detecting and treating VD under a proposed Public Health Bill. Although the provision for detecting syphilis in Africans through the pass laws distinguished Africans from whites, in practice, as mentioned in Chapter 4, Africans and whites were treated in the same lock or gaol hospitals and suffered similar neglect. This was now seen as demeaning for the white population, and alongside calls for voluntary and segregated treatment for whites came demands for compulsory VD examinations among the African population. This was not without precedent and had been implemented in Windhoek, then under South African martial law, in 1917, 1918 and 1920.[5]

Dr J. A. Mitchell, then assistant MOH for the union, suggested that a system of compulsory examination could be applied 'with discretion and with reasonable discrimination as regards race and circumstance ... it is undesirable to introduce racial distinctions in the Bill, all that is necessary in this connection can be done administratively'.[6] The government's concern to avoid open racial discrimination in legislation while accepting class differentiation reflected its Cape liberal, assimilationist antecedents. Jan Smuts, an eminent statesman and then prime minister, traced his segregationist ideas back to the protective and incorporationist elements of this tradition and opposed blatant racial legislation that might unnecessarily arouse the hostility of the African elite, or undermine their sense of economic and social privilege.[7]

The government chose to act cautiously and the Public Health Act of 1919 made free and voluntary treatment applicable to all races. However it was the Native Urban Areas Act (NUAA) of 1923 that proved to be the crucial legislation shaping the government's approach to African health and the control of VD, as well as underpinning policy on African influx and settlement in urban areas. It broadened the scope of the 'sanitation syndrome' from the local to the national level: it aimed to prevent contagious diseases in African rural areas from entering white urban areas by imposing pass medical examinations; and within urban areas its aims were to destroy the slums (metaphorically the wild, contaminating part of the city), to channel the respectable African population into approved, segregated housing, and to sift out 'dissolute' women who might infect male workers, and expel them, so creating morally clean urban settlements. The NUAA was also, as Mitchell had hinted earlier, a means to monitor VD in the African population in a more coercive way than was permissible for the white population, without introducing blatantly racially discriminatory health legislation.

VD detection and treatment, 1920–35

The government's segregationist tenets meant that it applied the Public Health Act differently for Africans. For the white population, the Act resulted in the development of voluntary, free, outpatient medical treatment where VD was treated as a disease rather than a moral crime, and great care was taken not to embarrass patients seeking treatment. For the African population, health services were based on the assumption that Africans were primarily migrants whose health was important only insofar as it determined their fitness for work and contact with the white population. This justified the restricted aims of health programmes for Africans, and the financial limitations that determined the quality of treatment.

The aims of the NUAA meant that medical services were concentrated in urban areas to ensure that the current workforce was healthy. The

Act sought to restrict the influx of African male jobseekers according to the labour needs of white urban areas. It intended to select only healthy workers and prevent unhealthy workers from entering the town. Before being registered as a jobseekers, men had to submit to a vaccination and medical examination for syphilis, tuberculosis and any other disease considered dangerous to public health. If found to be free from contagious diseases, the medical officer endorsed their permits to seek work or their service contracts with the words 'medically examined and vaccinated'. The registering officer would not register the service contract of an African who had not been examined or failed the examination.

The government was obliged to treat VD cases detected during pass examinations, yet the urban medical services remained meagre. In Johannesburg men continued to be sent to Rietfontein. However as late as 1932 Durban still had insufficient hospital accommodation for these cases.[8] As I discussed in Chapter 6, although local authorities' attempts to introduce medical examinations for women met with little success, they still considered women to be a priority. In 1931 the Johannesburg local authority built a clinic for African and coloured women, initially bearing the cost of the clinic itself when the government declined to do so, because it felt that treating women was 'one of the prime necessities'.[9] Johannesburg and Durban also introduced medical examinations at women's hostels, in 1929 and 1934 respectively, to monitor jobseekers.

The missions provided most of the medical services for urban Africans. On the Witwatersrand, from the late 1920s the Anglican and American Board missions set up a network of local clinics catering for maternal and infant health,[10] including VD treatment. The Anglicans also ran a VD clinic in Benoni – this had been built by the municipality in 1931 and by 1937 treated 100 patients a week.

The bulk of the African population lived in rural areas, where medical services were sparse even by urban standards. The government built a VD hospital at Taungs and assisted the missionary hospitals at Jane Furse, Elim and Bochem, but these were in areas where endemic syphilis was so widespread that it could not be ignored.[11] It refused to build VD hospitals in other areas, and Africans had to seek outpatient treatment from district surgeons. They often had to travel such huge distances that regular treatment was impossible, and once the lesions disappeared the patients assumed they were cured and ceased taking their medicine, which meant that the disease often just became latent.[12] Africans could also seek treatment at mission stations, but here the government refused to subsidise the cost of drugs and patients frequently could not afford treatment.[13]

The medication Africans received was also quite inadequate. The DPH and the mining industry considered that the new, quicker and more effective arsenic treatments were too expensive. Africans were given just enough medication to ensure that they were no longer infectious but not completely cured.[14] The secretary for public health stated in 1932 that mercurial treatment was 'the best that can be done. . . . The considerable expenditure involved in sending them to . . . hospital for a full course of treatment, would not be justified.'[15] This attitude was not unique. In Baltimore in the USA, for example, a similar measure deprived the poor, largely black population of a full cure.[16] However in South Africa, limited treatment also neatly matched the needs of employers who were dependent on migrant labour. The mining industry, for example, had argued from the mid 1920s that it would not reap the results of expensive but complete cures as its contract workers were all temporary.[17] The consequent inadequate treatment made a worker fit for work in the short term, but could lead to tertiary complications many years later. By then, however, a worker might have ended his migrant career so his health was of little concern to employers and the burden was borne by his family in a distant rural area.[18]

The process of detecting and treating VD among Africans was coercive and authoritarian. Africans with VD tended to be hospitalised and segregated from society, or deported to rural areas – in a very literal sense, 'cleansing' society of its contaminating elements. In Johannesburg, for example, Africans detected through the pass inspection, and especially domestic workers, were sent to Rietfontein for treatment. Although the hospital offered outpatient treatment it was too inaccessible to be practical: Africans were not permitted to travel on the tram line in that direction, and therefore had to walk, and workers who took time off to seek treatment risked losing their jobs. Employers tended to dismiss servants with VD, and without health certificates workers were ineligible for a pass and lost their right to live and work in the urban area.[19] Thus the pass system criminalised Africans with VD. Most rural districts and small towns had no accommodation for syphilitics and even voluntary patients were housed in or near the local gaol, which similarly connoted that VD was a criminal offence.[20]

In many country districts, magistrates advocated compulsory treatment and 'a proper system of rounding up patients' in the belief that Africans were indifferent to their own health.[21] In Pondoland, for example, police rounded up suspects in raids and then prosecuted the prisoners for failing to comply with the provisions of the Public Health Act. Offenders were sentenced to a fine of £25 or imprisonment, as the intention was to 'enable the District Surgeon to treat, house and control patients (prisoners) whilst under treatment for a month or six weeks'. The only drawbacks, the magistrates reckoned, were that this scheme was expensive and the districts occasionally ran out of prison accommodation. When Africans under treatment absconded to Johannesburg to look for work, the director of native labour alerted all pass offices to keep watch for the offenders so they could be tried under the Public Health Act for avoiding treatment, which was a criminal offence.[22]

In urban areas, by 1930 municipal native administration departments were crowing that the NUAA had achieved its purpose of preventing sick and diseased Africans from contaminating white towns. Medical examinations had had a 'moral effect' explained the medical officer for Durban's Native Administration Department: 'The fact that the Native is aware that he will be medically examined on seeking work in the Borough has a restraining influence upon ill-conditioned Natives seeking employment, with the result that a fairly healthy Native population is resident within the urban area.'[23] In Pietermaritzburg the municipal public health department claimed that the most important feature of its VD scheme was the 'examination at the gateway to the town', through which infectious cases 'have been caught . . . before they could import these diseases into the borough'.[24]

Yet the results of pass medical examinations were hardly impressive. In practice the number of African men rejected after a pass medical examination for being unfit was marginal. For example in Durban the percentage of jobseekers rejected for VD remained consistently under 1 per cent between 1923 and 1945.[25] This may reflect either the low incidence of VD in the workforce (though the incidence of VD in rural areas seems to have been relatively high – see Appendix 2, Table A2.4), or the ineffectiveness of the pass examination. The examination was intended to be a cursory visual inspection so that 'a large number can be examined in a comparatively short time'.[26] On the Witwatersrand in 1936, medical examinations were often sporadic or non-existent, and often jobseekers were registered and their service contracts endorsed without a medical examination.[27]

Despite white fears that African women were rife with VD, the raids detected relatively few who were infected. In Umtata, of the 134 women suspected of prostitution and arrested in a raid in 1929, only 13 (10 per cent) were infected, which although high was considerably below the frequently quoted figure of 80 per cent.[28] Burnside colliery in Natal treated 1 per cent of the female population resident in the location in 1928, and two years later, when the scheme was better established, it treated 4 per cent. The comparative figures for men detected and treated for VD were 2.5 per cent of the working population in 1928 and 3.5 per cent in 1930.[29]

The attempts to regulate the health of Africans on their entrance to and residence in urban areas, and even in rural areas, was characterised by coercive state regulation, rather than the surveillance and normalisation that characterised health services for whites. Vaughan suggests that African health was monitored through coercion and what she terms 'unitisation', the depersonalised codification of Africans into sick or healthy bodies.[30] This seems an apt description for the system of VD control in South Africa in the 1920s and early 1930s. The mass medical examinations for passes incorporated African men into the labour system and in a material way marked out their new status – 'labourer' – which ignored class or generational differentiation among Africans and reduced them to a homogeneous mass. The brief, impersonal assessment, oblivious to an individual's status or merits, simply categorised individuals as sick or healthy and capable of work. Similarly the raids were a head-counting exercise, monitoring the health and by implication the activities and status of women in peri-urban and urban areas. The detection and control of VD was a symbol of the absolutist, repressive power of the state over a population defined by its racial otherness. These assumptions also shaped the intentions of VD propaganda aimed at African audiences in the 1920s.

VD propaganda from 1920 to 1935

Initially some health officials believed that health education for Africans was pointless.[31] After the 1919 Public Health Act, local health departments and voluntary organisations began to take more interest in the matter. Chapter 4 discussed the gradual professionalisation of health education as the National Council for Combating Venereal Disease (NCCVD) and its successors, the Social Hygiene Council (SHC) and the Red Cross Social Hygiene Committee (RCSHC), incorporated more medical or social work personnel and gradually dispensed with the philanthropic Christian welfare workers. A similar shift was not evident for officeholders specifically concerned with the African population. These officeholders were selected for their 'expert' knowledge of 'the African', derived from religious welfare activities, anthropological studies or the holding of government office.

In the NCCVD they included H. S. Cooke (director of native labour and native commissioner for the Witwatersrand), J. D. Rheinnallt Jones and Reverend Bridgman.[32] The latter two were liberal Christian philanthropists dedicated to fostering a moderate African political voice and, through social welfare, cushioning the impact of urban life on Africans. Rheinallt Jones was a prominent liberal exponent of segregation and was involved in the establishment of anthropological studies at the University of the Witwatersrand. New organisations were brought into the SHC, including representatives from the Bantu Mens Social Centre, which had been set up by Bridgman, the Compound Managers Association and the Native Affairs Department (NAD).[33] The Red Cross absorbed the SHC in the mid 1930s and consisted of similar range of 'experts', including representatives from the Mine Medical Officers Association, the NAD, the WNLA and individuals such as Rheinallt Jones, H. Britten (a magistrate in Johannesburg) and Reverend Ray Phillips, an American Board Missionary also actively involved in social welfare for urban Africans.[34]

The different composition of 'experts' dealing with VD in the white and African populations was reflected in the different ways they viewed VD. For the white population, as discussed in Chapter 6, these organisations gradually came to construe VD as a sociological or psychological problem requiring social reform and individual rehabilitation. VD propaganda was a way of explaining the symptoms of VD, urging men and women to take responsibility for their own and the national health, inculcating appropriate attitudes towards sexuality and marriage, and defining racial and gendered identities. Africans were regarded as problem patients. Doctors frequently complained that African patients were irresponsible about seeking medical help unless forced to do so; they were too 'raw and ignorant' for self-administered medication; and they believed in indigenous healers' remedies or in witchcraft rather than medicine.[35] As a result VD services were defined as a problem of state regulation of the African population and of philanthropic welfare to offset the debilitating moral effects of exposure to urban life.

The NCCVD's approach to VD education for Africans was shaped by the new ventures into African social welfare organised by liberals and churchmen, following the pass protests and strikes of 1918 and 1919 and the radicalisation of educated, urbanised Africans.[36] The NCCVD's VD education was part of this broader project to moralise African leisure time in urban areas.

Liberals' assimilationist heritage made them sensitive to class differentiation in the African population, but they still tended to perceive all Africans as different from whites – as a homogeneous population defined by its tribal identity and morals, rather than as individuals with a moral conscience. This shaped the content of VD propaganda. For the migrant population, the NCCVD distributed posters for display in mine and industrial compounds in Johannesburg, in pass offices, on labour trains, in all the eating houses in Johannesburg and in mission stations. The aim of this publicity, like the NUAA, was to ensure that while in urban areas African migrants remained healthy, efficient workers. 'Money spent in securing the health of the worker', explained the NCCVD, 'has always proved a good investment for employers of every kind'.[37]

The NCCVD also showed to elite Africans, British VD films intended for white audiences. It screened *Whatsoever a Man Soweth* in 1921 to educated and middle-class Africans and also proposed showing it to the Native Mine Clerks Association and the Bantu Mens Club.[38] The RCSHC's audience during a lecture and film tour of the Northern Transvaal in 1935 was similarly elite, consisting of school teachers, ministers of religion and nurses. Although educationists realised that this audience was more sophisticated and educated than the working-class population, one RCSHC lecturer nevertheless considered that the films produced for a white audience were 'too advanced for the native mind and impossible for them to understand'.[39]

The educationists believed that films showing that whites did not live up to the ideals of purity and morality were not appropriate for any African audience, even the elite. Bridgeman stressed that the NCCVD 'must be careful to avoid lowering the status of the white man in the eyes of the native, [because] our reputation has already suffered to a large extent'.[40] The RCSHC lecturer similarly maintained that such films did 'not give the Native a good impression of moral standards amongst the Europeans'.[41] So the NCCVD and RCSHC censored the films they screened, cutting the story line and retaining only footage of laboratory scenes and the gross effects of VD on the genitalia and other parts of the body. The NCCVD and RCSHC also recommended that special films be made with African characters for an African-only audience to avoid the dilemma of publicising white moral shortcomings.[42] Nothing came of this proposal until the late 1930s. Educationists' belief that the African elite would be unable to understand educational films and should be barred from unsavoury views of white morality indicates that they regarded the elite as primarily African, bound by tribal origins and different from whites. Thus the messages about VD given to the elite and migrant audiences were similar.

The films, pamphlets and posters also depicted VD as a disease that only a medical doctor could understand and treat. The intention was to convince Africans of the superiority of biomedicine over traditional healing. NCCVD posters stressed the importance of proper treatment by a white doctor,[43] and DPH pamphlets the importance of clinical treatment rather than 'useless' or dangerous' native remedies.[44] Africans' acceptance of biomedicine was regarded as a sign they were rejecting the 'reactionary' and 'stagnant' aspects of their tribal system in favour of the 'advanced ideas of the civilised race' – part of the process of adaptation urged by the NEC.[45]

VD propaganda seems to have been directed solely at men, probably on the assumption that the urban African population was predominately migrant and male, and because Africans tended to be depicted as a homogeneous people, gender differences were subsumed under the principle racial difference. The health of women was addressed only insofar as it affected African men as potential fathers. Health propaganda warned that if a man contracted VD he could make his wife sterile. The DPH's pamphlets stressed that VD would 'prevent you [the husband] from having big, healthy children. If you have any at all they will be small, weak, deformed and perhaps covered with sores. If you go at once and get treatment, you will be cured and your wife will not get the disease and become sick. YOUR CHILDREN ALSO WILL BE HEALTHY AND STRONG.'[46] The RCSHC lecturer explained the consequences of VD to his African male audience in terms of *lobola*: when a husband 'purchased' his wife she became 'his property and the return of interest on the capital invested is the number of children born by the woman'. A woman rendered sterile due to VD, he explained, had 'no economic value' and was 'therefore useless to her husband and father alike'.[47] In the eyes of the educationists, the value of a wife for an African man was simply her ability to bear children, and his status as a man depended on the number and physique of his children.[48] The occasional poster proclaimed: 'Loose women give this disease', thus feeding off the predominant perception of urban women as prostitutes.

Educational propaganda subsumed gender and class differences among Africans under the principle of racial difference. It was as Africans they were addressed, not as individuals. It also presented VD as a threat to male social status and African custom, rather than as a moral problem requiring prescriptions for male and female sexual behaviour.

African reaction

In order to be registered, most African men had no choice but to undergo the medical inspection. Indirect evidence suggests that they resented the fact that medical examinations ignored class, generational and cultural differences and affronted their dignity. The Native Affairs Commission, for example, requested that the government 'observe Native custom when Natives are being medically examined at Pass Offices: that is to say, the young and the old should not be mixed'.[49] The Pedi, Xhosa, Basotho and certain Mozambican groups practiced male circumcision as part of their initiation rituals, signifying the transition to adult status. Strict social hierarchies, status and styles of social conduct marked off initiated men from uncircumcised 'boys', regardless of the latters' age. Uninitiated men were looked down on as inferior and were compared to women. The medical examination, during which all men regardless of status, had to strip in front of one another, was deeply insulting to circumcised men and broke the prohibition against nakedness between men and boys. As the examination was often cursory, the process marked the initiation of all men into urban life, where their value existed in terms of their capacity for labour.[50]

A union health officer, after inspecting Reef pass office medical examinations in 1936, commented that 'a growing number of educated and civilised non-Europeans . . . feel this class and race discrimination, and . . . are already on occasions giving voice to their resentment. These dislike not alone the discriminatory legislation but also the usual herd methods of examination, when all and sundry are stripped and examined in the mass.'[51] This suggests that urbanised Africans may have resented being assessed in a similar way to migrants. Similarly 'school' migrants, who had accepted 'civilised' Christian values ànd lifestyle, and had received some education, may have resented the indignity of being examined along with 'red' traditionalist migrants, whom they regarded as backward.[52]

African men who were parliamentary voters, property owners in proclaimed areas, professionals and certain government employees were exempt from carrying a pass and registering service contracts. They did have to apply for an exemption certificate, in effect a pass, but this did not entail a medical inspection.[53] In evidence to the NEC in 1930 they riled against the possibility that the examination might be extended to themselves, rejecting it as a 'painful thing' and an 'indignity'.[54] In Benoni in 1937, African male residents protested against a similar proposal. They declared that compulsory examination was an 'indignity', as well as 'unfair and unjust racial discrimination, a studied insult to our manhood and a shameful exploitation of authority', and 'repugnant to our feelings'.[55] Both sets of protestors suggested that if compulsory examination was necessary, it should be applied to Africans and whites, rather than treat Africans as particularly suspect. What especially rankled was that medical examinations ignored their status as an elite who had assimilated the norms of white society. The examinations reduced all to the rank of 'the African' and did not treat the elite with the respect they believed was their due as civilised men.[56]

Welfarism and new forms of control

By the mid 1930s some doctors had begun to criticise the coercive approach of health policy for Africans. In 1935 the government appointed H. S. Gear, a venereologist, as a union assistant health officer to help develop VD programmes.[57] Gear suggested that the pass examination went against a basic principle that health programmes should be based on the cooperation and trust of the public. Africans treated for VD would conclude that 'especially in its association with police, pass issues and other official relationships, . . . medical and health measures are not for the benefit of the natives, but for repressive and disciplinary purposes'.[58] The secretary for public health also argued that a health scheme that might 'antagonise or . . . intrude "police" methods' was of 'extremely doubtful utility'.[59] The Smit report similarly observed that coercion was undesirable.[60]

The Smit report still stressed the curative aspects of VD programmes, but some doctors tied their call for non-coercive treatment to the merits of preventive medicine and a socioeconomic explanation of ill-health. This approach had begun to be aired internationally, with many doctors citing as a model the Soviet Union, where prostitution was attributed to poverty and economic reforms were posited as the solution to VD.[61] One such doctor was George Gale, a former mission doctor who joined the DPH in 1938 as an expert on African health in rural areas, became secretary of public health between 1946 and 1952 and was a keen advocate of preventive healthcare.[62] The high incidence of VD, argued Gale, was caused principally by 'the destruction of normal family life and the disturbance of the old tribal social customs consequent upon the system of migrant labour. . . . Neither syphilis nor tuberculosis can be overcome by establishing clinics or building hospitals. . . . The overall campaigns must include radical changes in the socio-economic system under which non-European labour is recruited, housed and fed.'[63] Sexually transmitted diseases had to be recognised as sociomedical problems that could be solved by complementing the expansion of health services with housing programmes and education, all founded on 'securing the understanding and co-operation of the community'.[64] Sidney Kark, founder of the first preventive healthcare centre, agreed with this approach. More clinics and hospitals alone would not solve the 'social pathology' of VD. 'The first line of treatment', he advocated, should be 'to remedy the unhealthy social relationships which have emerged as the inevitable result of masses of men leaving their homes every year'.[65] Gale's ideas and support were central to the radical proposals outlined by the National Health Service Commission of 1944, which was headed by Dr Henry Gluckman. Additional 'doctoring' was insufficient to ensure good health, stated the commission, and attention had to be given to adequate wages, nutrition, education, exercise, industrial welfare and preventive health services accessible to all people regardless of colour.[66]

The new welfarism in VD programmes seems to have been restricted to the urban African population. This reflected the recognition by the NEC of 1932 and the Native Laws Amendment Act of 1937 that the existence of a permanent urban population was irreversible and had to be protected from undercutting by migrants through stricter influx control and measures such as higher wages and better housing. The government began to encourage urban local authorities to establish voluntary outpatient clinics, which the central government would partly subsidise and for which it would provide free drugs, as it had for white VD clinics. Several Reef local authorities and Durban also appointed full-time MOHs with the brief to develop VD schemes for the African population in their cities.[67] With a government subsidy forthcoming, local health departments now showed greater concern with the health of the resident African population, rather than simply monitoring the health of new arrivals to the city. Johannesburg tried to make treatment more accessible by running outpatient clinics in ten townships, which were certainly easier to reach than Rietfontein, but were understaffed and operated in cramped conditions.[68] In Durban the expansion of VD services coincided with the more effective racial segregation of health services.[69]

Despite the reformist ethos, the new urban VD services were coercive in a different way. The VD service introduced more extensive surveillance and control of the resident and working African population in urban areas, and this was more thorough than the pass examination of

Africans at their point of entry to the city. Thus as well as expanding the health services, health departments tried to ensure that outpatients attended regularly for a full course of treatment. Pietermaritzburg was the first town to use native health assistants to follow up patients who did not attend the clinic regularly, and for contact-tracing to bring in for treatment the person identified as the original source of infection. As a result attendance jumped from 1884 in 1932–33 to 4334 in 1933–34, and reached 10 111 in 1934–35.[70] Durban introduced a similar system in 1939, when it employed three full-time native health assistants and reported that this reduced defaulting among outpatients from 50 per cent to 5 per cent. Defaulters were traced by a health assistant, interviewed, given a pamphlet in Zulu and advised to resume attendance immediately. Johannesburg followed up defaulters only at the clinics in Western Native Township, Orlando and Pimville, but made antenatal screening for syphilis and gonorrhoea routine.[71] Durban also tried to survey its resident African population to detect cases of VD. In 1946 the city health department received frequent requests from industry and schools to screen workers and pupils, and it organised a mobile injection team.[72]

The contact and defaulter tracing and screening programmes made eminent medical sense as a way of detecting latent cases and ensuring that patients completed the full course of treatment. Similar programmes were in place in the USA and in Britain, but in South Africa the more effective monitoring of the health of urban Africans was still linked to the pass system, and thus tied to a more inquisitorial and authoritarian state.[73] Being labelled a VD patient or defaulter could result in an African losing his job and right to work in an urban area. In Durban, defaulting patients who could not be traced were blacklisted by the NAD and when they sought to reregister they were detained and sent to hospital.[74] Hospitalised patients who absconded were tracked down by the police.[75] In Umtata the names of intimate contacts of patients were passed on to the police, who then tracked them down for examination.[76] Doctors reported that Africans were becoming more 'hospital minded' as they were voluntarily seeking treatment, but when men feared retribution they gave a fictitious address in a large compound to avoid being tracked down.[77] For Africans the association between pass controls and VD treatment continued to reinforce the perception that disease was a crime.

In the absence of pass controls for women, the government suggested that employers, rather than the state, should police the health and sexual relationships of domestic workers. Reflecting the growing number of women entering domestic service, in the late 1930s the DPH and NAD recommended that employers 'encourage' their servants to seek an examination as a condition of service.[78] The NAD commented that employers could be 'made to realise fully that improvement in the position lies in their hands as they can refuse to employ anyone who does not produce proof of examination and freedom from disease'.[79] In 1944 Durban outlined a proposal for a nursemaid panel in line with this new philosophy. African women wanting to be engaged as 'nurse-girls' would need a medical certificate of health and periodic health checks in order to be eligible for registration with the panel. Since employers would be informed of their servants' health status, the scheme would allow far more intimate surveillance of women's health.[80] It would weed out African women with VD, whom the administration and employers assumed were sexually promiscuous and unlikely to make good servants.

The nursemaid panel was never set up but it seems that employers enforced the procedure themselves. According to the Durban council, many employers sent their servants for an examination before engaging them, and often for periodic check-ups too.[81] Likewise Johannesburg noted that the number of medical examinations of African women requested by employers was increasing. However, many domestic workers with VD avoided treatment even after detection. In 1939–40, of the 860 women examined in Johannesburg, 41.2 per cent were declared syphilitic but only 10 per cent submitted to treatment.[82]

The health department, it seems, tried to send male and female domestic workers to Rietfontein hospital as a matter of policy.[83] Similarly in Durban, although the emphasis was now on outpatient treatment and the number of inpatients had declined, between 1942 and 1955 the proportion of female patients hospitalised actually increased from 34 per cent to about 50 per cent, or about one third of all VD patients.[84] In this way potentially infectious workers were removed from white homes, and since servants who had VD were likely to lose their jobs the council continued to control their movement and prevent carriers from drifting into inner-city or peri-urban slums or finding a new job.

Schemes to detect and treat VD in the 1920s and early 1930s had relied on pass examinations to bar infected workers from the city, and on raids and the NUAA to sift out, imprison and repatriate economically independent women who were believed to be spreading VD. The schemes introduced from the late 1930s were based on the recognition that a permanently urbanised African population existed. Although the voluntary outpatient clinics and the practice of tracing defaulting patients and sexual contacts of patients resembled the schemes to control VD in the white population, this extended surveillance was underpinned by coercion. Public health officials believed that the white population was sufficiently responsible to seek treatment when necessary, but the African population had to be monitored through pass examinations or employers' requests for surveys and examinations. Urban Africans, especially women, were still regarded as a dangerous, potentially uncontrollable, diseased population.

New directions in education

Another outward similarity to the white VD service was a new aggressive propaganda programme under the aegis of municipal health departments. In comparison with the propaganda images of the 1920s, Africans were now presented in a more complex if contradictory way. Some VD propaganda stressed racial difference through cultural stereotypes of the tribal and urban African who lacked a moral conscience, while other propaganda tried to construct a moral subjectivity in the African audience, as did propaganda aimed at white audiences.

Durban's health education programme was extensive. From 1939, African health assistants gave lectures at factories, compounds, barracks and in the VD wards.[85] By 1943 the scheme had expanded and educators spoke to commercial, industrial, social, cultural and religious groups, night school students, the residents of townships and slum areas, and parent groups.[86] By 1945 the council had a routine programme of four daily lectures and a weekly film for males seeking registration at the pass office. It claimed that these drew audiences of 100 to 2000. The municipality also had a health van, which it sent to white suburban and industrial areas for open-air lectures that often attracted audiences of 500. The Durban Health Department began to screen health films at an open-air cinema. The first film was shown to an audience of 2000. The Health Department also distributed three new VD pamphlets and published weekly health columns in *Ilanga Lase Natal*, which in 1945 included three articles on VD.[87]

The explosion of activity in respect of African health propaganda coincided with a more energetic approach to African health education by the RCSHC. The Red Cross absorbed the Sex and Social Hygiene Committee of the New Education Fellowship in 1937. The latter had had close links with the British Social Hygiene Council and had focused its activities exclusively on Africans. The committee consisted of Christian philanthropists and liberal segregationists, such as the American Board missionaries Ray Phillips and Dexter Taylor. Phillips and his wife had lectured African audiences on social hygiene under the aegis of the New Education Fellowship and they became the nucleus of the Red Cross panel for African health education, with Phillips as the head. Phillips resigned in 1941 and was replaced by Dr P. A. Peall, a member of the Transvaal Mine Medical Officers Association, and the committee members were dispersed among white committees and instructed to adapt white propaganda to an African audience. Phillips' ideas and activities reveal the way in which African health problems and education were being perceived by the 1940s.

Since the 1920s VD educationists had called for separate educational materials for Africans. Phillips proposed that the Red Cross produce films, gramophone records, books and pamphlets about VD and wider health issues, translated into African languages and adapted to African conditions.[88] As a result the RCSHC, with the approval of the DPH, made a VD film, *The Two Brothers*, specifically for an African audience. (Phillips, along with other white health educationists, believed that Africans would understand medical propaganda better if it was delivered by African educators in an African setting.)[89] The film presented a fairly complex story to deliver its factual message, thus diverging from the widely accepted view that films aimed at Africans had to offer a simple, literal message.[90]

The Two Brothers was about Sifo and Nyati, who went to work in town to earn their *lobolo*. Nyati befriended a respectably dressed woman in a domestic worker's uniform, while Sifo visited a prostitute. Later the brothers discovered they both had syphilis. Sifo visited an *inyanga* (traditional healer), paying for the medicine he received. Nyati visited the clinic, where he was treated for free and warned not to marry until he was cured. The film showed the taking of blood for a Wasserman test, the weekly injection treatment and the gross deformities that resulted from lack of treatment. After a year the brothers returned home and Sifo decided to marry, despite Nyati's warnings. Nyati continued treatment until he was cured. Ten years later Nyati was happily married, had three healthy children and many cattle. Sifo's wife was dead, his only child was blind and he had sold his cattle to pay the *inyanga*. Sifo finally admitted he had been foolish and agreed to visit a clinic.

Analysis of *The Two Brothers* reveals a multitude of segregationist messages about morality, cultural difference and the process of 'civilisation', which reflected white perceptions of African society and disease.[91] Just as with the 1920s propaganda, the film did not raise moral questions about whether sex before marriage or adultery was sinful, or whether contracting VD was vengeance for the brothers' absence of chastity. It did not create stereotypes of sexually moral and amoral men and women, as did the films aimed at a white audience.

The film identified all urban women, regardless of their appearance, as the source of disease, implying that they were naturally promiscuous and diseased. It suggested that Africans lacked a sense of shame when it came to displaying their naked bodies and contracting VD. Doctors' belief that Africans 'had no shame' meant that they were often indifferent to the sensitivities of their African patients. The film depicted male patients being lined up against a wall in an open-air courtyard and instructed to drop their trousers, where upon two white doctors moved along the row injecting the exposed buttocks. While patient confidentiality was stressed at white clinics, at African clinics women patients were not always offered private undressing facilities or were examined in the company of male interpreters, while men were told to undress within the sight of women patients.[92]

The overarching message of *The Two Brothers* was not moral but medical: the aim was to show that European medical knowledge was superior to African knowledge. Phillips argued that 'any serious attempt ... to build an enduring edifice of sound physique and healthy-mindedness among the Non-Europeans' was dependent on an education programme that sought the 'conquest of witchcraft and the inculcating of a scientific attitude towards health'. So deeply was witchcraft embedded in the African mind 'that nothing short of ... "a reconstruction of their thought world" can eradicate it'.[93] *The Two Brothers* was an attempt to 'reconstruct' the African mind. By the film's conclusion Nyati had come to believe in Western medicine and absorbed some aspects of white culture. But he still retained elements of his own background: thus he wore a shirt over his skins, hiding his nakedness; he still lived in a kraal, but it consisted of white-washed rondavels with doors and windows rather than grass and mud huts. His acceptance of science had given him health, a family and cultural progress. Nyati had been 'civilised', without losing his tribal roots. The film clearly drew on segregationist views of Africans, emphasising the appropriateness of tribal culture and rural life for African well-being and health, and the dangers of urbanisation and detribalisation.

There is no evidence of how the film was received by African audiences. The Durban Health Department attributed the growing number of voluntary patients at its clinics to the success of its public education programme. African residents and workers presented themselves for examination following a health talk, or requested a blood test when they discovered their partners were receiving treatment, and women who had experienced a series of miscarriages or failed to bear children sought treatment for sterility.[94] Yet this does not mean that Africans subjectively identified with the characters or the segregationist message. When the film was shown in Lusaka the audience found the images of Africans either offensive or humourous. Officials blamed this on lack of ethnic identification, but Vaughan suggests that as the viewers were literate, middle class and educated, it was a lack of class identification with the characters that was probably responsible.[95] A similar lack of identification by the educated and working-class urban audiences in South Africa was possible. Educated Africans may have rejected the film as insulting, and found little to commend even the hero's lifestyle; while more traditional Africans may have seen the depiction of the *inyanga* as offensive, and considered themselves easily able to differentiate between illnesses requiring the help of an *inyanga* and those requiring a doctor. The film's attempt to convince its African audience of the superiority of 'scientific medicine' over 'superstition' was also of doubtful success, as even staunchly Christian African women with many years of exposure to missionary-run medical schemes for mothers and children continued to visit diviners, use protective medicine against sorcery and adhere to the traditional rituals connected with bodily pollution during menstruation and childbirth.[96]

In parallel with the universalist discourse, which focused on socioeconomic rather than cultural determinants of disease, a more complex perception of the African as a subject began to emerge. This was evident in educationists' new attention to Africans' moral values, and the maladjustment of individuals to 'normal' family and sexual life in urban settings – themes reminiscent of VD education for whites.

Rather than focusing simply on detribalisation as the cause of immorality, Phillips called for recognition of the economic and social factors leading to demoralisation. He was central to the establishment in 1941 of the School of Social Work at the University of the Witwatersrand to train social workers to deal with problems in the urban African community.[97] The course offered an amalgam of psychological theory on normalcy and maladjustment, segregationist ideas about detribalisation, and Christian edicts about morality and family life to explain the origins of and solutions to delinquency, crime and cohabitation.[98] Rheinallt Jones observed in 1943 that this new thrust was 'designed to help in the building up of a normal individual and family life for the Natives'.[99]

Phillips suggested that African customs decried by missionaries as immoral could be given a new Christian content. Initiation schools, for example, which were formerly seen as merely encouraging obscenity and promiscuity, also taught adolescents discipline, and Phillips felt that they could help solve the problem of widespread premarital pregnancy and illegitimacy. He recommended to the RCSHC that it arrange vacation schools modelled on initiation schools to inculcate the principles of hygiene and social hygiene.[100] The Holy Cross Hospital in Pondoland organised a week-long circumcision school for boys and planned to follow it up with another for girls, led by hospital nurses. During the former, initiates were circumcised by a medical doctor and then given a lecture by a teacher. The teacher emphasised that boys should 'first and foremost . . . look up to and respect women', that sensuality was base and the soul sublime, and that VD was the result of a 'downward and degrading' path. The initiates were warned about sex and their thoughts were 'directed to the highest channels'. Moral purity, the teacher emphasised, was borne of abstinence, chastity and the control of bodily impulses by the mind.[101] Thus initiation schools could deliver to African adolescents biomedical explanations of disease, and enforce Christian attitudes towards sexuality and the family.

For urban dwellers, who seemed to accept cohabitation, adultery and prostitution without qualm, Phillips emphasised the encouragement of marriage and the strengthening of the African home: 'More must be attempted by direct instruction to explain in attractive, compelling fashion, the Western ideals of marriage and the basic place which the home occupies in any civilised stable community. Africans should be encouraged to feel a pride in their new home in the urban areas.' He suggested that joint councils and social centres should offer lectures in the townships on monogamy and the centrality of a good home in children's development; and that films should be selected to display home life at its best.[102] The Christian Council declared a one-year 'crusade for the sanctity of Home Life' to encourage marriage among cohabiting couples.[103] Churches established young women's groups to encourage chastity before marriage, and to this end instilled the idea that it was marriage, rather than motherhood, that transformed girls into women.[104]

This focus on personal morality and conscience implied that Africans were individuals rather than just part of a homogeneous tribal group; that Africans had a subjectivity that could be guided along particular channels, so that each individual would be the guardian of his or her moral behaviour. This approach is evident in the VD propaganda of the

1940s distributed by missionary organisations, the RCSHC and the Durban Health Department. The Red Cross translated English posters on VD into Zulu, Sesotho and Xhosa and printed 1000 copies.[105] The wartime pamphlet 'Facts on Sex for Men', available in English and Afrikaans, was translated into Xhosa and Sesotho.[106] The pamphlet warned women to remain chaste before marriage, and defined freedom from VD as a national duty for men. A pamphlet published by the Durban Health Department in English and Zulu, and aimed at men and women, advocated 'a pure life' and avoidance of sexual relationships until marriage.[107] An article in the *South African Health Magazine*, aimed at an African audience, warned married men working away from their homes to stay away from 'bad girls' and 'remember your duty to your wife and family'.[108] Those doctors who advocated preventive medicine and a socioeconomic analysis of VD espoused a similar moral conservatism. Health centres planned to intervene directly in the home and remodel it on appropriate lines. Their advice was prescriptive and assumed that women were responsible for morality and family stability. The solution to a family's economic instability and poor health was to reform the 'maladjusted' woman.[109]

All the pamphlets gave explicit information about the symptoms of and cure for VD. This implies that the propagandists now assumed that Africans had a sense of personal responsibility, and like the white population could seek out appropriate treatment or follow instructions for a self-administered cure. These new themes in propaganda dealt with VD in moral terms – as resulting from premarital sex or adultery – and thus recognised Africans as individuals who made choices about their lives and relationships, rather than just as bearers of tribal customs.

Conclusion

Schemes to detect and control VD in the African population were motivated by state health officials' and industrialists' concern to monitor the health of migrants and the urban population. But the schemes were also shaped by predominant assumptions about the racial character of Africans, which predisposed them to VD and justified repressive state regulation.

For the white population, the system of voluntary VD clinics and VD propaganda allowed the state to protect the health of its citizens through health and welfare services while depending on individuals to monitor their own health voluntarily in their personal and the national interest. In contrast health policy for the African population was shaped by repressive rather than welfarist state measures in the 1920s, and even when a VD treatment network modelled on that for whites was established in the late 1930s and 1940s, welfarism was underpinned by coercion. VD surveillance and treatment schemes for the African population were shaped not by public health legislation but by influx control, in the attempt both to control the pace of African urbanisation and to protect the white population from the threat of disease.

VD education for Africans was also based on different assumptions from that for whites. VD propaganda aimed at whites defined notions of normal and abnormal sexuality, morality and gender that were central to notions of white identity, supremacy and civilisation, and attempted to mould individual subjectivity. Africans were regarded as a pathological, homogeneous group whose natural promiscuity became dangerous when removed from their natural tribal idyll and customs. The VD propaganda of the 1920s was influenced by this perception and ignored questions of good and bad morality, while trying to convince Africans of the superiority of Western medicine. The propaganda of the 1940s was ambiguous and ranged from depictions of the African as part of a tribal group bound by superstition, to representations of Africans as individuals who could make moral choices about their sexuality.

Fears about an epidemic of syphilis in Africans, cross-infection in white areas and the decline of the labour force were largely put to rest with the introduction of penicillin in the late 1940s. This new antibiotic meant that patients could be quickly and completely cured, so health propaganda now seemed to be less important.

8
Conclusion

In this study of syphilis in the white and African populations of South Africa during the past 150 years I have tried to mesh the strengths of two approaches: political economy and social constructionism. A political economy approach situates patterns of disease and the function of health services within wider patterns of socioeconomic change and class interests. However the perceptions that are held of disease carriers are as important in shaping medical and social explanations of the causes of disease. Thus I have drawn on a social constructionist approach to explore how fears about disease may reflect anxieties about the consequences of wider social change, rather than simply reflecting epidemiological patterns. I have examined how medical discourse is shaped by its political and intellectual context and also helps to shape perceptions about racial, gendered or class identities.

To suggest that fears about a disease may be socially constructed is not to deny the existence of VD and its relation to social change, but a way of recognising that the process of defining a disease and disease carriers as a problem is politically charged. This tension lies at the heart of this book, and through it I have explored three main themes. Firstly, I examined how the spread of VD in South Africa was associated with broader political, economic and social changes that led to the emergence of new patterns of sexual behaviour. Secondly, I discussed how fears about VD symbolised anxieties about changing relationships in respect of gender, race and class in times of social upheaval and the way in which medical debates about the identity of the VD carrier helped define gendered and racial identities and made differences explicit. And finally, I described how the medical services and educational propaganda reinforced these identities through medical practice, legislative edict and the

163

portrayal of what were considered to be appropriate mores and personal identities.

Political economy and social construction of VD

Sexually transmitted diseases were not indigenous to South Africa – their introduction and spread accompanied the wider process of European colonisation, incorporation into the colonial economy and industrial development. VD was first confined to port and garrison towns, and then spread inland with the army, the railroads and, with the discovery of gold and diamonds in the late nineteenth century, the migrant networks. It was not just venereal syphilis that migrants spread from urban to rural areas, but also endemic syphilis, which depended on poor personal and community hygiene. The late nineteenth century saw an epidemic of endemic syphilis across the north-western Transvaal, the northern Cape and Cape interior. By the 1930s this had begun to subside, and cases of venereal syphilis became more frequent.

Despite clinical evidence to the contrary, most doctors assumed that all syphilis was venereal syphilis and their views reflected the racial ideas of the time. In the late nineteenth century, doctors drew on ideas about racial evolution and hybridisation to explain the prevalence of syphilis among 'half-caste' and 'civilised' Africans, and to warn against the danger of growing racial interaction. Lower evolutionary development was associated with more bestial and promiscuous sexuality, and – in a period in which racial views were rigidifying – was regarded as a sign of the unbridgeable difference between Africans and Europeans. Poor whites in rural areas were also associated with endemic syphilis, but it was their dirt and poverty rather than their racial heritage that doctors associated with the disease. Doctors' explanations of syphilis in the late nineteenth century reinforced the scientific racist views that were becoming widely accepted as justification for colonial conquest and the beginnings of social segregation, and helped define racial identities.

The period between the 1920s and the 1940s was a time of massive social transformation for whites and Africans. Poor whites, usually Afrikaans speaking, abandoned their lives as small landowners or labour tenants and settled in cities in racially mixed slums, competing with Africans for low-paid, unskilled factory or mining jobs. Similarly Africans abandoned the drought-stricken, overpopulated, barren reserves or were evicted from white farms, which were gradually turning towards waged labour, and flooded into the cities.

Doctors' assumption that poor whites were more susceptible than middle-class whites to VD reflected eugenic concern about the quality of the white population, the uncertain foundations of white supremacy and the problem of incorporating poor whites into mainstream white society. Poor whites' 'preference' for slums, poverty, involvement in criminal activities, unemployment and acceptance of racially mixed relationships were seen as markers of their degeneration and a threat to social order.

Unmarried white working women were believed to bear a particular responsibility for spreading VD in their guise as the 'amateur prostitute'. Many families were dependent on the wages of wives or daughters who worked in the new manufacturing industries. In a period in which women's individual and national racial roles were tied to childbearing and caring for their families, women's rapid entry into the workforce seemed to threaten race and nation. Given high male unemployment, women's access to factory work and essential contribution to household incomes also threatened gender differentiation. Attitudes towards sexual relationships were also changing: easier access to contraception and new views about female sexuality in the context of the greater anonymity of a city meant that some betrothed couples cohabited before marriage. Welfare workers regarded sex outside marriage as akin to prostitution.

Doctors and social workers tried to evaluate the relative importance of genetic and socioeconomic factors that apparently predisposed poor whites to immorality and VD. They tended to emphasise the impact of migration and poverty on particular individuals, implying that poor whites as a group were not inherently immoral and could be rehabilitated in an economically stable, urban family environment. In a period of rapid social change, the amateur prostitute and the loafer threw into relief characteristics that might lead to the decline of the white population. The amateur prostitute was seen as disregarding propriety and national duty and indulging in animalistic sex for pleasure, a characteristic considered typical of Africans and thus suggestive of poor whites' degenerate status. VD in poor white men was usually associated with unemployment rather than abnormal sexuality. 'Civilised' morality, by contrast, affirmed the qualities of 'Europeanness' that would ensure the strength of the white polity.

Medical explanations of Africans' susceptibility to VD were similarly shaped by prevailing notions of racial difference and helped confirm these beliefs. Doctors drew on anthropological analyses of Africans to suggest that urbanised Africans were pathological and predisposed to disease. They believed that in their rural tribal environment, Africans were naturally promiscuous but were controlled by traditional customs and sanctions. In towns, however, Africans allegedly lost their tribal restraint, and promiscuity led to disease. Doctors were trying to explain very real changes in African social life as a result of proletarianisation and urbanisation, but they continued to insist that Africans were inherently different from whites and unsuited to urban life – conclusions that reinforced segregationist policies that restricted urbanisation, reinforced migration, and bolstered traditional authority. Only in the 1940s did some doctors develop a liberal critique of segregation. They argued that disease among both whites and Africans was due to socioeconomic rather than cultural factors. They recognised that many Africans had become permanently urbanised, and that migration was destructive of social relationships.

Although the urban working population was predominantly male, it was 'loose town women' who were considered the source of VD by administrators and African men. Women were exempt from the pass laws, and as conditions in rural areas worsened they began to migrate to towns, joining male kin or living independently, apparently beyond the control of African men. From the 1920s the number of women settling in towns escalated rapidly.

In towns, men and women often preferred to cohabit than to marry. This was a way for men to avoid the costs and obligations of marriage, and for women to escape the social restrictions and loss of economic independence associated with marriage. Presenting themselves as a couple married under customary law also meant that they were eligible for municipal housing. Administrators and philanthropists viewed informal relationships as a sign of African promiscuity due to 'detribalisation', and as the cause of VD. 'Town women' embodied the dangers associated with the influx of women into towns, cohabitation and the increasing numbers of urbanised families. Administrators and African men feared that these trends would lead to the collapse of rural society and traditional male authority.

The uncontrolled entry of women into the towns also undermined municipal hopes to restrict urbanisation and create moral order and stability in urban areas by demolishing the slums, providing supervised hostel and family housing and expelling the 'redundant' and 'dissolute' members of the population. Concern about contagion from African servants reflected white fears about the boundaries of intimacy within the household, while concern about VD and 'loose' town women encapsulated anxiety about the fragility of the social order in rural and urban areas. The problem of African immorality was one of a people out of place, rather than the abnormal sexuality of individuals. Medical discourse defined Africans as primarily tribal, and African women in particular were 'safe' only in the controlled environment of tribe and family.

Racial perceptions also shaped the implementation of health policy for VD. In the Cape Colony in the nineteenth century, the government introduced the Contagious Diseases Act to control prostitution in port and military towns, and more importantly to control the spread of syphilis among the poor in the rural hinterland. The legislation did not differentiate between the white and black poor, but the way in which it was implemented complemented the move towards social segregation and the emergence of more rigid racial ideas. Syphilitics, particularly Africans and coloureds, were hunted down and incarcerated in gaols or lock hospitals, thus reinforcing the association between poverty, disease, criminality and immorality. In the Transvaal, from the outset legislation differentiated between white and black and, reflecting the importance of the mining industry, attempted to link the detection of VD cases to pass controls. The Cape and the Transvaal state bureaucracies were rudimentary and unable to implement their schemes on the scale they envisaged, nevertheless they laid the basis for the racially differentiated VD detection and treatment schemes that were introduced in the early twentieth century.

The Public Health Act of 1919 marked a shift towards a medicalised and welfarist approach to VD. In the case of whites, VD became a disease that threatened national health and political supremacy. The state was deemed responsible for the health of its citizens, and was thus obliged to offer medical and welfare services. Individuals were also regarded as being sufficiently responsible to seek treatment and protect their own health, and thereby the health of their families and the 'race'. Medical treatment for whites shifted away from institutional incarceration and exclusion from society to voluntary outpatient treatment and public education. In medical institutions, whites were screened off from Africans to emphasise their racial difference. Education schemes defined norms of sexual behaviour and gender and tied normality to whiteness. Good health and good morals came to be associated with the strength of the white nation.

Africans were subject to the same health legislation as whites, but it was implemented differently. Initially African health was important only insofar as it affected the labour supply. The normal African was assumed to be promiscuous and potentially diseased, thus when health

legislation was tied to pass controls the intention was to screen potentially diseased workers from white cities and the labour market. Sick
Africans were institutionalised or sent to rural areas. In rural areas and
small towns, African slums were raided, suspects examined and those
with VD confined to lock hospitals or gaol. Educationists viewed
Africans as a homogeneous group rather than individuals, so education
ignored questions of individual choice and sexual and moral norms. For
Africans, medical intervention was largely associated with repressive,
public displays of state power. The intention of health policy was to
limit the contact between diseased Africans and whites, in other words
to protect white health.

In the late 1930s and 1940s local urban authorities began to
introduce a clinic system based on the white model, and launched
education campaigns. This reflected concern about the impact of
African ill-health on the labour market, and recognition of an established urban African population. The new welfarist orientation continued to be repressive, and defaulters were traced through the pass
system and confined to hospital. Educational propaganda was contradictory, shifting between segregationist views of healthy tribal and
diseased urban Africans, and representing Africans as individuals with
a moral conscience who could avoid VD through chastity and
monogamy.

In the late 1940s the introduction of penicillin offered a quick and
total cure for syphilis and marked the beginning of an era when VD,
though still considered a stigma, lost its place in the popular imagination as a metaphor for social and moral disorder. Treatment rather than
moral propaganda could now solve the VD problem, until of course the
acquired immuno-deficiency syndrome (AIDS) emerged. Melding the
political economy and social constructionist models of disease also
offers a useful approach to understanding how AIDS has spread, and the
way in which the disease was popularly represented from the 1980s to
the mid 1990s.

AIDS in South Africa

The first two AIDS cases in South Africa were diagnosed in December
1982.[1] The number of reported cases escalated rapidly and had reached
8784 by November 1995, made up of 3941 adult males, 3873 adult
females and 909 infants. Of these 1785 had died.[2] The number of
cases of HIV infection was higher. Annual national surveys of women
attending antenatal clinics reveal that the national prevalence among

women increased from 0.73 per cent in 1990 to 10.44 per cent in 1995. When the statistics are broken down regionally, the prevalence varied from 18.3 per cent in KwaZulu-Natal, and 12.03 per cent in Gauteng, to 6 per cent in the Eastern Cape and 1.66 per cent in the Western Cape, showing a gradient of infection from east to west, possibly indicating where the epidemic began. Based on this survey it was estimated that just over 1.8 million people (4.3 per cent of the total population) were infected with HIV by the end of 1995, of which 719 862 were male, 986 113 were female and 40 557 were infants.[3] Another study of the projected demographic impact of HIV and AIDS in South Africa estimated that by the year 2000 between 3.7 and 4.1 million people would be infected with HIV, and about 600 000 may have died of AIDS.[4]

Two patterns of transmission are apparent. In the white population HIV was initially confined to the male homosexual population although cases were gradually found among the heterosexual population. In the African population, HIV is contracted predominantly through heterosexual intercourse.

The AIDS and HIV epidemics are still relatively recent, but one sign of the potential scale of the disease in the African population is the high STD morbidity rate in the 1970s and 1980s. (STDs that are characterised by genital ulceration, such as syphilis and chanchroid, are also associated with greater susceptibility to HIV.) Table 8.1 shows that urban and rural inhabitants carry an equally heavy burden of STDS, and rural areas are also a source of infection. STDs are also an important health problem among migrants and have increased among mine workers since the mid 1970s. STD morbidity at gold mines in the Transvaal rose from 51.19 per 1000 employees per year in 1978 to 104.41 per 1000 in 1985, and in the Orange Free State from 39.61 to 76.11 per 1000.[5] The true figures may be even higher as many workers consult private practioners rather than mine doctors.[6]

Studies assessing high-risk environments for HIV have emphasised the importance of social, economic and political forces that make marginalised groups vulnerable to infection. Some studies have pointed to higher concentrations of HIV along transport networks, and also to the impact of population displacement due to political violence in Natal and the Reef, and to the return of 40 000 African National Congress guerillas who had been stationed in Angola, Tanzania, Uganda and Zambia, all of which are areas of high HIV prevalence.[7] Other studies tracing the progression of HIV from urban to rural areas have suggested that migrant labour is a significant factor in the nationwide spread of

Table 8.1   STD prevalence in the South African black population, 1969–94

Year	Sample frame	Sample description	STD prevalence
Urban population:			
1969–70	Urban hospital, Johannesburg	587 men and women	17% syphilis
1978	Urban family planning clinic, Johannesburg	186 women	10% gonorrhoea
1981	Urban antenatal clinic, Bloemfontein	1200 pregnant women	12% gonorrhoea
1981	Urban antenatal clinic, Durban	232 women	10% gonorrhoea
1985–86	Urban hospital antenatal clinic, Johannesburg	6287 pregnant women	6% syphilis
1994	Urban areas of the Orange Free State	120 women	16% syphilis
Rural population:			
1985–86	Urban hospital antenatal clinic, Johannesburg	1625 pregnant women, mostly rural wives of migrants	16% syphilis
1989	Rural hospital antenatal clinic, KwaZulu	193 pregnant women	12% syphilis 6% gonorrhoea
1994	Farm, Orange Free State	120 women	12% syphilis

Sources: Dogliotti (1971), p. 9; Hall and Whitcomb (1978), pp. 121–4; Welgemoed *et al.* (1986), p. 32; Hoosen *et al.* (1981), p. 828; Venter *et al.* (1989), p. 95; Farrell *et al.* (1989), p. 277; Cronjé *et al.* (1994), p. 602.

the disease.[8] As discussed earlier in this book, the migrant labour system and economic marginality was significant in shaping high-risk sexual behaviour among men and women, making them susceptible to syphilis. A similar situation prevails for HIV today.

Migrants' frequent and lengthy absences from home disrupt stable familial and sexual relationships. Living in lonely and hostile single-sex hostels, some men assuage their loneliness and anxiety about home and work by engaging in relationships with many partners.[9] A study of 240 migrant mineworkers attending an STD clinic in a Transvaal mining town in 1986 showed that 49 per cent had contracted an infection from a regular girlfriend, 33 per cent from casual sexual contacts and 15 per cent from local prostitutes. Ten per cent of the men had had more than one sexual partner in the previous month.[10] Attitude surveys of migrants, urban residents and urban and rural high school pupils show that condoms are seldom used as they are often associated with infidelity and distrust of a partner.[11]

The migrant labour system also ensures the rapid distribution of infection within urban areas, from urban to rural areas, within rural areas and across national boundaries.[12] In the study of migrant mine/workers mentioned above, 55 per cent of the men had acquired their STD infection locally, 20 per cent in Lesotho, 10 per cent in Botswana, 5 per cent in KwaZulu and 3 per cent in Transkei. The remaining 7 per cent had contracted their infection in Ciskei, Malawi, Swaziland and Johannesburg.[13] Another study of 429 mine workers found that 36.5 per cent had picked up an infection in neighbouring townships and 24.8 per cent in Transkei.[14]

Women have been affected differently but as severely by the migrant labour system. Long separations subject marriages to great strain and both partners may seek extramarital partners. Although urban and rural areas have similarly high rates of infection, migrant males are likely to be the main source of contact for STD infection. A study of pregnant rural women with STDs showed that while most had had between one and five partners in their lifetimes (the average age was 25.6 years), they had a very high incidence of STDs, which the researchers attributed to contact with male migrants.[15] Wives of migrants are dependent on the remittances sent home by their husbands, but long separations frequently result in divorce or abandonment, which deprives women of economic support. With access to few opportunities in the labour market, some women choose prostitution as the only means of economic survival.[16]

The high STD rates are matched by escalating HIV rates among migrant mine workers. The Chamber of Mines conducted an HIV screening programme in 1986 and tested almost 30000 specimens drawn from a larger pool of 300000. In the general mine-worker population HIV positivity was highest among those from Malawi (3.76 per cent) and Botswana (0.34 per cent), but relatively low among those from Lesotho and Mozambique (0.09 per cent), Swaziland (0.05 per cent) and South Africa (0.02 per cent), reflecting the southward movement of the disease. The overall prevalence was 0.45 per cent.[17] The Chamber of Mines also tested 1200 women living in areas around the mines, but all tested negative.[18] No further surveillance studies were conducted, but in 1996 mine doctors estimated that the prevalence among mine workers was over 15 per cent, and they noted that the incidence of tuberculosis over the preceding two years had doubled, reaching 1000–100 000 per year, which they attributed to HIV accelerating the transmission of opportunistic diseases.[19] A study of women living on farms in the Orange Free State in 1994 similarly showed that 0.4 per cent were HIV positive.[20] Thus for HIV, as for syphilis, there is evidence that economic and social disruption can lead to unsafe sexual practices, making particular groups more vulnerable to STDs.

However in popular representations HIV, like syphilis before it, became a symbol of the disintegration of white political power, economic vulnerability and the desegregation of society in the late 1980s and early 1990s.

The first reported AIDS cases affected white homosexual men. A newspaper headline announced 'Gay Plague Hits South Africa'[21] and intimated that homosexual men were polluting white society. Homosexuality was technically illegal in South Africa, and in the 1980s the gay community kept a low profile. South Africa had not been subject to the same public politicking around gay and feminist issues that had occurred in the USA and Europe, where the association between AIDS, 'corrupt' life-styles and 'unnatural' sexual behaviour came to signify the decline of moral society, and the need to preserve the family and heterosexuality.[22]

In South Africa there was a similar undercurrent of anxiety about the collapse of sexual morality and family life among whites. Educational propaganda for white schools aimed to cultivate 'a lifestyle based on high moral standards, chastity and being aware of the ideal sexual relationship: one man with one woman'.[23] AIDS was seen as a moral issue that required a moral solution. The talk of morality as the basis for a healthy society may have reflected political unease in the white community that apartheid was gradually unravelling. With the political future uncertain, a strong, virile and moral populace was essential.

The media focus soon shifted to the escalating number of cases among the African population, and as the disease seemed to be spread heterosexually all Africans were collectively labelled a 'risk group' and assumed to be sexually licentious. Throughout the 1970s and 1980s, as the country slipped into recession, the currency devalued and the union movement consolidated its strength, South Africa's economic vulnerability was of prime public concern. AIDS heightened the country's sense of economic crisis and anxiety about dependence on a volatile African labour force. Some reports warned that as the epidemic took hold it would curtail African population growth, and that by the year 2000, 50–70 per cent of Africans would have HIV or be dying of AIDS. This, it was prophesied, would lead to labour shortages, a fall in demand for consumer goods and an enormous medical burden that white tax-payers would have to fund. Thus AIDS would hasten South Africa's economic decline.[24]

Other images associated with AIDS embraced political tensions. The African National Congress (ANC) and the South African Communist Party were still banned in the 1980s, but their insignia, symbols and songs were part of the popular uprising during the mid 1980s. Stay-aways, boycotts and strikes became part of daily existence in large cities and small country towns. Umkhonto we Siswe, the guerila army of the ANC, began to infiltrate the country more successfully and the discovery of arms caches and bomb blasts in major cities were regular features of the national news. The revolt was followed by severe state repression.

In an attempt to discredit the ANC the government characterised HIV as the new '*swart gevaar*' (black peril), sweeping down from the north in the form of ANC guerillas.[25] A popular book warned that 'infected terrorists' could 'establish themselves in townships and infect prosti-tutes', leading to the spread of AIDS. Soweto, the largest township adja-cent to Johannesburg, was an obvious danger area.[26] Smear pamphlets distributed in Johannesburg in 1988 warned 'socialize with the ANC freedom fighters and cry and die from AIDS', in a crude attempt to discredit the ANC and scare potential supporters.[27] The association between AIDS and the ANC implied that the latter organisation and political protest were a disease that was spreading across the country and, unless rooted out and destroyed, could lead to an ugly and violent death. In 1990, when the ANC was unbanned, another smear pamphlet, bearing the name of a prominent ANC leader, warned the parents of ANC exiles that returnees would be quarantined and tested for AIDS.[28] Again the intention was to discredit the organisation.

White unease about racial desegregation also fed off myths about AIDS. From the early 1980s the government gradually removed its social segregation measures, for example blacks and whites were allowed to use the same entrance to liquor stores, and to visit the same cinemas and restaurants. By the late 1980s the extreme housing shortage had forced increasing numbers of blacks illegally to seek accommodation in white cities. Certain areas of Johannesburg became informal 'grey areas', that is, racially mixed. These changes were clear indications that apartheid was crumbling.

Other smear pamphlets, aimed at a white audience, claimed that all blacks would be infected with AIDS by 1992, and that the disease was spread by informal social contact such as sneezing and coughing or by mosquitoes. The pamphlet warned that 'to save the white race from extinction', whites should avoid visiting multiracial hotels, restaurants and churches and should regularly test their black domestic servants 'to safeguard your family'.[29] Newspapers reported that white madams (domestic employers) were testing their maids for HIV without their consent, and then dismissing them if the test proved positive – a cry-back to medical examinations for syphilis earlier in the century.[30]

During the 1990s, as the transition towards a democratically elected, multiracial government proceeded, newspapers reported on the escalating criminal and political violence that was now reaching into white suburbs. Between 1990 and 1994 there were an estimated 14000 deaths due to political violence, largely in Natal, where ANC and Inkatha fighters battled for control. The total number of murders during this period rose to 20000 a year, giving South Africa one of the highest rates in the world.[31] Higher walls guarded by armed security response teams or emigration were the two responses of white South Africans.

AIDS also had a role in fuelling Whites' fears. One newspaper carried reports of AIDS in Angola being 'a serious threat to South Africa' as South African mercenaries were based there. The subtext was an implicit warning that South Africa might follow the Angolan path if the elections collapsed and civil war ensued, resulting in AIDS wiping out the armed forces, famine and the collapse of industry.[32] Another commentator believed that AIDS represented the 'biggest threat to South African society', as increasing numbers of people falling ill put health workers at risk, especially surgeons, and this would 'lead to another wave of emigration', diminishing the pool of whites even further.[33]

The apartheid government's initial response was authoritarian – denying that a potential problem existed and introducing coercive legislation to prevent infection from entering the country. As in the 1920s, government and industry's main concern was maintaining a healthy, productive workforce. Foreign migrants seeking work in South Africa were blamed for importing the disease into the country. In 1987 the government introduced regulations for the compulsory testing of foreign labour recruits and the repatriation of all HIV-positive foreign workers.[34] Recruitment from Malawi, where the HIV prevalence was higher than in South Africa, came to a halt. This action was shortsighted as a preventive measure: it failed to deal with the cases that already existed in the local population, and by demonstrating that job loss and repatriation would follow detection, effectively forced HIV carriers underground and undermined the potential impact of any educational or outreach programmes. The mining industry initially intended to screen all prospective African mine employees routinely, and repatriate HIV-positive workers or those with AIDS who were no longer fit for work.[35]

The AIDS budget gradually grew from R10 million in 1985 to R5.4 million in 1990, and about R21 million in 1992 and 1993.[36] The government launched education programmes, but these were limited in outlook and impact. Educational material for whites emphasised the significance of long-term, monogamous relationships, while material aimed at the black population focused on debilitation and death. Many people were left more confused than informed about the causes and prevention of HIV.[37] The government was also reluctant to promote the use of condoms, believing that this would encourage promiscuity, and only from 1993 did it allow limited advertising for condoms on late-night TV.[38] As part of its AIDS prevention strategy the government made condoms freely available at family planning clinics. Africans viewed these efforts with suspicion, associating the clinics and contra-ception with racist attempts at population control. The authoritarian and moralistic views of clinic staff also hindered STD prevention programmes.[39]

The Chamber of Mines gradually changed its approach and invested in education and improved STD treatment for mineworkers. In 1996, however, it too acknowledged that its scheme had not been as success-ful as it had hoped. It found that miners were often reluctant to seek treatment at the free STD clinics, fearing that they would be discrimi-nated against in the workplace. Many men did not view STDs as a particularly serious ailment, or believed that they could be treated more effectively by traditional healers.[40]

The most creative preventive responses came from community groups. In 1987 the director general of the Department of Health stated publically that the department would do nothing to help the homo-sexual community as 'homosexuality is not accepted by the majority of the population' and it was the community's 'own affair'. The gay com-munity took matters into its own hands and modelled its network of education and support structures on the American movement.[41] In the townships and in workplaces, progressive groups tried to develop appropriate community-based educational and counselling services, aimed at workers, residents and healthworkers.[42] There were also attempts to draw traditional healers into the formal health education system in recognition of their importance in dealing with a range of health problems, including sexually transmitted diseases.[43]

In 1994 the ANC assumed power. Its election platform was tied to its vision of reconstruction and development, and the health service was seen as a prime target for restructuring. The government drew up a National AIDS Plan, called on the resources of international donors and health agencies, and in 1994 allotted a budget of R256.77 million to deal with AIDS.[44] Two years later the HIV directorate was discredited in a financial debacle and the Health Department was still struggling to restructure itself at the national, provincial and local levels. Insiders described the AIDS campaign as being in the doldrums.[45] Officials in the AIDs directorate admitted in mid 1997 that they had yet to spend half their R65 million budget from the previous year, which had been allotted from the Reconstruction and Development Programme, as they had not managed to create an institutional framework or overcome bureaucratic wrangling.[46]

By the mid 1990s health researchers were warning that the opportunity to restrict the impact of the AIDS epidemic had been lost, and with the epidemic in East and Central Africa being 10 years ahead of that in South Africa, South Africans could begin to look to these countries for signs of their possible future.[47] The demographic, economic and social impact of AIDS in developing countries is grim. The epidemic has hit the economically active population and greater absenteeism (for funerals or caring for sick relatives) has resulted in lower productivity. In rural areas where women are subsistence farmers, their illness or death can deprive a family of food, and force children to leave school to take over the farm. The growing number of orphans is placing a burden on already hard-pressed states, and usually on families that are already under pressure after losing one or more income earners. Finally, the direct medical costs of treating AIDS and opportunistic infections have the potential to undermine the health services.[48]

Health workers and policy makers are gradually recognising that preventive measures have to go beyond simple informational campaigns. The most effective educational strategies have drawn on a broad range of civil groups – trade unions, management associations, community and civic organisations, government and local health authorities – that can take into account the cultural, economic and social constraints of sexual activity and tailor health messages appropriately. This broad base can also link HIV education to other significant community issues such as teenage pregnancy, migrant labour, population displacement and rapid urbanisation, placing health and sexuality in a more political context.[49]

Conclusion

HIV and AIDS have an historical precedent in the hold that syphilis took amongst whites and Africans in the late nineteenth and early twentieth centuries as rural society began to decline and men and women settled in the cities or became temporary migrants. The fears about AIDS also resonate with the way in which VD metaphorically represented fears about social disorder and class, racial and gender identities. The parallel between HIV and syphilis also extends to the efficacy of medical cures. As yet there is no cure for HIV or AIDS. Similarly, until 1950, when penicillin was introduced, doctors relied on mercury and arsenic treatments, which might render a patient non-infectious but resulted in latent syphilis. Thus doctors saw public education as the best means of prevention.

If this study of the causes of VD, the social construction of its carriers and the limitations of treatment and educational services over half a century ago has any lessons for today, they are, firstly, that health personnel need to be sensitive to the fact that their own moral and racial perceptions may influence their interpretations of the causes of AIDS and HIV and the 'neutral' educational messages they try to put across. And secondly, that planners and educationists need to view AIDS and HIV in a political and socioeconomic context, as addressing these disparities are a priority in dealing with all health problems in South Africa.

In 1996 new billboard posters tied HIV prevention to 'health for all', but the task will be immense. The government faces not only an escalating number of cases of HIV and AIDS, with their attendant medical and social costs, but also a broad range of preventable diseases that are endemic in the country due to poverty. So it will have to decide on its priorities. The problem with HIV, as with many other diseases, is that its cause is as much social as natural. The spread of HIV, like that of syphilis in the twentieth century, will be influenced by the economic and social disruption that accompanies institutionalised migrancy, urban and rural poverty and massive unemployment, and these problems, though easy to pinpoint, are difficult to solve.

Appendix 1

Today four treponemal infections are recognised: venereal syphilis, endemic syphilis, yaws and pinta. The first three coexist in Southern Africa, but endemic syphilis is confined to the arid south and central regions, and yaws to the humid north and east.[1] The agents that cause each syndrome are morphologically similar and provoke the same antigenic response. Hence the syndromes are usually differentiated according to their epidemiology and certain clinical symptoms.

In the primary stage of venereal syphilis a single sore or hard chancre usually appears at the point of innoculation on the genitals after an incubation period of three weeks. A period of latency follows after healing. A primary chancre is rare in endemic syphilis, though common in yaws. The secondary stage of venereal syphilis is characterised by a rash of contagious lesions appearing anywhere on the body. Endemic syphilitic lesions can resemble this but more common are mucous patches in the mouth and lesions in the axillary and genital areas. The tertiary stage of syphilis appears after twenty years of latency only in a third of cases and is characterised by cardiovascular, neurological and visceral complications. These do not seem to occur in endemic syphilis, which is characterised in 25–50 per cent of cases by destructive ulcers of the nasopharynx, skin and bone, which disable and deform an individual but seldom cause death.

Venereal syphilis is transmitted through sexual intercourse, and thus usually occurs in the adult, sexually active population. It can also be transmitted perinatally from mother to child, and in such cases spontaneous abortion, stillbirth or premature birth are likely.[2] A newborn baby born with congenital syphilis may appear healthy at first but later develops secondary and tertiary symptoms simultaneously. A child may die from a lesion in a vital organ or, if it survives, develop characteristic deformities, including protruding brows, abnormalities of the upper jaw, saddle nose, saber shins and the Hutchinson triad (peculiarly shaped teeth, blindness and deafness). Infection of a foetus by endemic syphilis is theoretically possible, but rare, because many pregnant women have very low levels of pathogenic treponemes in their bloodstream due to the long period between treponemal infection in childhood and becoming pregnant in adulthood.

Non-sexual transmission is typical of endemic syphilis and yaws. It occurs through direct lesion-to-skin contact, or indirect contact with fingers or objects contaminated with saliva containing treponemes. Transmission of venereal syphilis through indirect contact is rare, though possible. The reservoir of infection for endemic syphilis and yaws consists of latent cases and children between the ages of two and 15. Venereal syphilis can coexist with endemic syphilis or yaws, though the latter two provide cross-immunity to venereal syphilis.[3]

Appendix 2

Table A2.1 Examination of prostitutes under part I of the CDPA, 1889–1908

Year	White women	Black women	Total women	Total no. of examinations	No. of diseased	Percentage diseased	Total expenditure (£)
1889	n.a.	n.a.	510	3957	170	33.3	4161
1890	n.a.	n.a.	456	4028	140	30.7	3599
1891	n.a.	n.a.	482	4418	114	23.7	3308
1892	n.a.	n.a.	528	4969	290	54.9	3944
1893	n.a.	n.a.	543	5827	250	46.0	3763
1894	n.a.	n.a.	561	1091	228	40.6	4002
1895	93	503	596	7158	246	41.3	4007
1896	190	510	700	6642	250	35.7	4594
1897	279	470	749	7040	254	33.9	4187
1898	333	448	781	7337	278	35.6	4104
1899	318	421	739	7244	255	34.5	4312
1900	98	465	763	6081	277	36.3	4244
1901	370	559	929	6612	334	36.0	4692
1902	308	501	809	6126	233	28.8	4620
1903	116	396	512	4258	146	28.5	4075
1904	84	310	394	3911	122	31.0	3777
1905	29	319	348	3076	125	35.9	3211
1906	55	393	448	4567	179	40.0	3328
1907	52	356	408	3786	162	39.7	3111
1908	47	408	455	3655	189	41.5	3089

Sources: G 19-94, pp. xv, 140; G 74-96, pp. lxxiv, lxxv, lxxvii; G 05-97, p. xcii; G 35-1904, pp. ciii–civ; G 39-1906, p. xciii, A72; G 40-1907, p. 113; G 33-1908, p. 83; G 43-1909, p. 9.

Table A2.2 Examination of black and white paupers under part II of the CDPA, 1889–1908

Year	White males	White females	Total whites	Black males	Black females	Total blacks	Total whites and blacks	Expenditure (£)
1889	n.a.	n.a.	n.a.	n.a.	n.a.	n.a.	n.a.	9103
1890	n.a.	n.a.	n.a.	n.a.	n.a.	n.a.	n.a.	10063
1891	n.a.	n.a.	n.a.	n.a.	n.a.	n.a.	n.a.	8696
1892	n.a.	n.a.	n.a.	n.a.	n.a.	n.a.	n.a.	8310
1893	75	71	146	943	861	1804	1950	8656
1894	n.a.	n.a.	n.a.	n.a.	n.a.	n.a.	n.a.	n.a.
1895	65	68	133	895	842	1737	1870	9092
1896	55	47	102	730	757	1487	1389	11092
1897	83	60	143	896	875	1771	1914	12170
1898	95	72	167	1013	1113	2126	2293	14366
1899	57	64	121	692	703	1395	1516	8470
1900	73	63	136	809	810	1619	1755	10086
1901	60	60	120	861	798	1659	1779	11498
1902	44	64	108	878	868	1746	1854	12132
1903	61	41	102	942	979	1921	2023	14666
1904	64	38	102	1006	1140	2146	2248	12067
1905	68	41	109	970	1211	2181	2290	8990
1906	70	60	130	1077	1173	2250	2380	9799
1907	94	41	135	1510	1613	3123	3258	11198
1908	74	53	127	1777	2138	3915	4042	8996

Sources: G 19-94, p. xix; G 74-96, pp. lxxxi, lxxxv–vi; G 05-97; p. cvi; G 35-1904; pp. cx–cxii, cxvi; G 39-1906, pp. A64–7; G 40-1907, pp. 114–17; G 33-1908, pp. 84, 86–7; G 43-1909, pp. 12–13.

Table A2.3 Incidence of syphilis in males examined for recruitment, 1914–37[1]

Year	Sample population	Number	Percentage
Jan. 1914–Sept. 1916	35 370 males at Pretoria pass office	259	0.730
1930	1100 recruits for New Tendega colliery	2	0.180
Jan. 1932	1143 males at pass examination in Pietermaritzburg	23 78	(2)[2] (6.800)[3]
1920–33	33 308 males examined at Kingwilliamstown	44	0.150
1936	300 000 males examined at WNLA recruiting depot	135 (286)[2]	0.045 0.095
Jan.–July 1937	13 928 mine recruits examined by NRC in Basutholand	179	1.290

Notes:
1. The low incidence of syphilis among new male recruits examined by the Native Recruiting Corporation and Witwatersrand Native Labour Association in rural areas, and on arrival in urban areas by pass medical officers, suggests that the incidence of sexually transmitted diseases was still low in rural populations. However it is possible that men with clearly visible lesions or in chronic ill-health due to sequelae of the disease, may have excluded themselves from recruitment, and the screened populations probably included first-time and returning migrants. Screening was also very peremptory.
2. Syphilis or gonorrhoea in contagious form.
3. Evidence of old STD infection.
Sources: Pijper (1919), p. 324; HPW, AD1438, Box 2, 'Health and Child Welfare Natal, pp. 1160–2523', Vryheid sitting, 20 September 1930: evidence of Dr M. Kuper, district surgeon for Vryheid and medical officer for New Tendega colliery, p. 32; NAB, 3/DBN 188, vol. 7, South African Health Officials Association, report on the proceedings of the 8th congress, held in Pietermaritzburg on the 5–8 June 1933, address by Dr C. C. P. Anning, 'Municipal Health Problems of the Non-European Population', p. 20; Burton (1934), p. 327; Central Mining-Rand Mines Group Health Department, *Report for the Year 1936*, p. 42; COMA, 2211:2033, J. F. Young, Medical Officer, to General Manager, Native Recruiting Corporation, 1 October 1937.

Table A2.4   Incidence of syphilis among Africans in urban and rural areas, 1921–46

Year	Sample population	% positive
Urban areas:		
1921	500 outpatients and friends, Pretoria clinic	47.80
1938	712 outpatients, Germiston dispensary	44.40
1938	227 women at antenatal clinic, Germiston	40.50
1938–44	2828 women at antenatal clinic, Springs	23.97
1940	381 women at antenatal clinic, Alexandra	39.40
1940	105 maternity cases, Alexandra	37.00
1943	Random testing among Kimberley abattoir employees	32.00
1943	Antenatal clinic, Kimberley	46.00
1946	715 antenatal cases at Edendale, Natal	20.10
Rural areas:		
1930	235 men attending a chief's meeting at Flagstaff, Pondoland	12.10
1943	1184 maternity cases at hospital, Umtata, Transkei	11.40
1943	57 antenatal cases, St Barnabas Mission, Transkei	19.20
1941–6	930 pregnant women, Polela, Natal	35.30

Note: The high Transvaal and Orange Free State urban rates may have been skewed by the presence of endemic syphilis in labour-supply areas. The Wasserman serodiagnostic test cannot differentiate between endemic and venereal syphilis.

Sources: Pijper (1921), p. 304; Rauch and Saayman (1938), p. 885; 'Abstracts. Venereal Diseases' (1944), p. 190; Medical Officer of Health report, Springs, cited in Kark (1949), p. 78; Landau (1946), cited in Kark (1949), p. 78; Drew, cited in UG 22–32, p. 214; Tobias (1944), p. 142; unpublished reports by the Medical Officer-in-Charge, Polela Health Unit, to Chief Health Officer (1941–6), cited in Kark (1949), p. 78; HPW, AD843 B2.1.1, Alexandra Health Committee, Medical Officer of Health's report for the year ending 30 June 1940, p. 9.

Table A2.5 STD morbidity of workforce at gold mines and collieries, 1936–46

Year	Population	No. with syphilis	Cases per 1000	No. with gonorrhoea	Cases per 1000
1936	269 540	1528	5.67	252	0.94
1936	300 000	618	5.85	n.a.	n.a.
1937	300 000	721	6.88	n.a.	n.a.
1938	300 000	659	6.19	n.a.	n.a.
1943	Gold mine	n.a.	6.71	n.a.	1.91
1943	Colliery	n.a.	5.50	n.a.	3.70
1946	Gold mine	508	5.38	144	1.53

Sources: COMA 2080:1704, General Manager, Gold Producers Committee, to Dr A. I. Girdwood, Chief Medical Officer, Witwatersrand Native Labour Association, 2 December 1936; *Central Mining-Rand Mines Group Health Department Report for the Year 1938*, p. 12; Allen (1943), p. 60; *Central Mining-Rand Mines Group Health Department Report for the Year 1946*, p. 5.

Notes and References

Introduction

1 Garrett (1995), ch. 11.
2 Chirimuuta and Chirimuuta (1989); Hunt (1989), Panos Dossier (1988).
3 For example Beck (1970); Burrows (1958); Laidler (1971).
4 Burke and Richardson (1978); de Beer (1984); Marks and Andersson (1985, 1992); Philip (1987, 1990); World Health Organisation (1983).
5 Bassett and Mhloyi (1991); Dawson (1988); Hunt (1989); Jochelson *et al.* (1991).
6 Bozzoli (1991); Jochelson (1995); White (1990).
7 Cohen (1972), pp. 9–10.
8 Bland (1982, 1985); Davenport-Hines (1991).
9 Brandt (1987); Hobson (1987), pp. 184–99; Jones (1981), chs 2–3.
10 Altman (1986); Sontag (1988), pp. 25–6, 46; Watney (1987).
11 Parry (1983); Schreuder (1976); Trapido (1980).
12 Dubow (1987, 1991, 1992); Marks and Trapido (1987).
13 Bank (1994); Dubow (1995).
14 Chisholm (1989); Deacon (1996); Swartz (1995).
15 Jacobus *et al.* (1990); Russett (1991); Weeks (1977, 1985).
16 Eckart (1988), pp. 85–7, 90–91; Marcovich (1988), pp. 106–7; Nicolson (1988), p. 67; Vaughan (1991).
17 Foucault (1980, 1987, 1991).
18 Vaughan (1991), pp. 10–12.

1 Tracking Down the Treponema

1 G 19-87, p. 9.
2 G 03-86, p. 10.
3 Chatterjee (1996); Decker (1996); Manderson (1997).
4 G 67-84, pp. 6–7.
5 G 03-86, p. 7.
6 G 13-88, p. 9.
7 G 67-84, p. 7.
8 G 67-84, p. 30.
9 G 03-86, pp. 18–19; G 04-89, pp. 14, 17; CDC (1906), p. 13, para. 28.
10 G 35-1904, pp. lvii–lviii; G 39-1906, pp. xcv–xcvi; G 40-1907, p. xlv.
11 A 13-88, p. 46.
12 G 13-88, p. 29.
13 G 17-90, p. 11; see also G 13-88, p. 29; G 04-89, pp. 20, 47.
14 G 19-87, p. 6.
15 G 19-94, p. xxiii.
16 G 03-86, pp. 18–19.
17 TAB, SS R1250/96, 'Landrost Pretoria zendt in rapporten van veldcornetten ... re sifilis lyders', pp. 132, 165, 172, 177, 187, 190, 207.

18 Transvaal Public Health Department, *Annual Reports for the Year Ended 30 June 1905*; *Annual Reports for the Year Ended 30 June 1906*.
19 Gelfand (1976), pp. 24–6.
20 CDC (1906), p. 13, para. 25.
21 Ibid., paras. 26, 28.
22 Ibid., p. 14, para. 37.
23 Ibid., p. 19, paras. 4–5; see also TAB, CS 578 2614A, G. Liegme, MOH Swiss Mission, Elim to MOH for the Transvaal, June 1906, p. 6; TAB, CS 910 17857, First report of the district MOH for the year ending 30 June 1907, p. 3
24 SAB, NTS 5760 15/315, MOH for the Northern Transvaal to Secretary for the Interior, 4 May 1913, p. 1.
25 G 03-86, p. 33; G 13-88, pp. 48–9; G 33-1908, pp. 46–52.
26 TAB, CS 965 19784 (9149/1898), Synopsis of Opinions of Magistrates, District Surgeons and City Health Officers re Prevalence of Syphilis, 1899; (1344/1899), District Surgeon to Magistrate, Ingwavuma, 30 December 1898; District Surgeon, Lower Umfolozi to Magistrate, Eshowe, 4 January 1899.
27 Delius (1980); Harries (1982); Kimble (1982); Turrel (1987), ch. 2; Worger (1987), pp. 65–107.
28 Turrell (1987), p. 19.
29 Van Onselen (1982a), p. 2.
30 Harries (1994), pp. 109–10.
31 Jeeves (1985), pp. 265–7.
32 Turrell (1987), pp. 19, 242.
33 Van Onselen (1982a), p. 104, Harries (1994), p. 114.
34 Van Onselen (1982a), pp. 104, 106–14.
35 Ibid., pp. 108–9.
36 Harries (1994), pp. 55–6.
37 Turrell (1987), p. 19.
38 Shillington (1982); Worger (1987), pp. 80–1, 88–9, 93–6.
39 Eales (1991), pp. 24–7, 33; Harries (1994), p. 114.
40 Eales (1991), pp. 25, 28–9.
41 Bonner (1990), pp. 228–9, 235–6.
42 G 19-85, p. 2; A 13-88, p. 16.
43 G 19-85, p. 21.
44 CDC (1906), annexure D, p. 30; see also G 19-94, p. xxii; G 35-1904, pp. lvii–lviii.
45 CDC (1906), p. 13, para. 28; G 19-94, p. xxii.
46 TAB, SS R1250/96, 'Landrost Pretoria zendt in repporten van veldcornetten . . . re syphilis lyders', pp. 132, 165, 172, 177, 187, 190, 207.
47 CDC (1906), p. 10, para. 12.
48 TAB, CS 965 19784 (1344/1899), Resident Magistrate to Chief Magistrate and Civil Commissioner, Eshowe, 4 January 1899; District Surgeon to Magistrate, Ngutu, 2 January 1899. For other cases see (9129/1898), letter from Magistrate, Upper Umkomanzi, 1898; (1344/1899), Resident Magistrate, Entonjaneni to Chief Magistrate, Eshowe, 5 January 1899; (9149/1898 (W1050/1898)), District Surgeon to Magistrate, Weenen, 11 January 1899; (I1645/98), District Surgeon to Resident Magistrate, Ixopo, 20 January 1899.

49   TAB, CS 965 19784 (9149/1898 (UT610/98)), District Surgeon to Magistrate, Upper Tugela, 19 December 1899.
50   Parsons (1988), p. 3.
51   Stone (1993), pp. 151, 155, 230.
52   Ibid., p. 174.
53   Ibid., pp. 217–20.
54   Ibid., p. 21; Transvaal Public Health Department, *Annual Reports for the Year Ended 30 June 1905*, pp. 12–16; Transvaal Public Health Department, *Annual Reports for the Year Ended 30 June 1906*, pp. 18–24; TAB, CS 221 283/03, Resident Magistrate to Colonial Secretary, 8 January 1903.
55   G 67-84, p. 23.
56   CDC (1906), pp. 13–14, paras. 26, 28, 34.
57   G 67-84, pp. 7, 23; see also MacArthur and Thornton (1910), p. 164.
58   G 03-86, p. 19.
59   Melle (1935).
60   G 04-89, p. 18.
61   G 19-85, p. 14.
62   CDC (1906), p. 9, para. 12.
63   G 67-84, p. 23.
64   G 04-89, p. 18; TAB, CS 909 17855, report on tour of medical inspection and vaccination through Pokwanie and north of Middelburg district, 1909, pp. 7–8.
65   TAB, CS 910 17857, District Surgeon to Resident Magistrate, Pietersburg, 6 September 1909.
66   G 67-84, p. 41.
67   G 03-86, p. 17.
68   G 03-86, p. 21; see also G 19-94, p. xviii; TAB, CS 578 2614A, G. Liegme, MOH Swiss mission, Elim to MOH for the Transvaal, June 1906, pp. 2–3, 6.
69   G 67-84, p. 29; G 04-89, p. 15; G 19-94, p. xviii.
70   G 19-85, p.14.
71   G 67-84, pp. 6, 12, 13, 15, 23, 27, 29, 32, 37, 41.
72   G 03-86, p. 17; G 67-84, pp. 6, 15.
73   McArthur and Thornton (1910), p. 163.
74   G 04-89, p. 84.
75   G 04-89, pp. 16, 20–1; TAB, CS 221 283/03, District Surgeon Nylstroom to Resident Magistrate, January 1903.
76   Willcox (1951), pp. 559, 560.
77   Gelfand (1976), pp. 24–6.
78   Murray, Merriweather and Freedman (1956), pp. 984–5.
79   Du Toit (1969); Scott and Lups (1973); Taylor (1954); van Beukering (1965).
80   Murray (1957).
81   Steyn and Henneberg (1995).
82   Rothschild *et al.* (1996).
83   G 04-89, p. 18.
84   Ricono (1911), p. 210.
85   Ibid.
86   G 04-89, p. 18.
87   TAB, CS 578 2614A, G. Liegme to MOH for the Transvaal, June 1906, p. 6.
88   CDC (1906), p. 16, para. 51.

89 TAB, CS 965 19784 (9149/1898 (W1050/1898)), District Surgeon to Magistrate, Weenen, 11 January 1899.
90 Kark (1949), p. 77.
91 TAB, CS 965 19784 (1344/1899), District Surgeon to Resident Magistrate, Ndwandwe, 23 December 1898; (9149/1898), District Surgeon to Resident Magistrate, Ixopo, 20 January 1899; District Surgeon to Chief Magistrate, Estcourt, 21 January 1899; NAB, DPH 30 57/1908, District Surgeon, Ingwavuma to Board of Health, 1 February 1908.
92 TAB, CS 965 19784, minute papers 9129/1898; R4395/1907; SAB NK 157, report of the Select Committee (no. 15, 1890) on the Contagious Diseases Prevention Bill (no. 19, 1890), Sixth Session, Twelfth Legislative Council, pp. 1, 5, 17.
93 Transvaal Public Health Department (1905), pp. 10–12.
94 CDC (1906), p. 9, para. 11.
95 Transvaal Public Health Department (1904), p. 7, (1905), p. 6, (1906), p. 9.
96 CDC (1906), p. 10, para. 11.
97 Ibid., p. 11, para. 17.
98 Ibid., p. 11, para. 18.
99 Packard (1989), pp. 68–73.
100 Morris (1988), p. 723.
101 G 13-88, p. 42.
102 G 03-86, pp. 18–19.
103 Cockburn (1963), ch. 7; Hackett (1963); Hudson (1965).
104 Packard (1989), pp. 75–6; Turrell (1987), pp. 160–2.
105 Harries (1994), p. 60; Katz (1994), p. 10; Packard (1989), p. 49; Worger (1987), pp. 31, 97, 134, 143, 172.
106 Hackett (1953), p. 160; Scott (1933, 1939).
107 Hackett (1953), pp. 159–66, (1957), pp. 159–60; Hudson (1965), p. 889.
108 Scott (1933), p. 49.
109 Garrett (1995).
110 G 67-84, p. 6.
111 G 04-89, p. 17.
112 G 67-84, p. 23; G 55-96, p. 124.
113 TAB, CS 909 17855, report on medical inspection and vaccination through Pokwanie and north of Middelburg district, 1909, p. 7.
114 Vaughan (1991), ch. 6, (1992); Callahan (1996) on central Africa; Dawson (1983), ch. 4, (1987) on Kenya; Callahan (1992) on Zimbabwe.
115 Jones (1981), chs 2, 3; Willcox (1960), pp. 82–3.
116 G 03-86, pp. 18–19.
117 G 04-89, pp. 17–18, G 03-86, p. 19.
118 G 04-89, pp. 14, 17, 54–7; G 19-94, p. xvii; G 39-1906, p. xciv.
119 CDC (1906), p. 16, para. 46.
120 A13-88, p. 5; G 04-89, p. 64.
121 Parry (1983); Schreuder (1976); Trapido (1980).
122 Bank (1994); Dubow (1995), pp. 25–32.
123 Lees (1985), pp. 107–11; Williams (1985), p. 221.
124 Lorimer (1978), pp. 144–7. On Social Darwinism see Jones (1980), esp. ch. 8.
125 Cited in Bickford-Smith (1995), pp. 77–83.

126   Ibid., pp. 118–19; Bickford-Smith (1981).
127   G 19-85, p. 2; G 13-88, p. 49; G 04-89, pp. 8, 47. See also CDC (1906), p. 14, para. 32, p. 15, para. 41.
128   G 04-89, p. 47.
129   G 19-87, p. 10. For similar comments by the district surgeon of Graaff-Reinet, see G 04-89, p. 47.
130   G 04-89, p. 29.
131   TAB, CS 965 19784 (9129/1898), A. A. Rouillaw to Town Clerk, Ladysmith, 3 January 1899.
132   Stepan (1982), pp. 104–6; ch. 4.
133   Bank (1994), p. 13.
134   Bickford-Smith (1995), pp. 118–19.
135   Dubow (1995), pp. 20–6; Gilman (1986), p. 237.
136   G 04-89, p. 91.
137   G 19-85, p. 42.
138   A 13-88, p. 31, quoting William Saunders, a doctor in Cape Town and former district surgeon at Fraserburg and Prince Albert.
139   Comaroff and Comaroff (1991), pp. 95–7, 274–5; Mostert (1992), pp. 177–9; Streak (1974).
140   A 13-88, p. 32; Stepan (1982), ch. 4. For later beliefs about the effects of colonial climates on settler health, see Dubow (1995), pp. 176–9; Kennedy (1987), ch. 6.
141   Van Heyningen (1991), pp. 131–2.
142   A 13-88, p. 24.
143   G 04-89, pp. 16, 20–1.
144   G 04-89, p. 66; Bickford-Smith (1995), pp. 114–15.
145   Bickford-Smith (1995), pp. 50, 61–2.
146   C 05-95, appendix, pp. viii–ix.
147   Woods Hutchinson (1897), pp. 133–5.
148   A 30-06, p. 137.
149   TAB, GOV 32/115/02, Jonathan Hutchinson to Colonial Secretary of State, 29 August 1902.
150   Mathias (1910), 1911, pp. 64, 174.
151   McArthur and Thornton (1910), pp. 164–5.
152   Ibid., p. 171; McArthur and Thornton (1911), pp. 29–30.
153   McArthur and Thornton (1910), pp. 164–5, 171, (1911), pp. 29–30.
154   Walker (1911).
155   TAB, CS 578, 2614A, G. Liegme, Elim to MOH for Transvaal, June 1906, pp. 6–7.
156   Transvaal Public Health Department, Annual Reports for the Year Ended 30 June 1906, p. 26.
157   SAB, NTS 5760 15/315, MOH for Northern Transvaal to Secretary for Interior, 4 May 1913.
158   McArthur and Thornton (1911), p. 21, (1910), p. 163.
159   McArthur and Thornton (1910), p. 164, (1911), pp. 23–4.
160   TAB, CS 909 17855, report on tour of medical inspection and vaccination through Pokwanie and north of Middelburg district, 1909, pp. 7, 9.
161   SAB, NTS 5760 15/315, MOH for Northern Transvaal to Secretary for Interior, 4 May 1913.

162 SAB, GG 916 33/453, G. O. Robertson to Government Secretary, Mafeking, October 1913.
163 Gilman (1986), p. 250.
164 McArthur and Thornton (1911), p. 20.
165 Packard (1987).
166 McArthur and Thornton (1910), p. 163.
167 McArthur and Thornton (1911), p. 30, comments by Dr Tomory, Dr H. A. Spencer.
168 A 30-06, p. 71.
169 Gaitskell (1982).
170 SANAC (1903–05), p. 40, paras. 282–4, 286.
171 Dubow (1995), pp. 130–2, 169, (1989), pp. 23–5; Rich (1980), pp. 176–7.
172 De Vos Hugo (1911, 1915); Mathias (1910, 1911b); Ricono (1916).
173 Mathias (1910), p. 102, (1911), p. 174.
174 Mathias (1911), p. 64.
175 Ricono (1911).

2 From Paupers to Pass Laws

1 Van Heyningen (1984).
2 Van Heyningen (1991), pp. 131–2; Bickford-Smith (1981).
3 Bickford-Smith (1995), pp. 28–9.
4 Ibid., pp. 118–19; Bickford-Smith (1981).
5 Bickford-Smith (1995), pp. 121–2.
6 Ibid., pp. 99–100, 117, 119–20; Bickford-Smith (1981); van Heyningen (1991), p. 133.
7 Saunders (1984), pp. 166, 168–9, 172–3. On the infection metaphor and segregation, see also Marks and Andersson (1984); Swanson (1976, 1977, 1983); Caldwell (1991).
8 Levine (1994), p. 580.
9 Van Heyningen (1984), pp. 174–6.
10 KAB, GH 23/36 62, p. 446, Governor Frere to Secretary of State, 8 March 1880; G 19-85, p. 11; A 13-88, p. 2; van Heyningen (1984), p. 178.
11 A 30-06, p. 86.
12 C 05-95, appendix, pp. viii–ix.; see also A 30-06, p. 48.
13 A 13-78; A 14-78.
14 G 19-85, p. 20.
15 Bundy (1980), pp. 211–15.
16 G 13-88, p. 29.
17 G 17-90, p. 11.
18 G 67-84, pp. 12, 32; G 19-85, p. 1; G 03-86, pp. 36–7.
19 Van Heyningen (1984), p. 177.
20 G 19-85, p. 6.
21 G 19-85, pp. 28, 30; G 03-86, p. 26; see also G 67-84, pp. 6, 30.
22 G 19-85, pp. 4, 33; G 67-84, pp. 4–5, 12.
23 A 13-88, p. 24.
24 Worger (1987), pp. 80–1, 92–6.
25 G 03-86, pp. 4–5.
26 G 67-84, p. 6.

27   G 67-84, pp. 5, 9, 14, 18, 29.
28   Trapido (1980).
29   Levine (1994); Warren (1990), pp. 363, 365.
30   Bickford Smith (1995), p. 93.
31   G 03-86, pp. 4–5, 14; G 19-87, pp. 11, 22, 26; G 13-88, p. 29.
32   Van Heyningen (1984), p. 179.
33   KAB, CO 7906, F127C, Colonial Secretary, Circular No. 52, 1904; G 39-1906, p. xcix; A 30-06, pp. 72–3.
34   Van Heyningen (1989), pp. 469–71.
35   Ibid., pp. 462–6; Bickford Smith (1995), pp. 39–40.
36   G 19-85, p. 26.
37   G 15-91, p. 26; G 19-87, pp. 44–5; G 67-84, p. 19; G 04-89, p. 4.
38   G 17-90, pp. 21–2; G 19-87, pp. 44–5.
39   G 17-90, pp. 38, 43.
40   Bickford Smith (1995), p. 31.
41   Ibid., pp. 40–2, 48–9; Giliomee (1979, 1989a, 1989b).
42   Bundy (1980), p. 217.
43   G 17-90, pp. 18, 50; G 20-92, p. 23.
44   Van Heyningen (1989), p. 466; Schreuder (1976), p. 290.
45   Van Heyningen (1989), pp. 466–8.
46   A 13-88, p. 29.
47   G 04-89, pp. 12, 63, 84; G 03-86, p. 15.
48   A 13-88, p. 11.
49   G 67-84, p. 7.
50   G 17-90, pp. 11, 37–99, 225; G 56-1900, p. 189.
51   G 04-89, p. 45.
52   G 17-90, p. 19.
53   G 17-90, p. 38; G 04-89, pp. 5, 39.
54   G 17-90, p. 7.
55   G 19-87, p. 39. For similar cases see G 55-96, pp. 24, 95, 184; G 19-87, pp. 44–5; G 17-90, p. 25.
56   G 03-86, p. 14; G 19-87, pp. 11, 26; G 04-89, p. 8; G 17-90, p. 11; G 55-96, p. 184.
57   G 04-89, p. 11.
58   Vaughan (1991), pp. 33–5, 38–40; Worboys (1988).
59   Van Heyningen (1984), pp. 188–9.
60   Hallett (1979), pp. 5, 7.
61   G 20-92, pp. 56–7.
62   KAB, MOH 310, C117B, report by the Assistant MOH for the Colony into the Working of the CDA in East London, 24 April 1902, pp. 3–4; KAB, MOH 311, C117B, the CDPA: East London and Kingwilliamstown, 1907, p. 1; G 43-1909, p. 8.
63   C 01-69, pp. 1–2, 6, 9.
64   Walkowitz (1980), pp. 58–9.
65   G 04-89, p. 40.
66   G 19-85, p. 39; G 55-96, p. 29.
67   KAB, CO 7403, 360, Vryburg Syphilitic Hospital.
68   CDC (1906), p. 17, para. 54; Annexure D, p. 29.
69   G 04-89, pp. 5, 32.

70 G 19-87, pp. 44–5; G 20-92, p. 23; G 17-90, p. 28.
71 G 04-89, p. 63.
72 G 17-90, pp. 22, 27.
73 Deacon (1996); Bickford Smith (1995), pp. 99–105; Swartz (1995), pp. 399–400.
74 Chisholm (1989), pp. 30, 33, 39, 47; Deacon (1996), pp. 305–7.
75 KAB, MOH 310, C117B, 'Report . . . into . . . the CDA in East London', 24 April 1902, pp. 3–4.
76 KAB, CO 7508, 629, report on an Enquiry into the Working of the Cape Town Lock Hospital and the Operation of the Act No. 39 of 1885, March 1898.
77 A 13-88, p. 47.
78 G 19-87, pp. 44–5; G 13-88, p. 29; G 04-89, p. 121.
79 KAB, MOH 310, C117B, report on the Working of the CDPA, 1885, Cape Town District, November 1904, p. 2; report on Lock Hospital and working of CDPA, 1885, Port Elizabeth, 28 December 1904, pp. 1–2.
80 KAB, MOH 311, C117B, The CDPA: East London and Kingwilliamstown, 1907, p. 10.
81 KAB, MOH 310, C117B, 'Report . . . into . . . the CDA in East London', 24 April 1902, pp. 3–4; KAB, MOH 311, C117B, The CDPA: East London and Kingwilliamstown, 1907, p. 1; G 43-1909, p. 8.
82 G 04-89, p. 122; G 55-96, p. 77.
83 TAB, SS R1250/96, 'Circulaire aan Landrosten en Mijncommissarissen CB 21/95', June 1985, and attached reports.
84 Hilton Barber (1907), pp. 69–72.
85 Contagious Diseases Law No. 12 of 1895, section 36 (b), (c), (e), (h), (i).
86 World Health Organisation (1983), pp. 87–8.
87 TAB, SS R1250/96, District surgeon, Barberton to Landdrost, Barberton, July 1895; TAB, PW 129 AR371/96, District surgeon to Cipier, Ermelo 28 February 1896, Cipier to district surgeon, Ermelo, 2 March 1896; TAB, SS R8585/97, 'Landdrost Piet Retief . . . lydende aan syphilis', June 1897.
88 TAB, SS R6135/98, 'Veldkornet Wyk 3 Carolina bericht dat een kaffer lydende aan syphilis . . .'
89 TAB, SS R423/86, 'Landdrost Ermelo heeft Dr. Everard een kraal . . .'; SAB, LD637 AG934/04, Resident Magistrate Ermelo to Secretary to the Law Department, 1 March 1904; Director of Prisons to Secretary for Law Department, 9 March 1904; MOH for the Transvaal to Secretary to the Law Department, 5 April 1904; TAB, CS 908 17847, Secretary to the Law Department to the MOH, Pretoria, 25 March 1904.
90 TAB, SS R1250/96, 'Rapport over het geneeskundige onderzoek der naturellen wonende in de Wyk Middelburg, ZAR', September 1896-March 1897; TAB, SS R3013/85, District Surgeon to Landdrost, Pretoria, 16 March 1885.
91 Richardson and van-Helten (1982), p. 83; Jeeves (1985), pp. 37, 46.
92 Jeeves (1985), pp. 44–5.
93 Marks and Trapido (1981), pp. 63–4; Warwick (1980), pp. 13–14; Richardson and van Helten (1980), pp. 31–4.
94 Richardson and van Helten (1980), p. 31; Jeeves (1975), pp. 11–12.

95   Hilton Barber (1901), pp. 58–9; Hindson (1987), p. 23; Jeeves (1985), pp. 42–3.
96   Marks and Trapido (1981), pp. 63–4.
97   Ibid.; Jeeves (1985), pp. 51–3, (1975), pp. 12–15, 17–18; Katzenellenbogen (1980).
98   TAB, CS 578 2614, C. A. Wheelwright to Secretary of Native Affairs, [1906?]; CDC (1906), p. 14, para. 38; see also TAB, SNA 100 NA291/03, W. N. Bolton, Resident Magistrate, Pietersburg, to MOH for the Transvaal, 30 September 1904.
99   TAB, CS 910 17857, first report of the District MOH for the year ended 30 June 1907, pp. 3, 5. See also TAB, CS 578 2614A, minute paper 2614(a), 19 September 1905.
100 TAB, SD 2614 D, Commission re syphilis amongst natives.
101 CDC (1906), p. 18, para, 58–63.
102 SAB, NTS 2863 10/303, Acting Under Secretary for Native Affairs to Secretary for Native Affairs, 8 November 1910.
103 SAB NTS 2891 (119/303), report concerning the native hospital at Elim, Spelonken, 10 August 1904, p. 1.
104 TAB, SNA 100 NA291/03, G. Liegme to Major W. N. Bolton, Resident Magistrate for Zoutpansberg, 19 November 1902, p. 6; TAB, CS 578 2614, C. A. Wheelwright to Secretary of Native Affairs, 3 March 1906, C. A. Wheelwright to Secretary of Native Affairs, no date [mid-March 1906]; TAB, CS 910 17857, G. Liegme, 'Diseases among Natives', 1905, p. 17.
105 TAB, CS 908 17845, 'Report of Tour for Inspection of Natives as regards Syphilis and Vaccination', no date (July/August 1909).
106 TAB, CS 910 17857, report on vaccination and syphilis tour, July 1909 to September 1910.
107 TAB, CS 908 17843, Special Anti-Syphilitic Measures, Circular No. 4, 15 April 1909.
108 TAB, CS 908 17843, Circular Minute CSO 42/18524, 8 April 1910.
109 TAB, CS 910 17857, Resident Magistrate Piet Retief to Assistant Colonial Secretary, 21 April 1910; District Surgeon Pilgrims Rest to Assistant Resident Magistrate, 18 June 1910.
110 TG 08-10, exhibit 'A'.
111 SAB, NTS 5760 15/315, MOH for Northern Transvaal to Secretary for Interior, 4 May 1913, p. 1.
112 TAB, CS 910 17857, Acting MOH for the Transvaal to District MOH, Northern Transvaal, 18 February 1908.
113 TG 28-10, p. 1.
114 Van Onselen (1982a), p. 146; Eales (1991), pp. 35–40.
115 TG 28-10, p. 2.
116 Moroney (1982), pp. 261–2; Eales (1991), p. 39.
117 Moroney (1982), pp. 263–4; Eales (1991), pp. 36–7.
118 TAB, CS 908 17848, Assistant Colonial Secretary to Resident Magistrates at Middelburg (in respect of Witbank Collieries), Johannesburg, Benoni, Boksburg, Germiston, Krugersdorp, Roodepoort, 5 November 1909.
119 TAB, CS 908 17848, C. Moller, District Surgeon to Resident Magistrate, Germiston, 25 October 1909.

120 TAB, CS 908 17850, Resident Magistrate, Johannesburg to Assistant Colonial Secretary, 23 November 1909.
121 TAB, CS 909 17855, Assistant Colonial Secretary to Resident Magistrate, Middelburg, 5 December 1909.
122 TAB, CS 908 17850, 'Control and Treatment of Syphilitic Natives', Circular no. 1 (CSA 3/18524), 15 January 1910, Annexure 1, part II, paras 14–23.
123 *Johannesburg City Council Minutes*, 26 April 1911, pp. 1917–18.
124 SAB, NTS 5760 15/315, Director of Labour to Under Secretary for Native Affairs, 27 May 1914.
125 TAB, CS 909 17853A, Acting Assistant Colonial Secretary to Resident Magistrate, Lichtenburg, 29 January 1910.
126 Millar (1909), p. 163.
127 TAB, CS 910 17857, first report of the District MOH for the year ended June 30th 1907, p. 3.
128 TAB, CS 578 2614A, G. Liegme, Elim to MOH for the Transvaal, June 1906, pp. 2, 4, 7; TAB, CS 910 17862, District Surgeon, Report on Syphilis Tour, July 1909.
129 TAB, CS 578 2614, C. A. Wheelwright to Secretary of Native Affairs, no date [mid-March 1906].
130 SAB, NTS 2863 10/303, R. Franz, Bochem to Administrator of the Transvaal, 6 February 1912.
131 Warwick (1983), pp. 165–9.
132 Ibid., pp. 175–8; Odendaal (1984).
133 TAB, CS 910 17857, first report of the District MOH for the year ended 30 June 1907, p. 2.
134 TAB, CS 910 17862, District Surgeon to Resident Magistrate, Report on tour 23–9 June, 8 July 1909.
135 SAB, NTS 5760 15/315, MOH for Northern Transvaal to Secretary for Interior, 4 May 1913; Sub-Native Commissioner, Pietersburg to Native Commissioner, Pietersburg, 17 January 1914.
136 TAB, CS 910 17857, District Surgeon, Duiwelskloof to Resident Magistrate, Pietersburg, 29 September 1909.

3 VD and the 'Poor White' Problem

1   Leipoldt (1920), p. 25.
2   'The National Prevention and Treatment of Venereal Disease', *Medical Journal of South Africa*, vol. 11 (1916), p. 211.
3   Brock (1917), p. 20.
4   Leipoldt (1920), p. 27.
5   UG 47-28, p. 47.
6   O'Malley (1940), p. 459; 'The Treatment and Prevention of Venereal Diseases in Reef Towns and Pretoria', *Proceedings of the Mine Medical Officers Association*, vol. XVII, nos 201, 202 (1938), p. 136.
7   Grosskopf (1932), p. vii.
8   van Onselen (1982b), pp. 111–17.
9   Brink (1987), p. 178; Grosskopf (1932), p. 57.
10 Stals (1986), pp. 11, 15.
11 Berger (1992), pp. 50, 309; UG 32-27, p. vi.

12   Brink (1987), p. 180, (1986), pp. 45, 48.
13   Berger (1992), pp. 30–1, 57, 311, footnote 42.
14   Bozzoli (1981), pp. 176–7. In 1915 there were 10 500 unionists; by 1920 this had risen to 132 000 members of 90 recorded unions.
15   On the Afrikaner nationalist movement see Giliomee (1987, 1989a, 1989b).
16   Davenport (1991), pp. 255–6, 289.
17   Bozzoli (1981), p. 157; Davenport (1991), pp. 257, 259–62; Davies (1979), ch. 5.
18   Bozzoli (1981), pp. 134, 165.
19   Ibid., pp. 161, 234–6, 244.
20   Kagan (1978), pp. 17–21.
21   *The Star*, 5 November 1917, cited in Kagan (1978), pp. 47–50; see also TP 1-22, p. 45, para. 260.
22   'Johannesburg Slums. Light on the Conditions', *The Star*, 8 July 1916.
23   TP 1-22, p. 46, para. 260.
24   SAB, JUS 805 1/600/23 part 1, Divisional CI Officer, Witwatersrand Division to Magistrate, Johannesburg, 8 October 1925; G. A. Godley, Acting Secretary for Native Affairs to Secretary for Justice, 1 November 1923; 'Cohabiting of White Men with Native Women, Resume of Replies', no date.
25   TAB, MJB, (4/2/145) A739, Deputy Commissioner commanding Witwatersrand division to Town Clerk, Johannesburg, 6 December 1922. For similar statements see 'Editorial: Johannesburg's Slums', *Rand Daily Mail*, 14 January 1916; Frack (1943), p. 73.
26   Gray (1937), p. 492; see also McNeil (1935), p. 743.
27   UG 42-29, pp. iii–iv, 153, table CLVIII.
28   Block (1934), p. 490.
29   Leipoldt (1937), p. 45.
30   Anning (1937), pp. 493–7.
31   On eugenic thought and nation building, see Stepan (1991).
32   'Killing Disease. Value of Johannesburg's clinics', *Sunday Times*, 27 February 1921.
33   Wells (1919), pp. 390–1.
34   'Killing Disease . . .', op. cit.
35   IADJ, SGJ, Box 200, File 59/4, MOH, Johannesburg to the Town Clerk, 6 April 1926; report of the proceedings at a round table talk called by the Transvaal SHC and held at the YMCA on Wednesday, 24 March 1926.
36   IADJ, SGJ, Box 200, File 59/4, Henry Gluckman, 'Report on the working of the venereal clinic', 24 September 1925. Gluckman eventually became the Minister of Public Health and oversaw the National Health Commission of 1944 discussed in Chapter 9.
37   IADJ, SGJ, Box 200, File 59/4, 'Report . . . Transvaal SHC . . .', 24 March 1926; Jochelson (1993), p. 215.
38   Freed (1949), p. 54.
39   Ibid., pp. 51, 111.
40   Ibid., pp. 143, 179–80.
41   Ibid., pp. 179–81.
42   Ibid., pp. 24–60; SAB, ARB 2017, CF 13, 'Prostitution and Houses of Ill-Fame in Johannesburg', report by V. P. Steyn, probation officer at Johannesburg Social Welfare Office, 12 May 1939, p. 1.

43 Stals (1986), p. 31.
44 Pollak (1932), pp. 266–7.
45 Grosskopf (1932), pp. 214, 216–17.
46 Pollack (1932), p. 268.
47 Brink (1986), p. 36.
48 Pollack (1932), pp. 145, 268.
49 Berger (1992), p. 76.
50 Freed (1941), pp. 260, 268.
51 Leipoldt (1937), p. 309.
52 HPW, AD843 B22.7, 'Report of . . . Transvaal SHC', 9 June 1926.
53 Albertyn (1932), pp. 26–7.
54 De Klerk (1925), p. 27.
55 Cited in Stals (1986), p. 42.
56 HPW, FAB329 HIGSON, confidential report of Miss Higson's Tour, 1932, p. 7.
57 Soloway (1982a), pp. 208, 211–15.
58 Russell (1988).
59 HPW, AD843 B22.7, report of the Third Round Table Talk, called by the Transvaal SHC on 9 June 1926.
60 Freed (1941), p. 316.
61 Ibid.
62 Pollack (1932), p. 210; SAB, K139, Box 3, Evidence of Fanny Klenermann, September 1925, p. 1219.
63 UG 28-38, p. x; Freed (1949), p. 117.
64 HPW AD843 B22.7, 'Report of . . . the Transvaal SHC', 9 June 1926.
65 Pollak (1932), Appendix, p. 58.
66 Stals (1986), p. 31.
67 Hofmeyr (1987), p. 113; Walker (1990b), p. 320.
68 Cited in Brink (1990), p. 281.
69 Bozzoli (1981), pp. 200–1, 208.
70 Walker (1990), pp. 337–40.
71 Porter, Mathew (1920), p. 109.
72 'Dogters van ons volk', *Die Huisgenoot*, vol. v, no. 49 (1920), pp. 6–8; van Heerden (1925), p. 43.
73 'Die Status van 'n Huisvrou', *Die Huisgenoot*, vol. ix, no. 148 (1925), p. 31; 'As die Sonnetjie Skyn', *Die Huisgenoot*, vol. ix, no. 165 (1925), pp. 32–3.
74 Rothmann (1932), pp. 171–2.
75 Pollak (1932), pp. 277–80.
76 Brink (1986), p. 151.
77 Van Niekerk (1988), p. 80.
78 Pollak (1932), pp. 182, 275.
79 Freed (1949), p. 193; Pollack (1932), pp. 153–4.
80 SAB, K139 Box 3, Evidence of Fanny Klenermann, September 1925, p. 1210.
81 SAB, K139 Box 10, Statement 130, Evidence of Mrs E. C. Steenkamp, p. 9.
82 Berger (1992), pp. 54, 83; Pollak (1932), pp. 95, 97–8.
83 Berger (1992), pp. 95–6; see also Lewis (1984), pp. 64–6.
84 Perks (1925), p. 33.
85 Kestell (1929), cited in Brink (1986), p. 16.
86 Freed (1941), p. 286.

87   Brink (1987), p. 177.
88   Fraser (1921), p. 62.
89   SAB, JUS 805 1/600/23 part 1, Divisional CI Officer, Witwatersrand Division to Magistrate, Johannesburg, 8 October 1925; TAB, MJB, 4/2/145 A739, Deputy Commissioner commanding Witwatersrand division to Town Clerk, Johannesburg, 6 December 1922.
90   TP 1-22, p. 46, para. 261.
91   *Hansard*, vol. 6, 3 March 1926, pp. 1891, 1894–6, vol. 8, 2 February 1927, p. 36.
92   *Hansard*, vol. 12, 15 February 1929, pp. 664, 729, vol. 15, 13 May 1930, p. 4057.
93   Wilcocks (1932), pp. xix, 62–3; see also Wilcocks (1930), p. 242.
94   SAB, MNW, Box 425, File 2036/18, Superintendent and Chief Inspector of White Labour to Chairman, Select Committee on Transvaal Liquor Laws, 1 March 1918, p. 3; D. Steyn, Inspector of White Labour to Superintendent and Chief Inspector of White Labour, 18 April 1918, p. 6; D. Steyn to Superintendent and Chief Inspector of White Labour, 6 May 1918, p. 5; Superintendent and Chief Inspector of White Labour to Secretary for Mines and Industries, 21 May 1918, p. 2.
95   SAB, MNW, Box 425, File 2036/18, Superintendent and Chief Inspector of White Labour to Chairman, Select Committee on Transvaal Liquor Laws, 1 March 1918, pp. 4–5, 7.
96   *Hansard*, vol. 8, 22 March 1927, pp. 1691, 1696.
97   'Agricultural Placement and Rehabilitation', *The Social and Industrial Review*, vol. 2, no. 6 (1926), p. 451; TP 1-22, p. 10, para. 21, pp. 13–14, paras 43–51.
98   Berger (1992), p. 59.
99   Freed (1949), pp. 116–21.
100 Dubow (1995), ch. 4; Klausen (1997), p. 31.
101 Searle (1976), pp. 6–8; Stepan (1991), pp. 22–4.
102 Searle (1976), pp. 20–6, 45–6; Soloway (1982b).
103 Bland (1985); Davin (1978); Dyhouse (1981); Searle (1976), pp. 9, 25–6.
104 Bidwell (1928), p. 143; Oosthuizen (1929), pp. 134–5.
105 Oosthuizen (1929), pp. 131–2; see also Frack (1943), pp. 55–62, 73–4, 84, 89.
106 Dubow (1991), pp. 152–6.
107 Ibid., pp. 159–60; Chisholm (1989), pp. 167–77; Grosskopf (1932), pp. vi, viii, xxiv–xxv.
108 Jurriaanse (1935), pp. 709–10; Oosthuizen (1929), pp. 131–2; *Hansard*, vol. 12, 18 March 1929, p. 1420.
109 Frack (1943) p. 84.
110 Dubow (1995), pp. 133–6, 184, (1991), p. 170.
111 Coetzee (1987).
112 *Hansard*, vol. 1, 21 March 1924, p. 1025.
113 'BMA News: Pretoria Branch', *Medical Journal of South Africa*, vol. 12 (1916), pp. 64–5; see also Dubow (1995), p. 148.
114 Bidwell (1928), p. 145.
115 Ibid., p. 146; SAB, GES 2281 85/38 vol. 1, Newman, 'Sterilisation of the Unfit', no date, p. 7.
116 Oosthuizen (1929), pp. 131–5; Frack (1943), p. 189.

117 SAB, GES 2281 85/38, vol. 1, Newman, 'Sterilisation of the Unfit', no date, p. 16.
118 SAB, GES 2281, 85/38, vol. 1, Race Welfare Society Constitution (Johannesburg, 1930).
119 IADJ, SGJ, Box 35, File 2/25/2, RWS (Johannesburg), Report of Executive Committee for the Eighteen Months ended 30 June 1936.
120 Laidler (1934), p. 823; Oosthuizen (1929), pp. 133–4.
121 Tonkin (1926), pp. 414–17.
122 IADJ, SGJ, Box 200, File 59/4, report of the Proceedings at a Round Table Talk called by the Transvaal SHC and held at the YMCA on Wednesday, 24 March 1926.
123 SAB, K139, Box 3, Evidence of Fanny Klenermann, September 1925, p. 1233.
124 'Ons Dogters', *Die Huisgenoot*, vol. x, no. 206 (1926), p. 39.
125 SAB, K139, Box 3, Evidence of Fanny Klenermann, September 1925, pp. 1227, 1235; see also Box 10, Statement 130, Evidence of Mrs E. C. Steenkamp, p. 7.
126 IADJ, SGJ, Box 200, File 59/4, 'Report of . . . the Transvaal SHC', 24 March 1926.
127 SAB, K139, Box 3, Evidence of Fanny Klenermann, September 1925, p. 1218.
128 UG 14-23, p. 220.
129 Higgins (1935), p. 527.
130 TAB, MJB, 4/2/145 A739, minutes of meeting between members of Central Housing Board and Parks and Estates Committee, 17 August 1923, p. 13.
131 Porter (1991), p. 171, develops a similar argument about public health ideology in Edwardian Britain.
132 IADJ, SGJ, Box 200, File 59/4, report of the Proceedings at a Second Round Table Talk called by the Transvaal SHC and held at the YMCA on Tuesday 25 May 1926.
133 Freed (1949), pp. 27, 31, 37, 41 (cases 11, 22, 50, 67).
134 Ibid., pp. 28–9, 31–3, 36–8, 45 (cases 15, 18, 20, 22, 23, 24, 27, 32, 38, 40, 66).
135 Ibid., pp. 47–8.
136 Burt (1926a, 1926b); Hobson (1987), pp. 191–2.
137 Clarry (1927), p. 342.
138 The idea of retarded emotional development also has resonances with the late-nineteenth-century theory of recapitulation. Gould (1981), pp. 114–18.
139 Clarry (1927), p. 342.
140 Ibid.; see also Norman's comments in IADJ, SGJ, Box 200, File 59/4, 'Report of the . . . Transvaal SHC . . . May 1926'.
141 Hobson (1987), pp. 139, 155–6; Miller (1993, 1994).
142 Freed (1949), pp. 19–20.
143 Ibid., p. 220.
144 Ibid., pp. 20, 153–5.
145 Ibid., pp. 174, 179.
146 Grosskopf (1932), p. 222; Wilcocks (1932), p. 83.
147 Grosskopf (1932), pp. ix–x.

148 Albertyn (1932), pp. 6, 21; Grosskopf (1932), p. xvi; Rothmann (1932), pp. 173, 195; Wilcocks (1932), p. 52.
149 On similar ideas in other colonies see Kennedy (1987), ch. 6; Stoler (1991), pp. 72–6.
150 Stoler (1991), pp. 76–7.
151 Albertyn (1932), pp. 26–7.
152 Davies (1979), pp. 107–12, 224–8.
153 Report of the Wage Board . . . 1929, cited in Pollak (1932), p. 191.
154 Cited in Berger (1987), p. 129.
155 Berger (1992), pp. 33–4, 56; Pollak (1932), pp. 251–2.
156 Parnell (1987, 1988, 1989); Proctor (1979).
157 Hart and Parnell (1989), pp. 25–31.
158 Johannesburg Housing Utility Company (JHUC), (1933–34?), p. 39; Parnell (1987), pp. 81–3.
159 Address by Lionel Leveson to 31st Annual Congress of Municipal Association of Krugersdorp, 1939, cited in Parnell (1987), p. 70.
160 JHUC (1933), p. 29.
161 IADJ, SGJ, Box 200, File 59/4, minutes of the fourth round table talk called by the Transvaal SHC and held in the YMCA on 20 August 1926; 'Social Welfare Work on Witwatersrand', *The Social and Industrial Review*, vol. 8, no. 44 (1929).
162 SAB, ARB 2017, CF 13, 'Prostitution . . .', report by V. P. Steyn, 12 May 1939, p. 13.
163 R. P. H. West, *Facts About Ourselves for Growing Boys and Girls* (Johannesburg Public Health Department and South African Red Cross Society (Transvaal), no date [1933–34?], pp. 26–7.
164 'Sosiale Werk, Kaapstad'. Eendrag Meisiesklub of Soutrivier', *Die Huisgenoot*, vol. x, no. 194 (1925), p. 51.
165 'Rehabilitation of Slum Dwellers. Response to City's Housing Schemes', *The Star*, 15 February 1938.
166 Higgins (1929), p. 299.
167 *Hansard*, vol. 23, 8 May 1934, p. 3315.
168 Chisholm (1989), pp. 301–11; Coetzee (1991), pp. 10–12; Dubow (1995), pp. 270–5.
169 Coetzee (1988), chs 3–4.

4 VD Treatment and Educational Propaganda for Whites

1 IADJ, SGJ Box 200, File 59 vol. II; 'Fighting Venereal Diseases', *Rand Daily Mail*, 26 February 1921.
2 Marks and Andersson (1988), pp. 191–2; Philip (1990), pp. 203–6.
3 Klausen (1997).
4 'Editorial: Control of Venereal Diseases', *South African Medical Record*, vol. 12 (1914), pp. 281–3; 'Editorial: The Anti-Contagious Diseases Act Agitation', *South African Medical Record*, vol. 15 (1917), p. 131.
5 'Editorial: Male Sexual Continence' *South African Medical Record*, vol. 15 (1917), p. 146; 'Discussion on the Control of Venereal Diseases', *South African Medical Record*, vol. 12 (1914), pp. 236, 242.
6 Van Heyningen (1984), pp. 187–91, 195.

7 NCCVD pamphlet, cited in 'Editorial: The Anti-Contagious Diseases Act Agitation' (1917), op. cit., p. 129.
8 Lieut.-Col. Moffat, speaker at the first NCCVD (Cape) meeting, quoted in 'Editorial: The Anti-Contagious Diseases Act Agitation' (1917), op. cit., p. 129.
9 See also JPL; S 176.5; Aletta Jacobs, *To the Women of South Africa* (no publisher, no date [1913?]); International Federation for the Abolition of State Regulation of Vice, Report of Hon. Sec. at First Annual Meeting of the South African Branch, 1913, Cape Town; David Kerr Cross, *Social Hygiene by a South African Physician* (no publisher, 1912); TAB, GNLB 183 915/14/103, NCCVD (Transvaal), Memorandum to the Minister of the Interior on the Provision of Chapter IV Public Health Bill for the Transmission to the Select Committee Appointed to Consider the Bill, p. 1.
10 Walker (1990).
11 Brandt (1987), pp. 96–121; Davenport-Hines (1991), pp. 193–4; Towers (1980), pp. 76–7.
12 Brandt (1987), p. 40.
13 TAB, GNLB 183 915/14/103, NCCVD (Transvaal), Memorandum to the Minister of the Interior on the provision of . . . Public Health Bill . . . , p. 1; 'Discussion on the Control of Venereal Diseases' (1914), op. cit., pp. 238, 240, 242, 244.
14 TAB, GNLB 183 915/14/103, NCCVD (Transvaal), Memorandum to the Minister of the Interior on the provision of . . . Public Health Bill . . . , p. 1.
15 'Discussion on the Control of Venereal Diseases' (1914), op. cit., p. 236.
16 Ibid., p. 240.
17 NAB, 3/DBN 188B, Minutes of Proceedings of the Public Health Conference, held at Bloemfontein on 16, 17 and 18 September 1918, pp. 51, 53, 54.
18 'Editorial: Sexual "Enlightenment"', *South African Medical Record*, vol. 15 (1917), pp. 227–8.
19 Davenport-Hines (1991), pp. 222–3.
20 Parnell (1993).
21 IADJ, SJG, Box 149, File 9728, Municipal Council of Johannesburg, *Special Report by the Medical Officer of Health on the Prevention and Treatment of Venereal Diseases*, 28 August 1916, p. 6; Evidence of C. Porter on Public Health Bill in parliament, session 1919.
22 IADJ, SJG, Box 149, File 9728, Municipal Council of Johannesburg, *Special Report . . . on . . . Venereal Diseases*, 28 August 1916, p. 6.
23 IADJ, SJG, Box 149, File 9728, Evidence of C. Porter on Public Health Bill in parliament, session 1919, p. 6.
24 IADJ, SGJ, Box 149, File 9728, Union of South Africa, *Bill To Make Provision for the Public Health*, C 606-'2-'19, s66, 67.
25 UG 04-20, cited in Philip (1990), pp. 71–4, 217, Philip (1987).
26 Bonfa (1917), p. 372.
27 SAB, NTS 6716 23/315; 'Rietfontein Hospital. Indictment by Select Committee', *Rand Daily Mail*, 11 September 1914.
28 SAB, NTS 6716 23/315; 'What's Wrong at Rietfontein? Amazing Conditions in the Lazaretto', *Sunday Times*, 29 August 1915.

29 SAB, GES 1155 6/18, Medical Superintendent, Rietfontein Lazaretto to MOH, 25 March 1918.
30 SAB, NTS 6716 23/315; 'Rietfontein Hospital. Indictment by Select Committee', *Rand Daily Mail*, 11 September 1914; 'What's Wrong at Rietfontein? Amazing Conditions in the Lazaretto', *Sunday Times*, 29 August 1915.
31 Ibid.
32 SAB, NTS 6716 23/315; 'Rietfontein Hospital. Indictment by Select Committee', *Rand Daily Mail*, 11 September 1914.
33 SAB, GG 8/297, Rietfontein Hospital Ordinance, 1915; Minute 18 February 1915, signed 'FA' (F. Arnold).
34 SAB, GES 1153 1/18, Medical Superintendent, Rietfontein to Secretary for Public Health, 22 November 1922.
35 Chisholm (1989), pp. 177–8, 189.
36 Stoler (1989), p. 150, (1991), p. 75.
37 SAB, GES 1153 1/18A, Secretary for Public Health to Secretary for Finance, 19 November 1928.
38 SAB, GES 1153 1/18A, Secretary for Public Health to Secretary for Public Works, 31 August 1927, pp. 1–3.
39 SAB, GES 1154 18/18B, Rietfontein VD Hospital, Note of Inspection on 27 November 1929, p. 1.
40 UG 47-28, p. 47.
41 IADJ, SGJ, Box 2, File A6340, Dr Henry Gluckman, 'Special Treatment Centre', 1930, p. 4; Porter (1920), p. 154.
42 IADJ, SGJ, Box 2, File A6340, Gluckman, 'Special Treatment Centre', 1930, p. 7.
43 TAB, GNLB 183 915/14/103, Constitution of the Transvaal Council for Combating Venereal Diseases (1921).
44 The office-holders of the Cape NCCVD are listed on the mastheads of the following letters: NAB, 3/DBN 188E vol. 1; NCCVD Honorary Secretary to Town Clerk, 26 November 1917; NCCVD letter accompanying pamphlets, 20 December 1918; JPL, S 176.5, International Federation . . . (1913), p. 12.
45 Officeholders and representatives are listed in IADJ, SGJ, Box 200, File 59/4, SHC (Transvaal), Aims and Objects, no date.
46 HPW, AD843/RJ/Ka28, SHC (Transvaal), minutes of meeting of the executive on 30 September 1927.
47 SAB, GES 1991 49/33A, E. H. Thornton to Minister of Public Health, 22 August 1933.
48 For a comparative study of British material see Bland (1982), p. 378; Mort (1987), part 4.
49 TAB, MBP 165 P4-28, Municipal Council of Johannesburg, 'VENEREAL DISEASES'; TAB, GNLB 183 915/14/103, Constitution of the Transvaal Council for Combating Venereal Diseases.
50 'Editorial', *Health And Medicine*, vol. 1 (1946), p. 5.
51 IADJ, SGJ, Box 199, File 59, NCCVD, list of slides and text of public lecture 'Love–Marriage–Parenthood', no date [1923?], p. 3.
52 Mrs Wright, Johannesburg district nursing assistant, cited in IADJ, SGJ, Box 200, File 59/4, minutes of the fourth round table talk called by the SHC (Transvaal) and held at the YMCA on Friday, 20 August 1926; Higgins (1935), p. 530; UG 43-35, p. 44.

53　TAB, GNLB 183 915/14/103, NCCVD (Transvaal), minutes of meeting, 27 October 1920.

54　HPW, AD843 B22.7, NCCVD (Transvaal), minutes of meeting of the executive on 25 November 1925.

55　SAB, UOD 773 E23/5/1, South African Red Cross Society, National Council for Health Education, report on the health propaganda activities of the committee to 30 November 1939.

56　HPW, AD843 B22.7, SHC (Transvaal), minutes of meeting of the executive, 28 May 1926.

57　NAB 3/DBN 188E, MOH to Town Clerk, Durban, 6 June 1921.

58　IADJ, SGJ, Box 199, File 59, Deputy Commissioner, Witwatersrand Division to . . . SAP Tvl, . . . Borough Police, Durban, . . . CI Department, Pretoria, 7 February 1923.

59　Freed (1949), p. 331.

60　SAB, UOD 773 E23/5/1, South African Red Cross Society . . . Report of the health propaganda activities . . . to 30 November 1939, p. 5.

61　IADJ, SGJ, Box 199, File 59, Deputy Commissioner, Witwatersrand Division to . . . SAP Transvaal, . . . Borough Police, Durban, . . . CI Department Pretoria, 7 February 1923.

62　HPW, AD843/Rj/Na18.4 (file 5), R. P. H. West, *Facts About Ourselves for Growing Boys and Girls* (Johannesburg Public Health Department and South African Red Cross Society (Transvaal), no date [1933/34?]); SAB, UOD 773 E23/5/1, National Committee for Health Education, routine work sub-committee, minutes of the third meeting, 13 June 1939, p. 1.

63　IADJ, SGJ, Box 200, File 59/4, H. Gluckman: Report on the Working of the Venereal Clinic, 24 September 1925, p. 5.

64　West (1933/34), p. 3.

65　Fraser (1921), p. 64.

66　HPW, AD843/RJ/Na18.4 (file 5), report on lecture tour by Dr J. H. Rauch, January 1935, p. 2.

67　West (1933/34), pp. 26–7.

68　TAB, GNLB 183 915/14/103. NCCVD, 'Sex Morality' (for private circulation), no date, p. 1.

69　West (1933/34), pp. 26–7.

70　Ibid., p. 20.

71　Ibid., p. 21.

72　IADJ, SGJ, Box 199, File 59, NCCVD, 'Love–Marriage–Parenthood', p. 3.

73　Ibid., p. 7; see also Chubb (1935), pp. 76, 193.

74　IADJ, SGJ, Box 199, File 59, ' "The End of the Road". The story of a motion picture drama, authorised by the NCCVD with the approval of the Ministery of Health' (no date).

75　Kuhn (1985), pp. 96–132.

76　IADJ, SGJ, Box 199, File 59, Synopsis, *The Shadow*, no date [1923?].

77　Jacobs, (1913); Cross (1912), p. 10.

78　TAB, GNLB 183 915/14/103, Constitution of the Transvaal Council for Combating Venereal diseases; Lieut.-Col. Moffat, a member of the Cape NCCVD, cited in 'Editorial: The Anti-Contagious Diseases Act Agitation', *South African Medical Record*, vol. 15 (1917), p. 129.

79　West (1933/34), p. 21.

80   Ibid., p. 19. For similar themes in British VD literature see Mort (1987), p. 194.

5   **Migration, Prostitution and VD**

 1   *Sunday Times*, 2 October 1937, cited in Humphries (1938a), p. 630.
 2   *The Star*, 3 October 1935, cited in Phillips (1938), p. 116.
 3   Cited in Marks (1989), p. 229.
 4   SAB, NTS 5760 15/315, Chief Magistrate of Transkeian Territories to Secretary for Native Affairs, 4 July 1923; SAB, NTS 5761 15/315, vol. 3, Chief Magistrate of the Transkeian Territories to all the magistrates in the Transkeian Territories, circular no. 19 of 1935, 20 July 1935; United Transkeian Territories General Council Session, minute 77, 8 October 1941.
 5   See for example, UG 22-32, part III and addendum by Mr Lucas; Smit Report (1942), pp. 5–11; UG 30-44, ch. XIX; UG 28-48; pp. 35–42, paras 51–6.
 6   Marks and Andersson (1985).
 7   UG 14-23, p. 212; UG 09-24, p. 254.
 8   HPW, AD1438, Box 2, 'Health and Child Welfare, Transkei', pp. 2524–3960, Flagstaff sitting, 7 November 1930: evidence of Rev. A. Schweiger, p. 50; Dr F. S. Drewe, pp. 51–4; Umtata sitting, 14 November 1930: evidence of Dr M. R. Mahlangeni, p. 60.
 9   UG 22-32, p. 215, para. 264.
10   IADJ, SGJ, Box 201, File 59/5; 'Disease Prevalent in Union', *The Star*, 20 June 1946.
11   Hackett (1963), pp. 23–4, Appendix 1.
12   HPW A1212/Caf. Mitchell, undated [1920s?], 'Venereal Diseases in SA', p. 5.
13   HPW, AD1438, Box 4, Vryburg sitting, 27 February 1931: evidence of Dr Frank Adolphus James Brodziak, p. 5456.
14   Sax (1952).
15   UG 09-24, p. 254; UG 48-36, p. 51.
16   UG 09-24, p. 255; UG 21-26, p. 31; see also HPW, A1212/Caf. J. A. Mitchell, 'Venereal Diseases in South Africa', undated [1920s?], pp. 4–5.
17   IADJ, SGJ, Box 25, File A219, Minutes of . . . the Council of Public Health . . . 15 June 1921, p. 1.
18   For a comparative case, see Dawson (1983), ch. 4 (1987, 1988).
19   Schapera (1947), p. 39.
20   HPW, AD843 B41.2, Drs F. William Fox and Douglas Back (for the Chamber of Mines), 'Summary of conclusions and findings. Preliminary survey of the agricultural problems of the Ciskei and Transkeian Territories, 1938', p. 9.
21   Schapera (1947), p. 195.
22   G 03-86, p. 19.
23   Becker, cited in Grek (1950), p. 70.
24   Grek (1950), p. 70.
25   Elliot (1950), p. 96.
26   Laidler (1938), p. 663.
27   HPW, AD843 B2.1.1, Alexandra Health Committee, Medical Officer of Health's Report for the Year ended 30 June 1940, p. 3.
28   Smit Report (1942), p. 10, para. 120.

29 Kark (1949), p. 78.
30 SAB, NTS 5760 15/315, P. Targett Adams to the Secretary for Public Health, 22 March 1922.
31 Hunter (1961, first published 1936), p. 146.
32 Parsons (1988), p. 23; HPW, AD1438, Box 6, Durban sitting, 1 April 1931: evidence of Dr George Archibald Park Ross, pp. 6123–4.
33 UG 21-26, p. 31; see also HPW A1212/Caf. Mitchell, undated [1920s?], pp. 4–5.
34 SAB, NTS 5760 15/315, Assistant Health Officer for the Union to the Secretary for Public Health, 22 March 1922, pp. 1–2; see also, UG 14-23, p. 212.
35 SAB, NTS 5761 15/315, Part III, Annual Health Report: 1935–36, Additional District Surgeoncy of Sibasa, 22 July 1936.
36 Kark (1949), pp. 82–3; UG 08-45, p. 17; HPW, AD1438, Box 6, Evidence of Dr Park Ross, pp. 6123–4.
37 SAB, NTS 5760 15/315, Assistant Health Officer for the Union to the Secretary for Public health, 22 March 1922, p. 4. On similar correspondence with the manager of the New Jagersfontein Mining and Exploration Company between September 1924 and June 1925, and on rest camps at Matatiele between February and June 1932, see correspondence in SAB, NTS 5760 15/315 and SAB, NTS 7055 136/322 respectively.
38 Redding (1987), pp. 248, 249.
39 Maloka (1994).
40 SAB, NTS 5761 15/315, Magistrate Potgietersrust to Secretary for Public Health, 4 July 1928; G. J. M. Melle to Native Commissioner, Potgietersrust, 22 May 1929.
41 SAB, NTS 5761 15/315, vol 3, Director of Native Labour to Secretary for Native Affairs, 15 February 1943; Chief Medical Officer to General Manager, WNLA, 29 January 1943; COMA, 2080:1704, Native Labour Adviser to General Manager, Transvaal COM, 3 December 1936.
42 SAB, NTS 5760 15/315, W. Raymond, COM to Director of Native Labour, 29 May 1922. Similar views from local administrators are discussed in Chapter 8.
43 COMA, 2080:1704, WNLA to General Manager, COM, 7 December 1936.
44 Segal (1989), pp. 23–4, 34.
45 SAB, GNLB 110 1328/13, Director of Native Labour to Secretary of Native Affairs, 24 July 1925, pp. 1, 3.
46 SAB, GNLB 110 1328/13, Murray, 'Report on Investigation into Alleged High Incidence of Venereal Disease in Breyten Labour Area, 21 March 1925', 27 March 1925, p. 2.
47 Herbst Report (1937–38), p. 78, paras 458–9; UG 08-40, p. 19, para. 74.
48 SAB, NTS 5761 15/315, Inspector of Native Labour, Dundee to Minister for Native Affairs, 7 February 1930; Acting Chief Native Commissioner, Natal to Secretary for Native Affairs, 18 March 1930.
49 On the decline of the peasantry, see Bundy (1979); on the creation of a labour supply for the mining industry, see Jeeves (1985).
50 Simkins (1981), pp. 264, 266, 275.
51 Calculated from Table 4 in Beinart (1982), p. 172.
52 Murray (1981), p. 4.

53   Bradford (1987b), p. 298; on the transformation to capitalist agriculture and African reaction see Bradford (1987a); Keegan (1987).
54   Posel (1991), p. 29.
55   UG 21-44, p. 15, paras 202–3; p. 16, paras 207, 209; p. 55, Appendix I; UG 22-32, pp. 119–20, paras 816–17; p. 299, Annexure 2-III.
56   Schapera (1947), pp. 54–9.
57   Sibusiswe Makanya cited a case of two young girls who were orphaned: as relations refused to accept responsibility for them they left for an urban area. HPW, AD1438, Box 6, Durban sitting, 4 April 1931: evidence of Makanya, pp. 6312–14.
58   Hunter (1961), pp. 203–8.
59   Ibid., pp. 205–6.
60   Ibid., p. 204; Ashton (1967), p. 304.
61   HPW, AD1438, Box 12. H, Prozesky, missionary at Ntlopenkulu mission station, Nongoma, Zululand to Mr Roberts, 11 January 1931.
62   Bonner (1990), pp. 247–8; Coplan (1982), pp. 363–4, (1985), pp. 98–107.
63   HPW, AD843 B91.3.3, *Annual Report of the Raleigh Fitkin Memorial Hospital, Bremersdorp, Swaziland, for the year ending December 31st 1936*, p. 4.
64   HPW AD1756/Bf, memorandum submitted by the Umtata Native Welfare Society on the Questionnaire of the Native Laws Commission of Enquiry.
65   Bonner (1990), pp. 228–9; Walker (1990), p. 190; Wilson (1981).
66   Bonner (1990), p. 228; Harries (1994), p. 280, fn 34.
67   Murray (1981), p. 4.
68   Unless otherwise indicated, the discussion on the reasons for women migrating is drawn from Bonner (1990), pp. 235–40; Walker (1990), pp. 187, 189, 192–3; HPW, AD1756/A30, Vol 30, Native Laws Commission of Enquiry, Minutes of evidence, 22 November 1946 at Maseru; evidence of M. B. Smith, member of the Basutoland Chamber of Commerce, pp. 2140–1.
69   Bonner (1990), pp. 235–6; Wilson (1981), pp. 138–9.
70   Wilson (1981), p. 136.
71   Hunter (1961), pp. 203–8.
72   Walker (1990), p. 190; Bonner (1990), pp. 228–9; Janisch (1941), p. 4; Hellmann (1934).
73   Levin (1947), p. 62; Moodie (1983), pp. 164–8; see White (1990) on prostitution as a form of domestic service.
74   Hellman (1934), pp. 55, 58.
75   Palmer (1931), p. 49.
76   HPW A1756/A36, Durban, 9 January 1947: minutes of evidence of Mrs W. A. Willgoose, Child Welfare Society, Durban, p. 2505.
77   Bonner (1988), p. 243; Eales (1991), pp. 115, 182, 186.
78   Bonner (1988), p. 395; Janisch (1941), pp. 2, 8, 9.
79   Krige (1936), p. 14.
80   Ibid., pp. 16–17, 21; Levin (1947), p. 20.
81   Krige (1936), pp. 16–17; Levin (1947), p. 9; HPW, AD1438, Box 7, Minutes of evidence, Henry Britten, Magistrate of Johannesburg, p. 7346.
82   Phillips (1938), pp. 91–2.
83   Krige (1936), p. 10.
84   Levin (1947), pp. 61–2.

85 Hellmann (1935a), p. 53; Janisch (1941), pp. 7–8; Levin (1947), pp. 27, 58.
86 HPW, AD1438, Box 5, 'Health and Child Welfare, Urban Areas', pp. 5458–6526, Grahamstown sitting, 23 March 1931: evidence of Dr Ella Miriam Britten, pp. 108–9; Findings of the Juvenile Native Delinquency Conference, Johannesburg, October 1938, cited in Janisch (1941), p. 8; Ballinger (1938), pp. 335–7.
87 Hellmann (1937), p. 420, (1948), pp. 80–1.
88 Gaitskell (1982), pp. 340–1, 344; Hunter (1932), p. 681, (1961), pp. 166, 174, 180–3; Krige (1936, 1937); Schapera (1933), pp. 60, 65–7, 73.
89 Gaitskell (1982), p. 342.
90 Hunter (1961), pp. 183–4; Kark (1954), Part B, pp. 59–60; Levin (1947), p. 30.
91 Gaitskell (1982), pp. 340–1, 344–5; Hunter (1932), p. 686; Schapera (1933), pp. 65–7, 73.
92 HPW, AD1756/Bj, Statements by Prof. Z. K. Matthews and Dr M. Wilson, 'The Social Effects of Migrant Labour', p. 9; Hunter (1932), p. 685; Kark (1954), Part B, p. 313; Schapera (1933), p. 86, (1947), p. 173.
93 Dikobe (1973); Hellmann (1935), p. 50; Levin (1947), p. 30.
94 Delius (1989), pp. 586–8.
95 Kark (1954), part B, p. 314.
96 Beinart (1987), p. 294; Moodie (1988), pp. 240, 248–50.
97 Beinart (1987), pp. 294–5.
98 HPW, AD1438, Box 12, 'Memo "Homosexuality"', no author, no date [1930/31?], marked 'secret'.
99 Delius (1989), p. 588.
100 HPW AD1756/Bj, 'Personal evidence given by Rev. H. P. Junod on some of the points examined by the Native Laws Commission of Enquiry' (1946–48), p. 8.
101 Junod (1962), p. 61.
102 COMA, 1942:0861, 'Migrant Native Labour: The Case For', p. 2.
103 Beinart (no date), pp. 12, 21–2, 32, 37.
104 Harries (1994), pp. 114, 156.
105 Mager (1996), p. 15.
106 Bonner (1990), pp. 247–9, (1988), p. 406; Glaser (1990), pp. 19–26.
107 Mager (1996), pp. 16–17.
108 Gaitskell (1982, 1990), p. 267.
109 Gaitskell (1982), p. 345; Marks (1987), pp. 31–6.
110 Marks (1989), pp. 217, 224, 228–9.
111 Bozzoli (1991), pp. 111–13.

6 Moral Tribes and Corrupting Cities

1 UG 40-30, p. 47; UG 43-35, p. 44.
2 Bonner (1990), p. 231, Kark (1954), part B, p. 151.
3 Bonner (1990), pp. 231, 247; Couzens (1985), pp. 57, 60; Dikobe (1973).
4 Dubow (1989), p. 69.
5 SAB, GES 1991 49/33, J. A. Mitchell, 'Venereal Diseases in South Africa', address to Imperial Social Hygiene Congress, 7 September 1925, p. 14.

6   NAB, 3/DBN 167, vol. 3, Layman, manager of Durban Native Administration Department, to Town Clerk, 21 January 1925.
7   SC 03-23, Evidence of C. F. Layman, p. 132.
8   Vaughan (1991), pp. 21–2, ch. 6.
9   Hunter (1932), pp. 682–3; Levin (1947), pp. 9–11; Marks (1989), p. 226.
10 Hunter (1961), pp. 205–6.
11 UG 15-22, p. 6; UG 40-25, pp. 22, 24; UG 26-33, p. 16.
12 Bonner (1982).
13 Couzens (1985); Eales (1989), pp. 116–17, 121; Marks (1989), p. 221.
14 Eales (1989), pp. 116–18, Koch (1983), pp. 167–8.
15 IADJ, SGJ, Box 200, File 59, vol. II; 'Disease and the Labour Supply. Ravages of the Venereal Plague', *Rand Daily Mail*, 25 February 1921.
16 SAB, NTS 5761 15/315, Magistrate Potgietersrust to Secretary for Public Health, 4 July 1928; G. J. M. Melle to Native Commissioner, Potgietersrust, 22 May 1929.
17 Humphries (1938a), p. 637, (1938b), p. 127; Purcell (1940), p. 453; UG 40-34, p. 8.
18 SAB, NTS 5761 15/315, Inspector of Native Labour, Dundee to Minister for Native Affairs, 7 February 1930.
19 Jochelson (1993), p. 219.
20 Smit Report (1942), p. 10, para. 119.
21 Bonner (1982); Davenport (1991), p. 253.
22 Bradford (1987a).
23 Roux (1948), chs XII–XXI; Simons and Simons (1983), ch. 17.
24 Dubow (1989), pp. 40–1, 70–3; UG 22–32, pp. 99–100.
25 Dubow (1989), ch. 2.
26 Ibid., p. 39.
27 Ibid.
28 TP 1-22, evidence of Vowell, p. 45, para. 260; also p. 48, para. 273.
29 UG 41-22, p. 13, para. 57, p. 12, para. 47.
30 TP 1-22, p. 47, para. 268, p. 48, para. 273.
31 TP 1-22, p. 52, para. 296, p. 49, para. 279.
32 SC 03-23, Evidence of Beyers and Cook, Bloemfontein, p. 90.
33 SAB, NTS 5760 15/315, Acting Secretary for the Interior to Secretary for Native Affairs, 2 November 1916.
34 TP 1-22, Evidence of Colonel T. G. Truter, Commissioner of Police for Prospect Township, p. 46, para. 263.
35 HPW, AD1438, Box 2, 'Health and Child Welfare Natal', Vryheid sitting, 20 September 1930: evidence of Dr M. Kuper, District Surgeon, p. 32.
36 SC 03-23, Evidence of Beyers and Cook, Bloemfontein, p. 90; UG 47-28, p. 47.
37 UG 41-22, p. 14, para. 63; TP 1-22, p. 52, para. 296, p. 49, para. 279.
38 UG 41-22, p. 14, para. 58; TP 1-22, p. 49, para. 278.
39 NAB, 3/DBN 4/1/2/1175 359A, vol. 3, Secretary for Native Affairs to Secretary for Public Health, 7 January 1921.
40 Wells (1982), pp. 86–150, 185, 199; Wells (1983).
41 Cited in Eales (1989), pp. 198–9.
42 UG 40-25, pp. 22, 24.
43 UG 41-22, p. 14, paras. 57, 63; TP 1-22, p. 52, para. 296, p. 49, para. 279.

44 Eales (1989), pp. 119–20, 127–30.
45 Eales (1989), (1991), pp. 198–203.
46 Bishop of Pretoria, cited in TAB, GNLB 183 915/14/103, NCCVD (Transvaal), minutes of meeting held 29 April 1919.
47 SAB, NTS 5760 15/315, Acting Secretary for the Interior to Secretary for Native Affairs, 2 November 1916.
48 TP 1-22, p. 46, para. 263.
49 *The Star*, 5 November 1917, cited in Kagan (1978), p. 50.
50 Hindson (1987), pp. 39–41.
51 HPW, A1212/Caf, Dr Mitchell, 'Venereal Diseases in South Africa', undated [1920s?], p. 4.
52 SC 6A-29, Evidence of Ballenden, pp. 6–7; Evidence of H. S. Cooke, Director of Native Labour for the Union and Chief Native Commissioner, Witwatersrand, p. 52.
53 SC 6A-29, evidence of Ballenden, pp. 6–7; Eales (1991), pp. 112–21.
54 SAB, GNLB 388 33/58, E. Cluver to Secretary for Public Health, 18 February 1931; HPW, AD1438, Box 2, 'Health and Child Welfare Natal, pp. 1160–2523', Ladysmith sitting, 15 October 1930: evidence of T. G. Holmes, chief compound manager of Burnside No. 1 shaft, p. 44.
55 SAB, GES 1527 7/26A, Secretary for Native Affairs to Secretary for Public Health, 26 March 1930.
56 Eales (1991), pp. 112–18, 131–3; Proctor (1979). On efforts to segregate Durban see le Hausse (1984), ch. 3; Maylam (1990).
57 Redding (1987), pp. 249–52.
58 Cited in ibid., p. 241.
59 Segal (1989), pp. 130–3; TAB, GNLB 110 1328/13, Murray, 'Report on . . . alleged high incidence of VD in Breyten Labour Area . . . ', 27 March 1925, p. 1.
60 Segal (1989), p. 133.
61 Eales (1991), p. 131.
62 TAB, GNLB 110 1328/13, Director of Native Labour to Secretary of Native Affairs, 24 July 1925, p. 3; see also Segal (1989), p. 125.
63 TAB, GNLB 388 33/58, Cluver to Secretary for Public Health, 18 February 1931; HPW, AD1438, Box 2, 'Health and Child Welfare, Natal, pp. 1160–2523', Ladysmith sitting, 15 October 1930: evidence of Holmes, p. 44.
64 TAB, GNLB 110 1328/13, Director of Native Labour to Magistrate, Ermelo, 28 September 1925; SAB, NTS 5761 15/315 Part III, Under Secretary for Public Health to Magistrate, Newcastle, 30 December 1935.
65 UG 56-37, p. 3.
66 UG 47-28, p. 47.
67 Dubow (1987), p. 89; Dubow (1989), ch. 1.
68 Couzens (1982), p. 318; Dubow (1987), pp. 80–5; Schapera (1934).
69 Kuper (1984), pp. 194–5; Kuklick (1984, 1992); Kuper (1983), pp. 2–4, 32–4; Stocking (1984).
70 HPW, AD1438, Box 5, Port Elizabeth sitting, 24 March 1931: evidence of Dr Duncan Lamont Ferguson, MOH for New Brighton Location, Assistant MOH for Port Elizabeth, and Director of Venereal Disease Clinics in Port Elizabeth, pp. 5761–2; Ferguson (1932), p. 806; Burton (1934), p. 329; HPW,

AD1483, Box 9, Vryburg sitting, 27 February 1931: minutes of evidence of Clifford St. Quentin, Inspector of Vryburg Native Location, p. 5389.

71   Packard (1989), (1987), pp. 191–208.

72   Melle (1935), p. 56. See also HPW, AD1438, Box 2, 'Health and Child Welfare Natal, pp. 1160–2523', Nongoma sitting, 22 September 1930: evidence of Dr Haupt, district surgeon, p. 33.

73   SAB, NTS 5761 15/315, G. J. M. Melle to Native Commissioner, Potgieter-srust, 25 March 1929.

74   UG 09-24, p. 255.

75   HPW, AD1438, Box 2, 'Health and Child Welfare Natal, pp. 1160–2523', Vryheid sitting, 19 September 1930: evidence of Dr G. S. van der Merwe, practitioner with many African patients, p. 30.

76   Pijper (1921), p. 304.

77   SAB, NTS 5760 15/315, P. Targett Adams, Assistant Health Officer for the Union to the Secretary for Public Health, 22 March 1922, p. 2.

78   NAB 3/DBN 188E, vol. 4, G. H. Gunn, Acting MOH to Town Clerk, Durban, 8 April 1929; Gunn to Town Clerk, Durban, 10 December 1929.

79   Hindson (1987), p. 53.

80   Ibid., p. 42.

81   HPW, AD1438, Box 7, Statement by Henry Britten, Magistrate, Johannesburg, p. 5.

82   Hellmann (1934), pp. 56, 58.

83   Elliott Report (1942), pp. 11–12, para. 23.

84   HPW, AD843/RJ/Aa.12.14.23, Rev. E. E. Mahabane, 'Marital Conditions in Urban African Life', SAIRR, 20 June 1947.

85   UG 22-32, p. 103, para. 707.

86   UG 22-32, p. 7, para. 41.

87   Phillips (1938), p. 93; Shropshire (1970), pp. 70, 91, 93.

88   HPW, AD1438, Box 10, Fred Harvey, Town Clerk, Uitenhage, p. 9.

89   Dr Neil McVicar, cited in Janisch (1941), p. 4.

90   Gaitskell (1982), pp. 339–40; ABCFM, Box 47:22, 'The Rising Tide of Native Crime. An Address to the Rotary Club of Johannesburg on 7 May 1940, by Dr Phillips'; Hellman (1934), pp. 59–60.

91   Titus Mabaso, letter to *The Bantu World*, 17 December 1938, cited in Shropshire (1970), p. 30, see also pp. 17, 145.

92   Taylor (1931), p. 55.

93   Palmer (1931), p. 49.

94   SAB, GES 455 47/9B, Gunn to Under Secretary for Public Health, 24 June 1940, p. 6.

95   Bradford (1987b); le Hausse (1984), pp. 137, 139, 164–5, 198, 250, 288, 298.

96   Bonner (1990), pp. 221–6.

97   SAB, GES 455 47/9B, Gunn to Under Secretary for Public Health, 24 June 1940, p. 6.

98   Eales (1991) offers an excellent discussion of this process in Johannesburg, and her thesis and our discussions were helpful in shaping this chapter.

99   Jochelson (1993), pp. 136, 146, 149–51.

100 Quoted in UG 22-32, p. 140, para. 964.

101 NAB 3/DBN 4/1/3/1625 359c, vol. 1, draft amendments: native registration regulations, 24 June 1936, p. 2.

102 NAB, 3/DBN 4/1/3/1625 359c, vol. 1, Memo for Native Administration Committee, Amendment of Native registration regulations: entry of Native women into urban area of Durban, 7 May 1936. On Johannesburg see Eales (1991), pp. 141–2.
103 Bonner (1990), pp. 245–6; Eales (1991), p. 149.
104 NAB 3/DBN 4/1/3/1625 359c, vol. 1, draft amendments: native registration regulations, 24 June 1936, p. 2.
105 Herbst Report (1937–39), p. 79, para. 459.
106 Redding (1987), pp. 250–2.
107 Eales (1991), p. 150.
108 JC 1-37; UG 56-37, p. 28.
109 UG 56-37, p. 21.
110 Bonner (1990), p. 245. The Prison Department suspended the activities of the female section in November 1951, and finally closed the facility in mid 1954.
111 Eales (1991), p. 167.
112 HPW, AD843, B. 56.4, 'Conference on Urban Native Juvenile Delinquency, 10–12 October 1938', address by G. Ballenden, 'The situation as viewed by municipal authorities'.
113 HPW, AD1438, Box 12, Statement by the Native Administration Committee of . . . Durban, pp. 4, 14. For details of Durban's slum clearance and housing programme see le Hausse (1984); Maylam (1983, 1990).
114 NUAA Section 12 (1) (d), cited in Janisch (1941), pp. 1–2; NAB, 3/DBN 643/J/18, vol. 1, Memorandum for consideration by the Finance Committee, Land at Wentworth: establishment of Native village, p. 2.
115 Simons (1968), pp. 53–4; on the status of *lobola* in the different provinces, see pp. 43–4, and on earlier attempts to codify native law see pp. 46–7.
116 For a comparative study of traditional law and indirect rule see Chanock (1985).
117 Janisch, cited in Shropshire (1970), pp. 8–9.
118 NAB, 3/DBN 4/1/3/1625, vol. 1, 359c, Native Welfare Officer to Town Clerk, Durban, 9 March 1937.
119 Simons (1968), p. 209. On the protests against passes and registration see NAB, 3/DBN 4/1/3/1625, 359c, extract from minutes of Native Administration Committee, 15 March 1937, p. 995; Deputation of Native Women to the Native Commissioner, Durban, 18 March 1937; Pass Laws for Native Women – Mass Meeting at the Bantu Social Centre, Durban, 17 March 1937.
120 Le Hausse (1984), pp. 75, 296.
121 Eales (1991), p. 181.
122 HPW, AD1438, Box 12, Statement by the Native Administration Committee . . . of Durban, pp. 4, 14.
123 NAB, 3/DBN 325A, Medical Officer of Municipal Native Administration Department to its Manager, 16 March 1934, p. 10.
124 Couzens (1982); Eales (1991), pp. 188–93.
125 Le Hausse (1984), pp. 252–80.
126 Eales (1991), pp. 190–3; le Hausse (1984), pp. 264–5.
127 HPW, AD1438, Box 9, Statement by Ballenden, p. 2.

128   Berger (1992), pp. 62, 162. For different estimates see Phillips (1938), p. 13; UG 12-42, pp. 78–89, table 14; UG 41-54, pp. 208–19, table 14.
129   Le Hausse (1984), p. 333, appendix XXII.
130   UG 12-42, pp. 78–89, table 14; UG 41-54, pp. 208–19, table 14; le Hausse (1984), p. 320, appendix VI; HPW, A917, Broome Report, p. 18, para. 24.
131   HPW, AD1438, Box 9, Statement by Ballenden, p. 3; see also Box 7, Statement by Britten; Box 12. Statement by Lugg; Box 9, Minutes of evidence of Ballenden, p. 7711.
132   Suid Afrikaanse Vroue Federasie, cited in Elliott Report (1942), p. 21, para. 28.
133   HPW, AD1438, Box 7, Statement by Britten.
134   Dr Baumann in *Hansard*, vol. 24, 29 January 1935, col. 786.
135   NAB, 3/DBN 4/1/3/1625, 359c, vol. 3, G. H. Gunn to Town Clerk, 1 September 1948.
136   Jochelson (1993), pp. 191–3.
137   NAB, 3/DBN 4/1/3/1625, 359c. Gunn to Town Clerk, 7 September 1944, p. 2; Hansen (1989), pp. 124–7; Gaitskell (1983).
138   HPW, AD1438, Box 12, Statement by Palmer, p. 2.
139   HPW, AD1438, Box 9, Minutes of evidence of Ballenden, pp. 7711-2.
140   HPW SAIRR AD843/RJ/J4.8, minutes of Rotary meeting held in the Union Castle Board Room on 29 March 1939 at 5pm.
141   Eales (1991), p. 180.
142   Wells (1983).
143   Posel (1991), pp. 44–60.
144   COMA, 2150:1202, Statement No. 8, The Social Aspect of Migratory Labour as Opposed to Stabilised Native Mining Communities, p. 1; COMA, 1942:0861, Migrant Native Labour: The Case For, pp. 1, 2; COMA, 1942:0651, Transvaal Chamber of Mines Address to Students and Staff of the Department of Social Studies, University of the Witwatersrand, October 1945, p. 18.
145   COMA, 1942:0861, Migrant Native Labour: The Case For, p. 2; see also COMA, 2150:1202, Statement No. 9, The Medical Aspect of Migratory Labour as Opposed to Stabilised Native Mining Communities, p. 3. For a similar argument see Herbst (1944), p. 127.
146   Packard (1987), pp. 208–9.
147   Dubow (1995), pp. 164–5.
148   Ibid., pp. 189–96.
149   Gale (1950), p. 11; Gale, cited in UG 28-48, p. 40, para. 54.
150   Freed (1948), pp. 65–6.
151   UG 18-47, p. 1.
152   Gale, cited in UG 28-48, p. 40, para. 54; HPW, AD843B 27.4.3, Precis of Evidence to the Native Mine Wages Commission by G. W. Gale (1943), p. 1.
153   Kark (1949), p. 83, (1950), p. 37.
154   Kark (1949), pp. 82, 83.
155   HPW, AD1756/Bj, Statements by Prof. Z. K. Matthews and Dr M. Wilson: The Social Effects of Migrant Labour, pp. 8–9; HPW, AD843/RJ/Aa12.14.11, Evidence of the SAIRR to the Native Laws Commission of Enquiry, pp. 66, 72, 74.
156   Vaughan (1991), pp. 144–5, 151.

7 VD Treatment and Educational Propaganda for Africans

1 HPW, AD1438, Box 9, Statement of Dr Alfred Bitini Xuma, p. 9.
2 HPW, AD1438, Box 2, 'Health and Child Welfare, Natal, pp. 1160–2523', Dundee sitting, 17 September 1930: evidence of Rev. E. A. Mahamba, p. 28; HPW, AD1438, Box 2, 'Health and Child Welfare, Transkei, pp. 2524–3960', Port St. Johns sitting, 10 November 1930: evidence of B. S. Ncabena, p. 54.
3 Vaughan (1991), pp. 33–40; Worboys (1988).
4 Marks and Andersson (1984), Swanson (1976, 1977, 1983).
5 Wallace (1993), p. 1.
6 TAB, GNLB 183 915/14/103, J. A. Mitchell to Mrs Scandrett, NCCVD, 26 February 1919; on the African elite's self-perceptions see Eales (1989).
7 Dubow (1989), p. 44.
8 NAB, DPH 4/1/2/854, 188E/5, notes of sub-committee re medical examination of natives, 26 April 1932.
9 HPW, AD1438, Box 8, Evidence of Dr A. J. Milne, Medical Officer of Johannesburg, p. 7671.
10 Gaitskell (1992), pp. 180, 186–8, 195.
11 IADJ, SGJ, Box 25, File A219, Minutes of the fifth meeting of the Council of Public Health . . . on 3 May 1922, p. 16.
12 TAB, GNLB 110 1328/13, Acting Magistrate Ermelo to Director of Native Labour, 17 July 1925; SAB, NTS 5760 15/315, District Surgeon, Mafeking to Secretary for Public Health, 13 October 1920; UG 22–32, evidence of Dr D. Huskisson, District Surgeon, Sekukuniland, p. 215, para. 264; HPW, AD1438, Box 8, Evidence of Milne, p. 7670.
13 HPW, AD1438, Box 2, 'Health and Child Welfare Ciskei, pp. 3961–4633'. Kingwilliamstown sitting, 26 January 1931: evidence of Rev. A. C. Grant, warden of St Matthew's College and Church, p. 80.
14 SAB, NTS 5761 15/315, Native Commisioner, Ubombo to Secretary for Public Health, 4 November 1932; TAB, GNLB 388 33/58, E. H. Cluver, Assistant Health Officer to Secretary for Public Health, 18 February 1931.
15 SAB, NTS 5761 15/315, Secretary for Public Health to Native Commissioner, Ubombo, 18 November 1932.
16 Fee (1988), p. 126.
17 'General Discussion on Venereal Diseases', *Proceedings of the Traansvaal Medical Officers Association*, vol. IV, no. 8. (1924), pp. 3, 6.
18 UG 28–48, evidence of Gale, p. 39, para. 54.
19 *Johannesburg City Council Minutes*, 24 June 1930, p. 478.
20 HPW, AD1438, Box 2, 'Health and Child Welfare, Transkei, pp. 2524–3960', Port St John's sitting, 10 November 1930: evidence of E. J. P. Almon (for local Village Management Board), p. 55.
21 SAB, NTS 5760 15/315, Klipdam Magistrate to Secretary of Public Health, 9 December 1924.
22 SAB, NTS 5760 15/315, Adams, Assistant Health Officer for the Union to the Secretary for Public Health, 22 March 1922, pp. 2, 4; SAB, NTS 5761 15/315, C. H. Blaine, Magistrate, Groot Marico, 10 July 1930; TAB, GNLB 149 136/14, H. G. Falwasser, for Director of Native Labour to Native Sub-Commissioners and Pass Officers, Witwatersrand, 12 April 1927; SAB, GES

376 4/5B, extract from minutes of Council of Public Health held at Cape Town on 26 January 1939.

23   NAB, DPH 3/DBN 4/1/2/854, 188E/5, O. L. Shearer, submission to the NEC, 1931, p. 4.

24   HPW, AD843/RJ/Na.10, Pietermaritzburg Public Health Department to Mayor, Pietermaritzburg, 28 April 1936, p. 3.

25   Jochelson (1993), p. 220

26   SAB, GES 376 4/5B, 'Instructions issued 7 February 1925 on medical examination of Africans under the NUAA'.

27   SAB, GES 375 4/5A, NAD to H. S. Gear, Assistant Health Officer, 24 July 1936; 'The medical examination of male Natives at the Pass Offices on the Witwatersrand. Report of the inspection undertaken by Dr H. S. Gear on the instructions of the Secretary for Public Health, May 1937'.

28   Redding (1987), p. 251.

29   Jochelson (1993), p. 219.

30   Vaughan (1991), pp. 49–52.

31   SAB, NTS 5760 15/315, Medical Officer of Health for the Union to Secretary for Native Affairs, 29 July 1918.

32   TAB, GNLB 183 915/14/103, Constitution of the Transvaal Council for Combating Venereal Diseases, no date [1920?].

33   IADJ, SGJ, Box 200, File 59/4, SHC (Transvaal), Aims and Objects, no date.

34   SAB, UOD 773 E23/5/1, RCSHC, report on minutes of 28 February 1938.

35   HPW, AD1438, Box 2, 'Health and Child Welfare Ciskei, pp. 3961–4633', Aliwal North sitting, 14 January 1931: evidence of Dr W. Stevenson, Medical Officer of Health, p. 70; Burghersdorp sitting, 16 January 1931: evidence of Dr E. W. Low, Medical Officer of Health, p. 73; SAB, NTS 5761 15/31, Native Commissioner, Ubombo to Secretary for Public Health, 4 November 1932; NAB, 1/NGA 3/3/2/14, Part 1, District Surgeon, Nongoma to Magistrate, Nongoma, 4 September 1938.

36   Bonner (1982); Couzens (1982), pp. 320–2.

37   TAB, MBP 165 P4-28, Secretary NCCVD (SA) to Town Clerk, Brakpan, 15 November 1922.

38   TAB, GNLB 183 915/14/103, NCCVD (Transvaal), minutes of executive committee on 15 June 1921.

39   HPW, AD843/RJ/Na18.4, File 5, report on lecture tour by Dr J. H. Rauch organised by the Transvaal branch of the South African Red Cross Society on the subject of venereal disease, 14 January 1935, pp. 10, 12.

40   TAB, GNLB 183 915/14/103, NCCVD (Transvaal), minutes of meeting 27 October 1920; NCCVD (Transvaal), minutes, 19 January 1921.

41   HPW AD843/RJ/Na18.4, File 5, report on lecture tour by Dr J. H. Rauch ... on ... VD, 14 January 1935, p. 12.

42   TAB, GNLB 183 915/14/103, NCCVD (Transvaal), minutes of executive committee on 15 June 1921.

43   TAB MBP 65 P4-28, 'LOOK! PEOPLE BEWARE!', poster issued by NCCVD (Transvaal), no date [probably 1922]; 'BEWARE! A WARNING – From Your Friends!', NCCVD pamphlet.

44   JPL, S Pam 496.3442:64.s47uni, DPH, 'Instructions to Native Patients Suffering from Syphilis or Gonorrhoea', no date; IADJ, SGJ, Box 200, File 59, vol. III, DPH, 'Instructions to Natives Suffering from Syphilis', 1921.

45 UG 22–32, p. 10, para 61, p. 30, para 199.
46 JPL, S Pam 496.3442:64.s47uni, DPH, 'Instructions to Native Patients suffering from Syphilis or Gonorrhoea', no date; IADJ, SGJ, Box 200, File 59, vol. II, DPH, 'Instructions to Natives Suffering from Syphilis', 1921.
47 HPW AD843/RJ/Na18.4, File 5, report on lecture tour by Dr J. H. Rauch . . . on . . . VD, 14 January 1935, p. 5.
48 Phillips (1938), p. 73.
49 UG 17–27, p. 83.
50 Beinart (1987), p. 293; Moodie (1983), p. 190; Pitje (1950a), pp. 109–16, (1950b), pp. 194, 198; Turner (1915), p. 134.
51 SAB, GES 375 4/5A, 'The medical examination of male natives . . . Report . . . by . . . Gear . . . May 1937', p. 2.
52 Mayer (1980).
53 Hindson (1987), p 40.
54 HPW, AD1438, Box 2, 'Health and Child Welfare, Natal, pp. 1160–2523', Newcastle sitting, 16 September 1930: evidence of exempted Africans, Philemon Yeni, Mr. Tembe and Mr. Dhlamini, p. 26.
55 HPW, AD843/RJ/Na 7.6, Benoni Location Protest Committee to SAIRR, 22 March 1937.
56 On the African urban elite's self-perception, though with reference to night passes for women, see Eales (1989), pp. 105–40.
57 SAB, GES 375 4/5A, Acting Secretary for Public Health to the Minister, 18 May 1936.
58 SAB, GES 375 4/5A, 'The medical examination of male Natives . . . Report . . . by Gear . . . May 1937', p. 2.
59 SAB, GES 376 4/5B, Secretary for Public Health to Secretary for Native Affairs, 23 January 1939.
60 Smit Report (1942), p. 11, paras 122, 123.
61 Weindling (1993), p. 101.
62 Marks and Andersson (1992).
63 HPW, AD843 B8.1.6, Dr G. W. Gale, 'Health Services in the Union', no date [1946–47?].
64 SAB, GES 376 4/5B, Secretary for Public Health to Secretary for Native Affairs, 23 January 1939; SAB, NTS 5761 15/315, vol. 3, Secretary for Public Health to Secretary for Native Affairs, 27 November 1939.
65 Kark (1949), p. 83.
66 Marks and Andersson (1992).
67 City of Durban, *Annual Report of Borough Medical Officer of Health for the Year ending 30 June 1938*, p. 5; *Johannesburg City Council Minutes*, 25 April 1939, pp. 488–9.
68 IADJ, SGJ, Box 201, File 59/5, memorandum on venereal disease services existing at various centres under the control of the Johannesburg City Council, 13 March 1946.
69 SAB, GES 455 47/9B, Durban City MOH to Under Secretary for Public Health, 24 June 1940, pp. 1–2; NAB, 3/DBN 4/1/3/1625, 359c, City Venereologist to City MOH, 30 November 1943; Durban City MOH to Town Clerk, 5 January 1944, and 15 March 1945.
70 HPW, AD843/RJ/Na.10, Pietermaritzburg Public Health Department to Mayor, Pietermaritzburg, 28 April 1936, pp. 1–2.

71   IADJ, SGJ, Box 98, File A6153, 'Medical Services: Native Townships, VD clinics', 27 September 1941; IADJ, SGJ, Box 201, File 59/5, memorandum re management of cases of syphilis and gonorrhoea, 14 November 1941; Memorandum on VD services . . . under . . . the Johannesburg City Council, 13 March 1946.

72   City of Durban, *Mayors Minutes*, 1946, pp. 150–1.

73   On the USA, see Brandt (1987), pp. 149–54; Fee (1988), p. 132; on Britain and Scotland see Davidson (1993).

74   SAB, GES 455 47/9B, City MOH to Under Secretary for Public Health, 24 June 1940, p. 4.

75   City of Durban, *Annual Report of Borough Medical Officer of Health for the Year ending 30 June 1939*, p. 15.

76   KAB, 1/UTA 58 39B, memorandum to the Town Council from the MOH on the Treatment and Control of Venereal Diseases in Umtata, 28 May 1946.

77   SAB, GES 455 47/9B, City MOH to Under Secretary for Public Health, 24 June 1940, p. 4; IADJ, SGJ, Box 201, File 59/5, Memorandum on VD services . . . under . . . the Johannesburg City Council, 13 March 1946.

78   SAB, GES 376 4/5B, Secretary for Public Health to Secretary for Native Affairs, 23 January 1939; Secretary for Public Health to Municipal Association of the Transvaal, 31 January 1941; NAB, 3/DBN 4/1/3/1625, 359c, extract from City Council minutes, 10 November 1943; Secretary for Native Affairs to Town Clerk, Durban, 2 December 1943.

79   NAB, 3/DBN 4/1/3/1625, 359c, Secretary for Native Affairs to Town Clerk, Durban, 2 December 1943.

80   NAB, 3/DBN 4/1/3/1625, 359c, City MOH to Town Clerk, 20 February 1945.

81   NAB, 3/DBN 4/1/3/1625, 359c, vol. 3, City Venereologist to City MOH, 30 November 1943; E. Havemann, Manager, memorandum to Native Administration Committee, 2 November 1948.

82   UG 42–41, p. 24. The high percentage does not reflect the incidence among the female domestic worker population, as employers may only have demanded an examination if already suspicious about the health of their servants, rather than as a matter of course.

83   IADJ, SGJ, Box 201, File 59, Mrs R. Williams to Public Health Department, 21 May 1939; MOH to Mrs R. Williams, 23 May 1939.

84   Jochelson (1993), p. 221.

85   City Of Durban, *Annual Report of Borough Medical Officer of Health for the Year ending 30 June 1939*, p. 15.

86   City of Durban, *Mayors Minutes*, 1944, pp. 113–14.

87   City of Durban, *Mayors Minutes*, 1943, p. 113; City of Durban, *Mayors Minutes*, 1945, p. 132; Gunn (1948), p. 2.

88   HPW, AD843/RJ/Na18.4, File 8, Dr Ray Phillips, 'Types of Red Cross Work which could with advantage be carried out amongst non-Europeans', 1938, p. 3.

89   NAD 3/DBN 188, vol. 7, Anning, 'Municipal Health Problems of the Non-European Population', p. 22.

90   Vaughan (1991), pp. 185–96.

91   For another analysis of the film, see Vaughan (1991), pp. 180–2.

92   HPW SAIRR AD843 B22.7, report of the subcommittee of the Native Welfare Association of Pretoria on the actual medical assistance to natives in Pre-

toria and suburbs, no date; SAB, NTS 5761 15/315, Part II, Minutes of Enquiry held in the Native Dutch Reformed Church at the Municipal Native Location, Pietersburg on the 10 November 1933, 20 November 1933, 28 November 1933, pp. 3, 5, 9, 11, 12, 20.

93   HPW, AD843/RJ/Na18.4, File 8, Phillips, 'Types of Red Cross Work which could . . . be carried out amongst non-Europeans', 1938, p. 1.
94   City of Durban, *Mayors Minutes*, 1946, p. 124.
95   Vaughan (1991), p. 186.
96   Gaitskell (1992), p. 191.
97   On the development of social work see Cobley (1995).
98   ABC 15:4 (52) 2:13, 'The Jan Hofmeyr School of Social Work for the training of social workers among non-Europeans in South Africa, no date [received 1940]; Hofmeyr School for Social Work, report of first six months of work, January–June 1941, Course of Study.
99   HPW, AD843 B42.11, Rheinallt Jones, 'Missionary Co-operation', 24 November 1943.
100 SAB, UOD 773 E23/5/1, SA Red Cross Society . . . report of sub-committee appointed to recommend steps . . . with regard to non-Europeans, 1 April 1938.
101 HPW, AB1886/M3.15.2, Diocese of St John's, Holy Cross Hospital, 'What the teacher may do for the health of the Pondo people', no date.
102 Phillips (1938), p. 226.
103 HPW, AD843 B15.1, the Christian Council of South Africa, 'Statement issued by the executive committee on Home Life', no date.
104 Gaitskell (1983), pp. 247, 248, (1982), pp. 344, 348–9, 352.
105 SAB, UOD 773 E23/5/1, National Committee for Health Education, routine work sub-committee. Minutes of meeting of the third meeting . . . on 13 June 1939, p. 2.
106 HPW, AD843/RJ/Ng7.10, 'Facts on Sex for Men'.
107 SAB, GES 455 47/9B, 'Venereal Disease', pamphlet issued by City of Durban Public Health Department in English and Zulu.
108 Gunn (1948), p. 4.
109 Jochelson (1993), p. 201.

8   Conclusion

1   Ijsselmuiden *et al.* (1988), p. 457.
2   Department of National Health and Population Development (1995), p. 233.
3   Department of National Health and Population Development (1996), pp. 9, 11.
4   Doyle (1993), p. 103.
5   Jochelson *et al.* (1991), p. 159.
6   Ijsselmuiden *et al.* (1990), p. 521.
7   Karim (1993), Webb (1995), pp. 82, 89–90, 110–11, Zwi and Cabral (1991), p. 1527.
8   Jochelson *et al.* (1991); Webb (1995), p. 35.
9   Jochelson *et al.* (1991), pp. 163–6; Moodie (1983), pp. 181, 187–8.
10 Dangor *et al.* (1989), p. 339. In contrast to these findings, a study conducted for the COM (Ijsselmuiden, 1990, p. 522) showed that only 2.6 per cent of

migrants had more than one girlfriend, 2.1 per cent admitted to sexual contact with a bar girl or prostitute in the preceding month, 14.2 per cent had a girlfriend close to the mine and 34.7 per cent had a girlfriend at home.

11 Blecher *et al.* (1995), pp. 1283–4; Buga (1996), p. 526; Evian *et al.* (1990), p. 518; Mathews *et al.* (1990), pp. 513–14; 'Womens Fight Against That Invisible Little Virus', *Weekly Mail*, 30 November 1990.
12 Jochelson *et al.* (1991).
13 Dangor *et al.* (1990), p. 339.
14 Ijsselmuiden *et al.* (1990), p. 521.
15 Farrell *et al.* (1989).
16 Gaye (1980), ch. 3; Jochelson *et al.* (1991), pp. 167–8.
17 Brink (1987a).
18 Martino (1987).
19 Williams and Campbell (1996), p. 149.
20 Cronjé *et al.* (1994), p. 604.
21 Crewe (1992), p. 14.
22 Altman (1986); Sontag (1988), pp. 25–6, 46; Watney (1987).
23 Transvaal Education Circular Minute 70/88, cited in Crewe (1992), p. 75.
24 'AIDS a hazard "beyond concept"', *Business Day*, 6 June 1989; 'It will kill one in four blacks in SA – Sanlam', *Saturday Star*, 10 June 1989; 'AIDS is wiping out SA workers', *Saturday Star*, 21 January 1990; Crewe (1992), pp. 58, 65.
25 *The Star*, 9 August 1988.
26 K. Edelston, *AIDS: Countdown to Doomsday* (Media House, 1988), p. 186, cited in Crewe (1992), p. 58.
27 'Anti-AIDS campaign AIDS from freedom fighters', pamphlet, no date (1988), no publisher.
28 'Sisulu's name on fake "AIDS" leaflet', *Weekly Mail*, 5 October 1990.
29 Aids Information Distributing Society of South Africa, 'FACTS ON AIDS: Press Won't Print!! AIDS hushed – why???', pamphlet, Johannesburg, no publisher (1989); West Gossip, 'AIDS – Hushed – Why?? The Origins of AIDS', Johannesburg, no publisher (November 1989).
30 'Fired the Maid with HIV', *The Weekly Mail*, 12–18 June 1992, p. 5; 'Madams, Maids and AIDS', *Mail & Guardian*, 28 July–3 August 1995, p. 27.
31 Webb (1995), p. 89.
32 'Combat Zone', *Sunday Times*, 3/13[?] July 1995.
33 'Sunter's Chilling Scenario as AIDS Takes Root in SA', *Saturday Star*, 2 November 1996, p. 12.
34 *Government Gazette*, no. 11014, reg. nos. 2438, 2439. Pretoria, October 30, 1987.
35 Zwi and Bachmayer (1990).
36 Webb (1995), pp. 81, 84.
37 Crewe (1992), pp. 63, 75; Webb (1995), p. 82.
38 Webb (1995), pp. 82, 84.
39 Browne (1987); Crewe (1992), p. 63; Jochelson *et al.* (1991), pp. 168–9.
40 Green (1992); Williams and Campbell (1996), p. 1250.
41 Zwi and Bachmayer (1990), p. 321.
42 Ibid., pp. 323–4; Webb (1995), pp. 85–7.

43 Karim (1993).
44 Webb, (1995), p. 222; 'Finally the State Gets Serious About AIDS', *The Weekly Mail & Guardian*, 22–28 July 1994, p. 11.
45 'What AIDS Programme?', *Mail & Guardian Special Supplement*, 29 November–5 December 1996, pp. 1–2; Zuma's Revenge', *Mail & Guardian*, 25 July–1 August 1996, p. 14.
46 'Bureaucrats Dither as HIV Invades', *Mail & Guardian*, 2–8 May 1997, p. 6.
47 Campbell and Williams (1996), p. 55.
48 Danziger (1994); Webb (1995), pp. 221, 224.
49 'Editorial. Reassessing Priorities: Identifying the Determinants of HIV Transmission', *Social Science and Medicine*, Vol. 36, no. 5 (1993), pp. iii–viii; Williams and Campbell (1996), p. 1250; Zwi and Cabral (1991), p. 1528.

Appendix 1

1 Morris (1988), p. 723.
2 Grin (1956).
3 Perine *et al.* (1984), pp. 2, 13–14, 19–21.

Bibliography

Official archival sources

Central Archive Depot (SAB) and Transvaal Archive Depot (TAB), Pretoria

Archives of the Department of Public Health (GES)

SAB, GES 375 4/5A, Medical Examination of Natives, 1935–38.
SAB, GES 376 4/5B, Medical Examination of Natives, 1938–45.
SAB, GES 455 47/9B, Syphilis, VD, Durban, 1931–40.
SAB, GES 1153 1/18, miscellaneous correspondence, Rietfontein Hospital.
SAB, GES 1153 1/18A, miscellaneous correspondence, Rietfontein Hospital, 1925–9.
SAB, GES 1154 18/18B, reports and miscellaneous correspondence, Rietfontein Hospital, 1929–36.
SAB, GES 1155 6/18, Police, Rietfontein, on fencing in of Lazaretto.
SAB, GES 1527 7/26A, Native Act (Urban Areas) No. 21 of 1923, medical examination and vaccination of natives etc., 1927–35.
SAB, GES 1991 49/33, Imperial Social Hygiene Congresses, 1925–33.
SAB, GES 1991 49/33A, Imperial Social Hygiene Congresses, 1933–39.
SAB, GES 2281 85/38, vol. 1, Sterilization of the Unfit Genetics and Birth Control, 1929–39.

Archives of the Government Native Labour Bureau (GNLB)

TAB, GNLB 110 1328/13, Venereal Disease in Ermelo-Breyten District, 1925–28.
TAB, GNLB 149 136/14, Mhlakuvane Gumede of Chief Mtshakela of Ingwavuma Suffering from Venereal Disease Absconds to Johannesburg, 1927.
TAB, GNLB 183 915/14/103, Supply of Leaflets on Venereal Disease, 1928.
TAB, GNLB 388 33/58, Venereal Disease – Natal Labour Areas, 1928–31.

Archives of the Native Affairs Department (post-union) (NTS)

SAB, NTS 2863 10/303.
SAB, NTS 2891 119/303, Elim Hospital, 1912–46.
SAB, NTS 5760 15/315, Venereal Diseases, 1913–25.
SAB, NTS 5761 15/315, Venereal Diseases, 1926–33.
SAB, NTS 6716 23/315, Rietfontein Lazaretto, 1914–24.
SAB, NTS 7055 136/322, Native Beer Canteens and Brothels on the Matatiele Side of the Basutoland Border, 1932.

Archives of the Colonial Secretary (CS)

TAB, CS 221 283/03, Syphilitic Girl named Pretorius. Re Above and Forwarding Report from District Surgeon re Prevention of Syphilis Generally in Nylstroom District, 1903.

TAB, CS 578 2614, Syphilis spread in Zoutpansberg, 1905–6.
TAB, CS 578 2614A, Syphilis in Zoutpansberg.
TAB, CS 908 17843, Special Syphilitic Measures Belfast (and Waterval Boven), 1909–11.
TAB, CS 908 17845, Special Syphilitic Measures, Carolina, 1909–11.
TAB, CS 908 17847, Special Syphilitic Measures, Ermelo and Amsterdam, 1909–11.
TAB, CS 908 17848, Special Syphilitic Measures, Germiston, 1909–10.
TAB, CS 908 17850, Special Syphilitic Measures, Johannesburg, 1909–11.
TAB, CS 909 17853A, Syphilis Lichtenburg, 1909–11.
TAB, CS 909 17855, Special Syphilitic Measures, Middelburg and Witbank, 1909–11.
TAB, CS 910 17857, Special Syphilitic Measures, Pietersburg, Duiwelskloof, Haenertsburg, Louis Trichardt and Sibasa, 1910–11.
TAB, CS 910 17858, Special Syphilitic Measures.
TAB, CS 910 17862, Special Syphilitic Measures, Rustenburg, 1909–10.
TAB, CS 965 19784, Syphilis, General, 1897–1910.

Archives of the State Secretary (SS)

TAB, SS R423/86.
TAB, SS R1250/96, Rapport over het geneeskundige onderzoek der naturellen wonende in de Wyk Middelburg, ZAR, Sept. 96–Maart 97.
TAB, SS R3013/85, District dokter kijer, zendt in nummer van 't volksblad waarin artikel over syphilis. Beveelt lezing daarvan, 1885.
TAB, SS R6135/98, Veldkornet Wyk 3 Carolina vraagt instructies re een kaffer lydende aan syphilis, 1898.
TAB, SS R8585/97, Landdrost Piet Retief, vraagt ondersteuning voor de familie J. van der Merwe die aan syphilis lydt, 1897.

Municipal files

TAB, MJB 4/2/61 A456, Transvaal Municipal Association, 1925–7.
TAB, MJB 4/2/145 A739, White and Native Housing, 1921–23.
TAB, MBP 165 P4–28, Venereal Disease: Combating Of, 1921–6.

Miscellaneous files

SAB, ARB 2017, CF 13, Welfare and General Correspondence, 1934–41.
SAB, GG 8/297.
SAB, GG 916 33/453, G. O. Robertson to Govenment Secretary, Mafeking, October 1913.
SAB, GOV 32/115/02, work on yaws written by Jonathan Hutchinson, 1902.
SAB, JUS 805 1/600/23, part 1, Immoral Relations Between Europeans, Natives and Asiatics, 1920–25.
SAB, K139, Economic and Wages Commission.
SAB, LD637 AG934/04.
SAB, MNW, Box 425, File 2036/18, Superintendent and Chief Inspector, White Labour Department, Report on Liquor Laws and Illicit Liquor Selling, 1918.

TAB, PW 129 AR371/96, Landdrost Ermelo vraagt een bedrag van £4.0.0 voor het onder dak brengenvan een kamer voor syphilis lijders, 1896.

TAB, SD 2614 D, Commission re syphilis amongst Natives.

TAB, SNA 100 NA291/03, report suggesting establishment of a colony for native 'lepers' and syphilitic patients on a farm to be provided by government, 1903.

SAB, UOD 773 E23/5/1, South African Red Cross Society, Social Hygiene Committee (Educational Section), Parts I, II, III.

Intermediate Archive Depot, Johannesburg (IADJ). Archives of the Johannesburg City Health Department

IADJ, SGJ, Box 2, File A6340, Alterations to VD Clinic, 1925–40.

IADJ, SGJ, Box 25, File A219, Council of Public Health, 1919–22, 1923–24.

IADJ, SGJ, Box 35, File 2/25/2, Birth Control, 1931–60.

IADJ, SGJ, Box 98, File A6153, Medical Services in Native Townships, 1940–45.

IADJ, SJG, Box 149, File 9728, Public Health Bill, 1919.

IADJ, SGJ, Box 199, File 59, Venereal Disease, 1920–35.

IADJ, SGJ, Box 200, File 59, vols 2–5, Venereal Disease, 1920–45.

Cape Archive Depot (KAB)

Archives of the Colonial Office (CO)

KAB, CO 7403, 360, Vryburg Syphilis Hospital, 1899–1903.

KAB, CO 7508, 629, Cape Town Lock Hospital, 1901–4.

KAB, CO 7906, F127C, Administration of CDA, Closure of Hospitals 1904–6.

Archives of the medical officer of health for the colony (MOH)

KAB, MOH 310, C117B, Contagious Diseases Act, Cape Colony, 1902–5.

KAB, MOH 311, C117B, Administration, Contagious Diseases Act, Cape Colony, 1906–8.

Miscellaneous

KAB, GH 23/36 62, general dispatches relating to VD.

KAB, 1/UTA 58 39B, Infectious Diseases: Venereal, 1940–50.

Natal Archive Depot (NAB)

Archives of the Durban borough (3/DBN)

NAB, 3/DBN 167, vol. 3.

NAB, 3/DBN 188, vol. 7.

NAB, 3/DBN 188B.

NAB, 3/DBN 4/1/2/854 188E, Venereal Diseases.

NAB, 3/DBN 325A, reports by the Medical Officer of Health, Native Affairs Department.

NAB, 3/DBN 4/1/2/1175 359A, Registration of Natives.

NAB, 3/DBN 4/1/3/1625 359c, Proposed Compulsory Registration of Native Women.

NAB, 3/DBN 643/J/18.

Miscellaneous

NAB, 1/NGA 3/3/2/14, 13/1/5, part 1, Venereal Disease Tours in Nongoma District, 1937–9.

NAB, DPH 30 57/1908, District Surgeon Ingwavuma Reports that Certain Natives Residing Near the Magistracy are Suffering from Syphilis, 1908.

Johannesburg Public Library

JPL, S 176.5, miscellaneous pamphlets on morality.

JPL, S Pam 496.3442:614.s47uni, Union of South Africa Public Health Department, Venereal Diseases: Their Prevention and Treatment (1935).

Unofficial archival sources

University of the Witwatersrand, historical papers collection, William Cullen Library (HPW)

HPW, A917, The Broome Report, 1947.

HPW, AB1886, Diocese of St Johns.

HPW, AD843 B, archives of the South African Institute of Race Relations: B Boxes.

HPW, AD843/RJ, archives of the South African Institute of Race Relations: Rheinallt Jones Collection.

HPW, A1212, Dr Louis Franklin Freed, 1903–79.

HPW, AD1438, Native Economic Commission, Minutes of Evidence.

HPW, AD1756, Native Laws Commission of Enquiry, Fagan Commission evidence.

HPW, FAB329 HIGSON, Confidential report of Miss Higson's Tour, 1932.

Chamber of Mines Archives, Johannesburg (COMA)

COMA, 1942:0651, Native Labour, Miscellaneous, 1945.

COMA, 2080:1704, Health Conditions, 1936.

COMA, 1942:0861, Native Labour, Miscellaneous, 1945.

COMA, 2150:1202, Native Laws Commission 2, 1947.

COMA, 2211:2033, Native Labour Supply, Medical Exam.

American Board Of Foreign Mission, Hoover Library, Harvard University (ABC)

ABCFM, Individual Biographical Collection, Box 47:22, Mr and Mrs Ray E. Phillips.

ABC 15:4 (52) 2:13, Johannesburg Social Work.

Printed government publications

Cape colony government publications

A 13-88, Cape of Good Hope, *Report of the Select Committee on Reports of District Surgeons*.

A13-78, Cape of Good Hope, *Petition of the Chairman and Members of the Committee of the Burghersdorp Chamber of Commerce and Association for General Purposes.*

A14-78, Cape of Good Hope, *The Petition of the Inhabitants of the Town and District of Fraserburg.*

A 30-06, Cape of Good Hope, *Report of the Select Commmittee on the Contagious Diseases Act (1906).*

C 01-69, Cape of Good Hope, *Report of the Select Committee Appointed by the Legislative Council to Consider and Report on the Contagious Diseases Prevention Act.*

C 05-95, Cape of Good Hope, *Report of the Select Committee on the Contagious Diseases Act Amendment bill [CB8–95].*

G 67-84, Cape of Good Hope, *Report of the District Surgeon for 1883.*

G 19-85, Cape of Good Hope, *Report of District Surgeons for 1884.*

G 03-86, Cape of Good Hope, *Reports of the District Surgeons for 1885.*

G 19-87, Cape of Good Hope, *Reports of District Surgeons on Public Health for 1886.*

G 13-88, Cape of Good Hope, *Report of District Surgeons for 1887.*

G 04-89, Cape of Good Hope, *Reports of District Surgeons on Public Health and Special Reports on the Prevalence of Contagious Diseases.*

G 17-90, Cape of Good Hope, *Reports of District Surgeons on Public Health for 1889.*

G 15-91, Cape of Good Hope, *Reports on Public Health for 1890.*

G 20-92, Cape of Good Hope, *Reports on Public Health, 1892.*

G 19-94, Cape of Good Hope, *Reports on the Public Health for Year 1893.*

G 55-96, Cape of Good Hope, *Reports on the Public Health for the Year 1895 including Reports of District Surgeons, Local Authorities and Medical Inspectors.*

G 74-96, Cape of Good Hope, *Report of the Medical Officer of Health for the Colony for the Year 1895.*

G 05-97, Cape of Good Hope, *Report of the Medical Officer of Health for the Colony for the Year 1896.*

G 56-1900, Cape of Good Hope, *Reports on the Public Health for the Year 1899 including Reports of District Surgeons, Local Authorities and Medical Inspectors.*

G 35-1904, Cape of Good Hope, *Report of the Medical Officer of Health for the Colony on the Public Health and on the Government and State-Aided Hospital of the Colony together with the Annual Health Reports of District Surgeons and Local Authorities for the Year 1903.*

G 39-1906, Cape of Good Hope, *Report of the Medical Officer of Health for the Colony on the Public Health and Local Government and the Registration of Births, Deaths and Marriages for the Two Calendar Years 1904 and 1905.*

G 40-1907, Cape of Good Hope, *Report of the Medical Officer of Health for the Colony on the Public Health for the Calendar Year 1906.*

G 33-1908, Cape of Good Hope, *Report of the Medical Officer of Health for the Colony on the Public Health for the Calendar Year 1907.*

G 43-1909, Cape of Good Hope, *Report of the Medical Officer of Health for the Colony on the Public Health and Local White of Births, Deaths and Marriages, 1908.*

Natal colony government publication

SAB NK 157, *Report of the Select Committee (No 15, 1890) on the Contagious Diseases Prevention Bill (No 19, 1890)*, Sixth Session, Twelfth Legislative Council.

Transvaal colony government publications

Report of the Contagious Diseases Amongst Natives Commission (1906) (chairman: Godfrey Lagden), referred to as CDC.

Report of the South African Natives Commission, 1903–1905 (chairman: Lagden), referred to as SANAC.

TG 08-10, *Prevalence of Syphilis amongst Transvaal Natives and the Means Adopted to Deal with the Disease (1910).*

TG 28-10, *Prevalence of Syphilis among Transvaal Natives and the Means Adopted to Deal with the Disease.*

Transvaal Public Health Department, *Annual Reports for the Year Ended 30 June 1904.*

Transvaal Public Health Department, *Annual Reports for the Year Ended 30 June 1905.*

Transvaal Public Health Department, *Annual Reports for the Year Ended 30 June 1906.*

Union of South Africa government publications

JC 01-37, *Report and Proceedings of the Joint Select Committee on the Amendment of Native Laws.*

SC 03-23, *First Report of the Select Committee on Native Affairs April 1923.*

SC 6A-29, *Second Report of the Select Committee on Native Affairs on the Native (Urban Areas) Act 1923 Amendment Bill, March 1929.*

UG 15-22, *Report of the Native Affairs Commissioner for the Year 1921.*

UG 41-22, *Report of the Interdepartmental Committee on the Native Pass Laws, 1920* (chairman: G. A. Godley).

UG 14-23, Department of Public Health, report for the year ending 30 June 1922, in *Annual Departmental Reports (Abridged) No. 2 Covering the Period 1921–22.*

UG 09-24, Department of Public Health report for the year ending 30 June 1923, in *Annual Departmental Reports (Abridged) No. 3 Covering the Period 1922–23.*

UG 40-25, *Report of the Native Affairs Commission for the Year 1924.*

UG 21-26, *Annual Report of the Department of Public Health for the Year ended 30 June 1925.*

UG 17-27, *Report of the Native Affairs Commission for the Years 1925–26.*

UG 32-27, *Fourth Census of the Population of the Union of South Africa enumerated 4th May 1926. Part 1. Population, Number, Sex and Geographical Distribution of the European Population.*

UG 47-28, *Annual Report of the Department of Public Health, Year Ending 30 June 1928.*

UG 42-29, *Fourth Census of the Population of the Union of South Africa enumerated 4th May 1926. Part X. Fertility of Marriage (Europeans).*

UG 40-30, *Annual Report of the Department of Public Health, Year Ending 30 June 1930.*

UG 22-32, *Report of the Native Economic Commission, 1930–32,* (chairman: J. E. Holloway), referred to as NEC.

UG 26-33, *Report of the Native Affairs Commission for the Years 1927–1931.*

UG 40-34, *Annual Report of the Department of Public Health for the Year ended 30 June 1933.*

UG 43-35, *Annual Report of the Department for Public Health for the Year ended 30 June 1935.*

UG 56-37, *Notes on conference between Municipalities and Native Affairs Department held at Pretoria on 28th and 29th September 1937, to discuss the provisions of the Native Laws Amendment Act (No. 46 of 1937).*

UG 28-38, *Report on the Sixth Census of the Population of the Union of South Africa enumerated 5th May 1936. Vol II. Ages of the Europeans, Asiatics and Coloured Population.*

UG 08-40, *Report of the Committee to Consider the Administration of Areas which are becoming Urbanised but which are not under Local Government Control 1938–1939* (chairman: E. N. Thornton).

UG 42-41, *Report of the Native Affairs Commission for the Years 1939–1940.*

UG 12-42, *Sixth Census of the Population of the Union of South Africa enumerated 5th May 1936. Vol IX: Natives (Bantu) and Other Non-European Races.*

UG 30-44, *Report of the National Health Services Commission on the Provision of an Organised National Health Service for All Sections of the People of the Union of South Africa, 1942–44* (chairman: Lieut. Col. H. Gluckman).

UG 21-44, *Report of the Witwatersrand Mine Natives Wages Commission on the Remuneration and Conditions of Employment of Natives on Witwatersrand Gold Mines, 1943* (chairman: C. Lansdown).

UG 08-45, *Annual Report of the Department of Public Health, Year Ended 30 June 1944.*

UG 18-47, *Annual Report of the Department of Health for 1946.*

UG 28-48, Department of Native Affairs, *Report of the Native Laws Commission, 1946–48.* (chairman: H. A. Fagan).

UG 41-54, *Population Census 7th May 1946. Vol V: Occupations and Industries of the European, Asiatic, Coloured and Native Population.*

Unnumbered union government publications

Report of the Native Farm Labour Committee 1937–39 (chairman: J. E. Herbst).

Department of Native Affairs (1942), *Report of the Interdepartmental Committee on the Social, Health and Economic Conditions of Urban Natives* (chairman: D. L. Smit).

Report of the Committee appointed by the Honourable Ministers of Justice and Native Affairs, July 1942, to Investigate the Position of Crime on the Witwatersrand and Pretoria (chairman: S. H. Elliott).

Republic of South Africa government publication

Government Gazette, no. 11014, reg. nos 2438, 2439. Pretoria, 30 October, 1987.

House of Assembly debates (selected years)

Hansard, vol. 1, 1924.
Hansard, vol. 6, 1926.
Hansard, vol. 8, 1927.
Hansard, vol. 12, 1929.
Hansard, vol. 15, 1930.
Hansard, vol. 23, 1934.
Hansard, vol. 24, 1935.

Provincial publication

TP 1-22, *Report of the Local Government Commission (1921)* (chairman: C. F. Stallard).

Municipal publications

Johannesburg City Council, *Johannesburg City Council Minutes*, 1910–50.
Borough/City Of Durban, *Annual Report of Borough/City Medical Officer of Health*, 1928–55.
Borough/City of Durban, *Mayors Minutes*, 1910–55.

Books and articles

Albertyn, J. R. (1932) 'Sociological Report a) The Poor White and Society', in *Report of the Carnegie Commission. The Poor White Problem in South Africa. Part V*, Stellenbosch: Pro Ecclesia.
Allen, F. J. (1943) 'Morbidity and Mortality on Coal and Gold Mines for 1941', *Proceedings of the Transvaal Mine Medical Officers Association*, vol. XXIII, no. 256, pp. 59–70.
Altman, Denis (1986) *AIDS and the New Puritanism*, London and Sydney: Pluto.
Anning, C. C. P. (1937) 'Sterility and the Falling Birth Rate: the Public Health Aspect', *South African Medical Journal*, vol. 11, pp. 493–7.
Ashton, Hugh (1967) *The Basutho. A Social Study of Traditional and Modern Lesotho*, London: Oxford University Press (first published 1952).
Ballinger, M. (1938) 'Native Life in South African Towns', *Journal of the Royal African Society*, vol. 37, pp. 326–38.
Bank, Andrew (1994) 'Race as Science: Phrenology at the Cape, 1820–1850', Institute of Commonwealth Studies, University of London: The Societies of Southern Africa Seminar, 20 January 1994.
Bassett, Mary T. and Mhloyi, Marvellous (1991) 'Women and AIDS in Zimbabwe: The Making of an Epidemic', *International Journal of Health Services*, vol. 21, no. 1, pp. 143–56.
Beck, Ann (1970) *A History of the British Medical Administration of East Africa*, Cambridge, Mass.: Harvard University Press.
Beinart, William (1982) *The Political Economy of Pondoland 1860–1930*, Johannesburg: Ravan Press.
Beinart, William (1987) 'Worker Consciousness, Ethnic Particularism and Nationalism: The Experiences of a South African Migrant, 1930–1960', in Shula Marks and Stanley Trapido (eds), *The Politics of Race, Class and Nationalism in Twentieth Century South Africa*, New York and London: Longman, pp. 286–309.
Beinart, William (no date) 'The Origins of the Indlavini: Male Associations and Migrant Labour in the Transkei', unpublished paper.
Berger, Iris (1992) *Threads of Solidarity. Women in South African Industry 1900–1980*, London, Bloomington and Indianapolis: James Currey and Indiana University Press.

Bickford-Smith, Vivian (1981) 'Dangerous Cape Town: Middle Class Attitudes to Poverty in Cape Town in the Late Nineteenth Century', in Christopher Saunders, Howard Phillips, Elizabeth van Heyningen (eds), *Studies in the History of Cape Town, vol. 4*, History Department in association with the Centre for African Studies, University of Cape Town, pp. 29–65.

Bickford-Smith, Vivian (1995) *Ethnic Pride and Racial Prejudice in Cape Town*, Cambridge: Cambridge University Press.

Bidwell, C. Hugh (1928) 'Eugenics' (presidential address at the 22nd South African Medical Congress), *Journal of the Medical Association of South Africa*, vol. 2, pp. 143–8.

Bland, Lucy (1982) ' "Guardians of the Race" or "Vampires Upon the Nation's Health"?: Female Sexuality and its Regulation in Early Twentieth Century Britain', in Elizabeth Whitelegg, Madeleine Arnot, Else Bartels, Veronica Beechey, Lynda Birke, Susan Himmelweit, Diana Leonard, Sonja Ruehl and Mary Anne Speakman (eds), *The Changing Experience of Women*, Oxford: Martin Robertson and Open University Press, pp. 373–88.

Bland, Lucy (1985) ' "Cleansing the Portals of Life": The Venereal Disease Campaign in the Early Twentieth Century', in Mary Langan and Bill Schwarz (eds), *Crises in the British State, 1880–1930*, London: Hutchinson and CCCS, pp. 192–208.

Blecher, M., Steinberg, M., Pick, W., Hennick, M. and Durcan, N. (1995) 'AIDS – Knowledge, Attitudes and Practices among STD Clinic Attenders in the Cape Peninsula', *South African Medical Journal*, vol. 85, no. 12, pp. 1281–6.

Block, I. J. (1934) 'Observations from the Work of a Birth Control Clinic', *South African Medical Journal*, vol. 8, pp. 490–2.

Bonfa, A. (1917) 'Syphilis and Salvarsan in Country Practice', *South African Medical Record*, vol. 15, pp. 372–5.

Bonner, Phillip L. (1982) 'The Transvaal Native Congress 1917–1920', in Shula Marks and Richard Rathbone (eds), *Industrialisation and Social Change in South Africa. African Class Formation, Culture and Consciousness, 1870–1930*, London and New York: Longman, pp. 270–313.

Bonner, Phillip L. (1988) 'Family Crime and Political Consciousness on the East Rand, 1939–1955', *Journal of Southern African Studies*, vol. 14, no. 3, pp. 393–420.

Bonner, Phillip L. (1990) ' "Desirable or Undesirable Basotho Women?" Liquor, Prostitution and the Migration of Basotho Women to the Rand, 1920–1945', in Cheryll Walker (ed.), *Women and Gender in Southern Africa to 1945*, Cape Town and London: David Phillip and James Currey, pp. 221–50.

Bozzoli, Belinda (1981) *The Political Nature of a Ruling Class. Capital and Ideology in South Africa, 1890–1933*, London: Routledge and Kegan Paul.

Bozzoli, Belinda, with the assistance of Mmantho Nkotsoe (1991) *Women of Phokeng. Consciousness, Life Strategy and Migrancy in South Africa, 1900–1983*, London: James Currey.

Bradford, Helen (1987a) *A Taste of Freedom. The ICU in Rural South Africa 1924–1930*, Johannesburg: Ravan Press.

Bradford, Helen (1987b) ' "We Are Now the Men: Women's Beer Protests in the Natal Countryside, 1929', in Belinda Bozzoli (ed.), *Class, Community and Conflict. South African Perspectives*, Johannesburg: Ravan Press, pp. 292–323.

Brandt, Allan M. (1987) *No Magic Bullet. A Social History of Venereal Disease in the United States Since 1880*, New York and Oxford: Oxford University Press.

Brink, B. A. (1987a) 'The Epidemiology of HIV Infection in the Mining Industry', paper presented at the Conference on AIDS: Perspectives on the Problem and its Management, Johannesburg, 10 September 1987.

Brink, Elsabe (1986) 'The Afrikaner Women of the Garment Workers Union, 1918–1939', MA thesis, University of the Witwatersrand, Johannesburg.

Brink, Elsabe (1987) '"Maar 'n Klomp "Factory" Meide": Afrikaner Family and Community on the Witwatersrand during the 1920s', in Belinda Bozzoli (ed.), *Class, Community and Conflict. South African Perspectives*, Johannesburg: Ravan Press, pp. 177–208.

Brink, Elsabe (1990) 'Man-made Women: Gender, Class and the Ideology of the *Volksmoeder*', in Cheryll Walker (ed.), *Women and Gender in Southern Africa to 1945*, Cape Town and London: David Phillip and James Currey, pp. 273–92.

Brock, B. G. (1917) 'Syphilis and the Commonweal', *South African Medical Record*, vol. 15, pp. 19–26.

Browne, B. B. (1987) 'Facing the "Black Peril". The Politics of Population Control in South Africa', *Journal of Southern African Studies*, vol. 13, pp. 256–73.

Buga, G. A. B., Amoko, D. H. A. and Ncayiyana, D. J. (1996) 'Sexual Behaviour, Contraceptive Practice and Reproductive Health among School Adolescents in Rural Transkei', *South African Medical Journal*, vol. 86, no. 5, pp. 523–7.

Bundy, Colin (1979) *The Rise and Fall of the South African Peasantry*, London: Heinemann.

Bundy, Colin (1980) 'Peasants in Herschel: a Case Study of a South African Frontier District', in Shula Marks and Antony Atmore (eds), *Economy and Society in Pre-Industrial South Africa*, London and New York: Longman, pp. 208–25.

Burke, Gillian and Richardson, Peter (1978) 'The Profits of Death: A Comparative Study of Miners' Phthisis in Cornwall and the Transvaal, 1876–1918', *Journal of Southern African Studies*, vol. 4, no. 2, pp. 147–71.

Burrows, E. H. (1958) *A History of Medicine in South Africa up to the End of the Nineteenth Century*, Cape Town and Amsterdam: A. A. Balkema.

Burt, Cyril L. (1926a) 'The Contribution of Psychology to Social Hygiene', *Health and Empire*, vol. 1, no. 1, pp. 13–37.

Burt, Cyril L. (1926b) 'The Causes of Sex Delinquency in Girls', *Health and Empire*, vol. 1, no. 4, pp. 251–71.

Burton, A. W. (1934) 'Common Disorders among Adult Male Xosas and Fingoes in the Border Districts', *South African Medical Journal*, vol. VIII, no. 9, pp. 327–37.

Caldwell, Sharon (1991) 'Segregation and Plague: King William's Town and the Plague Outbreaks of 1900–1907', *Contree*, vol. 29, pp. 5–10.

Callahan, Brian (1992) 'Venereal Disease and the Rise of Medical Liberalism in Southern Rhodesia, 1900–1946', first-year paper, Comparative World History Seminar, Department of History, The Johns Hopkins University.

Callahan, Brian (1996) '"Veni, VD, Vici"? Reassessing the Ila Syphilis Epidemic, 1900–1963', paper delivered at the conference on Comparative Perspectives on the History of Sexually Transmitted Diseases, Institute of Commonwealth Studies, University of London, 26–8 April 1996.

Campbell, Cathy and Williams, Brian (1996) 'Academic Research and HIV/AIDS in South Africa', *South African Medical Journal*, vol. 86, no. 1, pp. 55–9.

Chanock, Martin (1985) *Law, Custom and Social Order. The Colonial Experience of Zambia and Malawi*, Cambridge: Cambridge University Press.

Chatterjee, Indrani (1996) 'Regulating Slavery: Recontextualising the Contagious Diseases Acts in Bengal in the Nineteenth Century', paper delivered at the conference on Comparative Perspective on the History of Sexually Transmitted Diseases, Institute of Commonwealth Studies, University of London, 26–8 April.

Chirimuuta, Richard C. and Chirimuuta, Rosalind J. (1989) *AIDS, Africa and Racism*, London: Free Association Books.

Chisholm, Linda (1989) 'Reformatories and Industrial Schools in South Africa: A Study in Class, Colour and Gender, 1882–1939', D. Phil thesis, University of the Witwatersrand, Johannesburg.

Clarry, E. (1927) 'The Probation System and the Juvenile Delinquent. Supervision and Care of Juvenile Offenders', *The Social and Industrial Review*, vol. 3, no. 16, pp. 339–43.

Cobley, Alan (1995) 'The "Professionalisation" of Social Work among Blacks in South Africa to 1960', Institute of Commonwealth Studies, University of London: The Societies of Southern Africa seminar series, 7 June 1995.

Cockburn, A. (1963) *The Evolution and Eradication of Infectious Diseases*, Baltimore, MD: Johns Hopkins Press.

Coetzee, J. M. (1987) 'Blood, Flaw, Taint, Degeneration: The Case of Sarah Gertrude Millin', in Charles Malan (ed.), *Race and Literature* (Pinetown, South Africa), pp. 26–47.

Coetzee, J. M. (1988) *White Writing. On the Culture of Letters in South Africa*, London and New Haven: Yale University Press.

Coetzee, J. M. (1991) 'The Mind of Apartheid: Geoffrey Cronjé (1907–)', *Social Dynamics*, vol. 17, no. 1, pp. 1–35.

Cohen, Stanley (1972) *Folk Devils and Moral Panics. The Creation of the Mods and Rockers*, London: MacGibbon and Kee.

Comaroff, Jean and Comaroff, John (1991) *Of Revelation and Revolution. Christianity, Colonialism and Consciousness in South Africa*, vol. 1, Chicago and London: University of Chicago Press.

Coplan, David (1982) 'The Emergence of an African Working Class Culture', in Shula Marks and Richard Rathbone (eds), *Industrialisation and Social Change in South Africa. African Class Formation, Culture and Consciousness, 1870–1930*, London and New York: Longman, pp. 358–75.

Coplan, David (1985) *In the Township Tonight! South Africa's Black City Music and Theatre*, Johannesburg: Ravan Press.

Couzens, Tim (1982) 'Moralising Leisure Time: The Transatlantic Connection and Black Johannesburg 1918–1936', in Shula Marks and Richard Rathbone (eds), *Industrialisation and Social Change in South Africa. African Class Formation, Culture and Consciousness, 1870–1930*, London and New York: Longman, pp. 314–37.

Couzens, Tim (1985) *The New African. A Study of the Life and Work of H. I. E. Dhlomo*, Johannesburg: Ravan Press.

Crewe, Mary (1992) *AIDS in South Africa. The Myth and the Reality*, London: Penguin.

Cronjé, H. S., Joubert, G., Chapman, R. D., Divall, P. and Bam, R. H. (1994) 'Prevalence of Vaginitis, Syphilis and HIV Infection in Women in the Orange Free State', *South African Medical Journal*, vol. 84, no. 9, pp. 600–5.

Dangor, Y., Fehler, G., Exposto, F. da L. M. P. P., Koornhof, H. J. (1989) 'Causes and Treatment of Sexually Acquired Genital Ulceration in Southern Africa', *South African Medical Journal*, vol. 76, no. 7, pp. 339–41.

Danziger, Renee (1994) 'The Social Impact of HIV/AIDS in Developing Countries', *Social Science and Medicine*, vol. 39, no. 7, pp. 905–17.

Davenport, T. R. H. (1991) *South Africa. A Modern History*, 4th edn, London: Macmillan.

Davenport-Hines, Richard (1991) *Sex, Death and Punishment. Attitudes to Sex and Sexuality in Britain Since the Renaissance*, London: Fontana.

Davidson, Roger (1993) ' "A Scourge to be Firmly Gripped": The Campaign for VD Controls in Interwar Scotland', *Social History of Medicine*, vol. 6, no. 2, pp. 213–36.

Davies, Robert H. (1979) *Capital, State and White Labour in South Africa, 1900–1960: An Historical Materialist Analysis of Class Formation and Class Relations*, Brighton: Harvester.

Davin, Anna (1978) 'Imperialism and Motherhood', *History Workshop*, vol. 5, pp. 9–66.

Dawson, Marc (1983) 'Socio-Economic and Epidemiological Change in Kenya: 1880–1925', PhD thesis, University of Wisconsin-Madison.

Dawson, Marc (1987) 'The 1920s Anti-Yaws Campaigns and Colonial Policy in Kenya', *The International Journal of African Historical Studies*, vol. 20, no. 3, pp. 417–35.

Dawson, Marc (1988) 'AIDS in Africa: Historical Roots', in N. Miller and R. C. Rockwell (eds), *AIDS in Africa. The Social and Policy Impact*, Lewiston and Queenstown: Edwin Mellon Press, pp. 57–69.

Deacon, Harriet (1996) 'Racial Segregation and Medical Discourse in Nineteenth Century Cape Town', *Journal of Southern African Studies*, vol. 22, no. 2, pp. 287–309.

de Beer, Cedric (1984) *The South African Disease. Apartheid, Health and Health Services*, Johannesburg: SARS.

Decker, Jody (1996) 'Who Gave It To Whom? A Geographical Analysis of the Distribution and Impact of Venereal Disease on Natives and Non-Natives in the Western Interior of Canada in the 18th and 19th Centuries', paper presented at the conference on Comparative Perspectives on the History of Sexually Transmitted Diseases, Institute of Commonwealth Studies, University of London, 26–8 April 1996.

de Klerk, J. T. (1925) 'Gesellige Kamer vir Meisies wat Werk', *Die Huisgenoot*, vol. IX, no. 159, p. 27.

Delius, Peter (1980) 'Migrant Labour and the Pedi, 1840–1880', in Shula Marks and Antony Atmore (eds), *Economy and Society in Pre-Industrial South Africa*, London: Longman, pp. 293–312.

Delius, Peter (1989) ' "Sebatakgomo": Migrant Organisation, the ANC and the Sekhukhuneland Revolt', *Journal of Southern African Studies*, vol. 14, no. 4, pp. 581–615.

Department of National Health and Population Development (1995) 'AIDS in South Africa. Reported AIDS Cases as on 30 November 1995', *Epidemiological Comments*, vol. 22, no. 10, pp. 233–4.

Department of National Health and Population Development (1996) 'Sixth National HIV Survey of Women Attending Antenatal Clinics of the Public

Health Services in the Republic of South Africa, October/November 1995', *Epidemiological Comments*, vol. 23, no. 1, pp. 3–17.

de Vos Hugo, D. (1911) 'Syphilis', *South African Medical Record*, vol. 9, pp. 41–2.

de Vos Hugo, D. (1915) 'Syphilis or Yaws', *South African Medical Record*, vol. 13, pp. 107–9.

Dikobe, Modikwe (1973) *The Marabi Dance*, London: Heinemann.

Dogliotti, M. (1971) 'The Incidence of Syphilis in the Bantu: Survey of 587 Cases from Baragwanath Hospital', *South African Medical Journal*, vol. 45, pp. 8–10.

Doyle, Peter (1993) 'The Demographic Impact of AIDS on the South African Population' in Sholto Cross and Alan Whiteside (eds), *Facing Up To Aids*, London and Basingstoke: Macmillan, pp. 87–112.

Dubow, Saul (1987) 'Race, Civilisation and Culture: The Elaboration of Segregationist Discourse in the Interwar Years', in Shula Marks and Stanley Trapido (eds), *The Politics of Race, Class and Nationalism in Twentieth Century South Africa*, London and New York: Longman, pp. 71–94.

Dubow, Saul (1989) *Racial Segregation and the Origins of Apartheid in South Africa, 1919–1936*, London and Basingstoke: Macmillan.

Dubow, Saul (1991) 'Mental Testing and the Understanding of Race in Twentieth Century South Africa', in Teresa Meade and Moore Walker (eds), *Science, Medicine and Cultural Imperialism*, London and Basingstoke: Macmillan, pp. 148–77.

Dubow, Saul (1992) 'Afrikaner Nationalism, Apartheid and the Conceptualisation of "Race" ', *Journal of African History*, vol. 33, no. 2, pp. 209–38.

Dubow, Saul (1995) *Scientific Racism in Modern South Africa*, Cambridge: Cambridge University Press.

du Toit, J. A. (1969) 'Endemic Syphilis in the Karoo', *South African Medical Journal*, vol. 43, pp. 355–8.

Dyhouse, Carol (1981) 'Working Class Mothers and Infant Mortality in England, 1895–1914', in Charles Webster (ed.), *Biology, Medicine and Society 1840–1940*, Cambridge: Cambridge University Press, pp. 73–98.

Eales, Katherine (1989) 'Patriarchs, Passes and Privilege. Johannesburg's African Middle Classes and the Question of Night Passes for African Women', in Philip Bonner, Isabel Hofmeyr, Deborah James, Tom Lodge (eds), *Holding Their Ground*, Johannesburg: Witwatersrand University Press and Ravan Press, pp. 105–40.

Eales, Katherine Anne (1991) 'Gender Politics and the Administration of African Women in Johannesburg, 1903–1939', MA thesis, University of the Witwatersrand, Johannesburg.

Eckart, Wolfgang (1988) 'Medicine and German Colonial Expansion in the Pacific: the Caroline, Mariana, and Marshall Islands', in Roy MacLeod and Milton Lewis (eds), *Disease, Medicine and Empire. Perspectives on Western Medicine and the Experience of European Expansion*, London and New York: Routledge, pp. 80–102.

Elliot, G. A. (1950) 'The Future of Disease and Health in the Bantu', *The Leech*, vol. 21, no. 1, pp. 95–8.

Evans, David (1992) ' "Tackling the Hideous Scourge": The Creation of the Venereal Disease Centres in Early Twentieth Century Britain', *Social History of Medicine*, vol. 5, no. 3, pp. 413–35.

Evian, C. R., Jsselmuiden, C. B., Padayachee, G. N., Hurwitz, H. S. (1990) 'Qualitative Evaluation of an AIDS Health Education Poster', *South African Medical Journal*, vol. 78, no. 9, pp. 517–20.

Farrell, N. O., Hoosen, A. A., Kharsany, A. B. M. and van den Ende, J. (1989) 'Sexually Transmitted Pathogens in Pregnant Women in a Rural South African Community', *Genitourinary Medicine*, vol. 65, pp. 276–80.

Fee, Elizabeth (1988) 'Sin versus Science: Venereal Disease in Twentieth Century Baltimore', in Elizabeth Fox and Daniel M. Fox (eds), *AIDS. The Burden of History*, Berkeley: University of California Press, pp. 121–46.

Ferguson, D. L. (1932) 'The Urbanisation of the Bantu', *South African Medical Journal*, vol. 6, pp. 802–6.

Foucault, Michel (1980) *Michel Foucault. Power/Knowledge. Selected Interviews and Other Writings, 1972–1977*, ed. Colin Gordon, Brighton: Harvester.

Foucault, Michel (1987) *The History of Sexuality. An Introduction*, London: Penguin.

Foucault, Michel (1991) *Discipline and Punish. The Birth of the Prison*, London: Penguin (first published 1977).

Frack, Isidore (1943) *A South Africa Doctor Looks Backwards and Forwards*, South Africa: Central News Agency.

Fraser, A. Reith (1921) 'Some Practical Observations on the Treatment of Acute Gonococcal Urethritis in the Male, with a Note on Prophylaxis and a Bibliography, *South African Medical Record*, vol. 19, pp. 62–75.

Freed, Louis Franklin (1941) 'The Problem of European Prostitution in Johannesburg. A Sociological Survey', D.Philthesis, University of Pretoria.

Freed, Louis Franklin (1948) 'The Social Aspect of Venereal Disease', *The Leech*, vol. 19, no. 2, pp. 55–69.

Freed, Louis Franklin (1949) *The Problem of European Prostitution in Johannesburg. A Sociological Survey*, Cape Town and Johannesburg: Juta.

Gaitskell, Deborah (1982) ' "Wailing for Purity": Prayer Unions, African Mothers and Adolescent Daughters 1912–1940', in Shula Marks and Richard Rathbone (eds), *Industrialisation and Social Change in South Africa. African Class Formation, Culture and Consciousness, 1870–1930*, London and New York: Longman, pp. 338–57.

Gaitskell, Deborah (1983) 'Housewives, Maids or Mothers: Some Contradictions of Domesticity for Christian Women in Johannesburg, 1903–1939', *Journal of African History*, vol. 24, pp. 241–56.

Gaitskell, Deborah (1990) 'Devout Domesticity? A Century of African Women's Christianity in South Africa', in Cherryl Walker (ed.), *Women and Gender in Southern Africa to 1945*, Cape Town and London: David Phillip and James Currey, pp. 251–72.

Gaitskell, Deborah (1992) ' "Getting Close to the Hearts of Mothers": Medical Missionaries among African Women and Children in Johannesburg between the Wars', in V. Fildes, L. Marks and H. Marland (eds), *Women and Children First. International Maternal and Infant Welfare, 1870–1945*, London and New York: Routledge, pp. 178–202.

Gale, G. W. (1950) 'National Health and the Bantu', *The Leech*, vol. 21, no. 1, pp. 9–11.

Garrett, Laurie (1995) *The Coming Plague. Newly Emerging Diseases in a World out of Balance*, London: Virago Press.

Gaye, Judy (1980) 'Basotho Women's Options: A Study of Marital Careers in Rural Lesotho', PhD thesis, University of Cambridge.

Gelfand, Michael (1976) *A Service to the Sick. A History of Health Services for Africans in Southern Rhodesia (1890–1953)*, Gwelo: Mambo Press.

Giliomee, Hermann (1979) 'The Growth of Afrikaner Identity', in H. Adam and H. Giliomee (eds), *The Rise and Crisis of Afrikaner Power*, Cape Town: David Philip, pp. 83–127.

Giliomee, Hermann (1987) 'Western Cape Farmers and the Beginnings of Afrikaner Nationalism, 1870–1915', *Journal of Southern African Studies*, vol. 14, no. 1, pp. 38–63.

Giliomee, Hermann (1989a) 'Aspects of the Rise of Afrikaner Capital and Afrikaner Nationalism in the Western Cape, 1870–1915', in Wilmot James and Mary Simons (eds), *The Angry Divide. Social and Economic History of the Western Cape*, Cape Town and Johannesburg: David Philip in association with the Centre for African Studies, University of Cape Town, pp. 63–79.

Giliomee, Hermann (1989b) 'The Beginnings of Afrikaner Ethnic Consciousness, 1850–1915', in Leroy Vail (ed.), *The Creation of Tribalism in Southern Africa*, London: James Currey, pp. 21–54.

Gilman, Sander L. (1986) 'Black Bodies, White Bodies: Towards an Iconography of Female Sexuality in Late Nineteenth Century Art, Medicine, Literature', in Henry Louis Gates Jnr (ed.), *"Race", Writing and Difference*, Chicago, Ill.: University of Chicago Press, pp. 223–61.

Glaser, Clive (1990) 'The Mark of Zorro. Sexuality and Gender Relations in the Tsotsi Sub-Culture on the Witwatersrand, 1940–1960', History Workshop, University of the Witwatersrand, Johannesburg, 6–10 February 1990.

Gould, Stephen (1981) *The Mismeasure of Man*, London: Penguin.

Gray, J. L. (1937) 'Sterility and the Falling Birth-rate', *South African Medical Journal*, vol. 11, pp. 491–7.

Green, Edward C. (1992) 'Sexually Transmitted Disease, Ethnomedicine and Health Policy in Africa', *Social Science and Medicine*, vol. 35, no. 2, pp. 121–30.

Grek, I. J. (1950) 'Venereal Disease in the Bantu', *The Leech*, vol. 21, no. 1, pp. 70–72.

Grin, E. J. (1956) 'Endemic Syphilis and Yaws', *Bulletin of the World Health Organisation*, vol. 15, pp. 959–73.

Grosskopf, J. W. F. (1932) 'Economic Report. Rural Impoverishment and Rural Exodus', in *Report of the Carnegie Commission. The Poor White Problem in South Africa. Part 1*, Stellenbosch: Pro Ecclesia.

Gunn, G. H. (1948) 'Successful Method of Health Education for Africans', *The South African Health Magazine*, p. 2.

Hackett, C. J. (1953) 'Extent and Nature of the Yaws Problem in Africa', *World Health Monograph Series*, no. 15, First International Symposium on Yaws Control, pp. 129–82.

Hackett, C. J. (1957) 'The Transmission of Yaws in Nature', *Journal of Tropical Medicine and Hygiene*, vol. 60, pp. 159–68.

Hackett, C. J. (1963) 'On the Origin of the Human Treponematoses (Pinta, Yaws, Endemic Syphilis and Venereal Syphilis)', *Bulletin of the World Health Organisation*, vol. 29, pp. 7–41.

Hall, S. M. and Whitcomb, M. A. (1978) 'Screening for Gonorrhoea in Family Planning Acceptors in a Developing Community', *Public Health (London)*, vol. 92, pp. 121–4.

Hallett, R. (1979) 'Policemen, Pimps and Prostitutes – Public Morality and Police Corruption', in Christopher Saunders (ed.), *Studies in the History of Cape Town*, vol. 1, History Department, UCT, pp. 1–41.

Hansen, Karen Tranberg (1989) *Distant Companions. Servants and Employers in Zambia 1900–1985*, Ithaca and London: Cornell University Press.

Harries, Patrick (1982) 'Kinship, Ideology and the Nature of Pre-Colonial Labour Migration. Labour Migration from the Delagoa Bay Hinterland to South Africa up to 1895', in Shula Marks and Richard Rathbone (eds), *Industrialisation and Social Change in South Africa. African Class Formation, Culture and Consciousness, 1870–1930*, London and New York: Longman, pp. 142–66.

Harries, Patrick (1994) *Work, Culture and Identity. Migrant Labourers in Mozambique and South Africa, c. 1860–1910*, Portsmouth, NH: Heinemann; Johannesburg: Witwatersrand University Press; London: James Currey.

Hart, C. P. and Parnell, Susan (1989) 'Church, State and the Shelter of White Working Class Women in Johannesburg Prior to World War Two', *South African Geographical Journal*, vol. 71, no. 1, pp. 25–31.

Hellmann, Ellen (1934) 'The Importance of Beer Brewing in an Urban Native Yard', *Bantu Studies*, vol. 8, pp. 39–60.

Hellman, Ellen (1935) 'A Johannesburg Slumyard', *Africa*, vol. 8, pp. 34–62.

Hellmann, Ellen (1937) 'The Native in the Towns', in Isaac Schapera (ed.), *The Bantu Speaking Tribes of South Africa: An Ethnological Survey*, London: Routledge and Kegan Paul, pp. 405–34.

Hellmann, Ellen (1948) *Rooiyard. A Sociological Survey of an Urban Native Slum Yard*, Rhodes-Livingstone Papers no. 13, Cape Town: Oxford University Press.

Higgins, T. Shadick (1929) 'Present Day Public Health Problems', *Journal of the Medical Association of South Africa*, vol. 3, pp. 299–303.

Higgins, T. Shadick (1935) 'The Housing Problem with Special Reference to the Slums Act', *South African Medical Journal*, vol. 9, pp. 527–30.

Hilton Barber, S. (trans.) (1907) *The Laws and Regulations etc etc Specially Relating to the Native Population of the Transvaal*, Pretoria: NAD.

Hilton Barber, S., Macfadyen, W. A. and Findlay, J. H. L. (trans.) (1901) *Laws, Volksraad Resolutions, Proclamations and Government Notices Relating to Natives and Coolies in the Transvaal*, Pretoria: Government Printing Works.

Hindson, Doug (1987) *Pass Controls and the Urban African Proletariat*, Johannesburg: Ravan Press.

Hobson, Barbara Meil (1987) *Uneasy Virtue. The Politics of Prostitution and the American Reform Tradition*, New York: Basic Books.

Hofmeyr, Isabel (1987) 'Building a Nation from Words: Afrikaans Language, Literature and Ethnic Identity, 1902–1924', in Shula Marks and Stanley Trapido (eds), *The Politics of Race, Class and Nationalism in Twentieth Century South Africa*, London and New York: Longman, pp. 95–123.

Hoosen, A. A., Ross, S. M., Mulla, M. J. and Patel, M. (1981) 'The Incidence of Selected Vaginal Infections Among Pregnant Urban Blacks', *South African Medical Journal*, vol. 59, pp. 827–9.

Hudson, E. H. (1965) 'Treponematosis and Man's Social Evolution', *American Anthropologist*, vol. 67, pp. 885–901.

Human Sciences Research Council (HSRC) (1987) *Dictionary of South African Biography*, vol. 5, Pretoria: HSRC.

Humphries, S. V. (1938a) 'Bantu Syphilis', *South African Medical Journal*, vol. 12, p. 630.

Humphries, S. V. (1938b) 'Syphilis – A Major Cause of Ill-Health in Native Labourers and Suggestions for Mass Treatment', *Proceedings of the Transvaal Mine Medical Officers' Association*, vol. XVIII, nos 201, 202, pp. 121–35.

Hunt, Charles W. (1989) 'Migrant Labour and Sexually Transmitted Disease: AIDS in Africa', *Journal of Health and Social Behaviour*, vol. 30, pp. 353–73.

Hunter, Monica (1932) 'Results of Culture Contact on the Pondo and Xhosa Family', *South African Journal of Science*, vol. XXIX, pp. 681–6.

Hunter, Monica (1961) *Reaction to Conquest. Effects of Contact with Europeans on the Pondo of South Africa*, London: Oxford University Press (first published 1936).

Ijsselmuiden, C. B., Steinberg, M. H., Padayachee, G. N., Schoub, B. I., Strauss, S. A., Buch, E., Davies, J. C. A., de Beer, C., Gear, J. S. S. and Hurwitz, H. S. (1988) 'AIDS and South Africa – Towards a Comprehensive Strategy. Part 1', *South African Medical Journal*, vol. 73, no. 8, pp. 455–60.

Ijsselmuiden, C. B., Padayachee, G. N., Mashaba, W., Martiny, O., van Staden, H. P. (1990) 'Knowledge, Beliefs and Practices among Black Gold Miners Relating to the Transmission of Human Immunodeficiency Virus and Other Sexually Transmitted Diseases', *South African Medical Journal*, vol. 78, no. 9, pp. 520–3.

Jacobus, Mary, Keller, E. Fox and Shuttleworth, Sally (1990) *Body/Politics: Women and the Discourses of Science*, New York and London: Routledge.

Janisch, M. (1941) 'Some Administrative Aspects of Native Marriage Problems in an Urban Area', *Bantu Studies*, vol. XV, pp. 1–11.

Jeeves, A. (1975) 'The Control of Migratory Labour on the South African Gold Mines in the Era of Kruger and Milner', *Journal of Southern African Studies*, vol. 2, no. 1, pp. 3–29.

Jeeves, Alan H. (1985) *Migrant Labour in South Africa's Mining Economy. The Struggle for the Gold Mines' Labour Supply 1890–1920*, Johannesburg: Witwatersrand University Press.

Jochelson, Karen (1991) 'HIV and Syphilis in South Africa: The Creation of an Epidemic', *African Urban Quarterly*, vol. 6, nos 1, 2, pp. 20–35.

Jochelson, Karen (1993), 'The Colour of Disease: Syphilis and Racism in South Africa, 1910–1950', D.Phil thesis, University of Oxford.

Jochelson, Karen (1995) 'Review Article – Women, Migrancy and Morality: A Problem of Perspective', *Journal of Southern African Studies*, vol. 21, no. 2, pp. 323–2.

Jochelson, Karen, Mothibeli, Monyaela and Leger, Jean (1991) 'Human Immunodeficiency Virus and Migrant Labour in South Africa', *International Journal of Health Services*, vol. 21, no. 1, pp. 157–73.

Johannesburg Housing Utility Company (JHUC) (1933/34?), *To Hell With Slums*, Johannesburg: JHUC.

Jones, Greta (1980) *Social Darwinism and English Thought. The Interaction between Biological and Social Theory*, Sussex: Harvester Press.

Jones, James H. (1981) *Bad Blood: The Tuskegee Syphilis Experiment*, New York: Free Press.

Junod, Henri A. (1962) *The Life of a South African Tribe*, vol. 2, New York, University Books (first published 1912, revised 1926).

Jurriaanse, A. (1935) 'Degeneration and its Remedy', *South African Medical Journal*, vol. 9, pp. 704–13.

Kagan, N. (1978) *African Settlements in the Johannesburg Area 1903–1923*, MA thesis, University of the Witwatersrand, Johannesburg.

Karim, S. S. Abdool (1993) 'Traditional Healers and AIDS Prevention', *South African Medical Journal*, vol. 83, no. 6, pp. 423–5.

Kark, Sidney L. (1949) 'The Social Pathology of Syphilis in Africans', *South African Medical Journal*, vol. 23, pp. 77–84.

Kark, Sidney L. (1950) 'The Influence of Urban–Rural Migration on Bantu Health and Disease', *The Leech*, vol. 21, no. 1, pp. 23–37.

Kark, Sidney L. (1954) 'Patterns of Health and Nutrition in South African Bantu being an Account of Investigations into the Relationship between Their State of Health and Way of Life and the Application of These Findings in the Development of a Family Health Project', thesis, University of Witwatersrand Medical School.

Katz, Elaine (1994) 'The Doctors' Dilemma. The Health Care of Workers on the Witwatersrand Gold Mines, 1892–1910', Institute of Advanced Social Research, University of the Witwatersrand, seminar paper no. 361.

Katzenellenbogen, S. E. (1980) 'Reconstruction in the Transvaal', in P. Warwick (ed.), *The South African War. The Anglo-Boer War, 1899–1902*, Harlow: Longman, pp. 341–61.

Keegan, Timothy (1987) *Rural Transformations in Industrialising South Africa. The Southern Highveld to 1914*, Basingstoke: Macmillan.

Kennedy, Dane (1987) *Islands of White. Settler Society and Culture in Kenya and Southern Rhodesia, 1890–1939*, Durham: Duke University Press.

Kimble, J. (1982) 'Labour Migration in Basutoland, c. 1870–1885', in Shula Marks and Richard Rathbone (eds), *Industrialisation and Social Change in South Africa*, London: Longman, pp. 119–41.

Klausen, Susanne (1997) ' "For the Sake of the Race": Eugenic Discourses of Feeblemindedness and Motherhood in the South African Medical Record, 1903–1926', *Journal of South African Studies*, vol. 23, no. 1, pp. 27–50.

Koch, Eddie (1983) ' "Without Visible Means of Subsistence": Slumyard Culture in Johannesburg 1918–1940', in Belinda Bozzoli (ed.), *Town and Countryside in the Transvaal*, Johannesburg: Ravan Press, pp. 151–75.

Krige, E. J. (1936) 'Changing Conditions in Marital Relations and Parental Duties Among Urbanised Natives', *Africa*, vol. 9, pp. 1–23.

Krige, E. J. (1937) 'Individual Development', in Isaac Schapera (ed.), *The Bantu Speaking Tribes of South Africa. An Ethnological Survey*, London: Routledge and Kegan Paul, pp. 95–118.

Kuhn, Annette (1985) *The Power of the Image: Essays on Representation and Sexuality*, London: Routledge.

Kuklick, Henrika (1984) 'Tribal Exemplars: Images of Political Authority in British Anthropology, 1885–1945', in George W. Stocking (ed.), *Functionalism Historicised. Essays on British Social Anthropology*, Wisconsin and London: University of Wisconsin Press, pp. 59–82.

Kuklick, Henrika (1992) *The Savage Within. The Social History of British Anthropology 1885–1945*, Cambridge: Cambridge University Press.

Kuper, Adam (1983) *Anthropology and Anthropologists. The Modern British School*, London and New York: Routledge & Kegan Paul.

Kuper, Hilda (1984) 'Function, History, Biography: Reflections on Fifty Years in the British Anthropological Tradition', in George W. Stocking (ed.), *Functionalism Historicised. Essays on British Social Anthropology*, Wisconsin and London: University of Wisconsin Press, pp. 192–213.

Laidler, P. W. (1934) 'The Practice of Eugenics', *South African Medical Journal*, vol. 8, pp. 823–34.

Laidler, P. W. (1938) 'The Unholy Triad: Tuberculosis, Venereal Disease, Malnutrition', *South African Medical Journal*, vol. 12, pp. 658–66.

Laidler, Percy Ward (1971) *South Africa and Its Medical History, 1652–1898. A Medical and Social Study*, Cape Town: C. Struik.

Lees, Andrew (1985) *Cities Perceived. Urban Society in European and American Thought, 1820–1940*, Manchester: Manchester University Press.

le Hausse, Paul (1984) 'The Struggle for the City: Alcohol, the Ematsheni and Popular Culture in Durban, 1902–1936', MA thesis, University of Cape Town.

Leipoldt, C. Louis (1920) 'Venereal Disease in Transvaal School Children', *Medical Journal of South Africa*, vol. XVI, pp. 25–31.

Leipoldt, C. Louis (1937) *Bushveld Doctor*, London: Jonathan Cape.

Levin, Ruth (1947) 'Marriage in Langa Native Location', Communications from the School of African Studies, *New Series*, no. 17.

Levine, Phillipa (1994) 'Venereal Disease, Prostitution and the Politics of Empire: the Case of British India', *Journal of the History of Sexuality*, vol. 4, no. 4, pp. 579–602.

Lewis, Jon (1984) *Industrialisation and Trade Union Organisation in South Africa, 1924–1955. The Rise and Fall of the South African Trades and Labour Council*, Cambridge: Cambridge University Press.

Livingstone, David (1857) *Missionary Travels and Researches in South Africa*, London.

Lorimer, Douglas A. (1978) *Colour, Class and the Victorians. English Attitudes to the Negro in the Mid-Nineteenth Century*, Leicester: Leicester University Press.

Mager, Anne (1996) 'Sexuality, Fertility and Male Power in the Eastern Cape, 1945–1959', The Societies of Southern Africa Seminar Series, Institute of Commonwealth Studies, University of London, 7 November.

Maloka, Tshidiso (1994) '"Khomo Lia Oela": "Canteens", Brothels and Labour Migrancy in Colonial Lesotho, 1900–1940', unpublished paper.

Manderson, Leonore (1997) 'Migration, Prostitution and Medical Surveillance in Early 20th Century Malaya', in L. Marks and M. Worboys (eds), *Migrants, Minorities and Health: Historical and Contemporary Studies*, London: Routledge, pp. 49–69.

Marcovich, Anne (1988) 'French Colonial Medicine and Colonial Rule: Algeria and Indochina', in Roy MacLeod and Milton Lewis (eds), *Disease, Medicine and Empire. Perspectives on Western Medicine and the Experience of European Expansion*, London and New York: Routledge, pp. 103–17.

Marks, Shula (1987) *Not Either An Experimental Doll*, London: The Women's Press.

Marks, Shula (1989) 'Patriotism, Patriarchy and Purity: Natal and the Politics of Zulu Ethnic Consciousness', in Leroy Vail (ed.), *The Creation of Tribalism in Southern Africa*, London, Berkeley and Los Angeles: James Curry and University of California Press, pp. 215–40.

Marks, Shula and Andersson, Neil (1984) 'Epidemics and Social Control in Twentieth Century South Africa', *The Society for the Social History of Medicine Bulletin*, vol. 34, pp. 32–4.

Marks, Shula and Andersson, Neil (1985) 'Diseases of Apartheid', in John Lonsdale (ed.), *South Africa in Question*, London: Cambridge African Studies Centre with James Currey, pp. 172–99.

Marks, Shula and Andersson, Neil (1988) 'Typhus and Social Control: South Africa, 1917–1950', in Roy MacLeod and Milton Lewis (eds), *Disease, Medicine and Empire. Perspectives on Western Medicine and the Experience of European Expansion*, London and New York: Routledge, pp. 257–83.

Marks, Shula and Andersson, Neil (1992) 'Industrialisation, Rural Change and the 1944 National Health Services Commission', in Stephen Feierman and John Janzen (eds), *The Social Basis of Health and Healing in Africa*, Berkeley: University of California Press, pp. 131–61.

Marks, Shula and Trapido, Stanley (1981) 'Lord Milner and the South African State', in Phillip Bonner (ed.), *Working Papers in Southern African Studies*, vol. 2, Johannesburg: Ravan Press, pp. 52–96.

Marks, Shula and Trapido, Stanley (eds) (1987) 'Introduction: The Politics of Race, Class and Nationalism', in *The Politics of Race, Class and Nationalism in Twentieth Century South Africa*, London and New York: Longman, pp. 1–70.

Martino, O. (1987) 'Prostitutes', paper presented at the AIDS Congress, Strategies for Southern Africa '88, Johannesburg, 29 April–1 May 1988.

Mathews, C., Kuhn, L., Metcalf, C. A., Joubert, G., Cameron, N. A. (1990) 'Knowledge, Attitudes and Beliefs about AIDS in Township School Students in Cape Town', *South African Medical Journal*, vol. 78, no. 9, pp. 511–16.

Mathias, J. (1910) 'Syphilis or Yaws', *South African Medical Record*, vol. VIII, no. 9, pp. 102–5.

Mathias, J. (1911) 'Correspondence – Syphilis and Yaws', *South African Medical Record*, vol. 9, pp. 64, 128, 174.

Mayer, Phillip (1980) 'The Origin and Decline of Two Rural Resistance Ideologies', in Phillip Mayer (ed.), *Black Villagers in an Industrial Society. Anthropological Perspectives on Labour Migration in South Africa*, Cape Town: Oxford University Press, pp. 1–80.

Maylam, Paul (1983) 'The "Black Belt": African Squatters in Durban, 1935–1950', *Canadian Journal of African Studies*, vol. 17, no. 3, pp. 413–28.

Maylam, Paul (1990) 'The Local Evolution of Urban Apartheid: Influx Control and Segregation in Durban c. 1900–1951', History Workshop Conference, University of Witwatersrand, 6–10 February.

McArthur, D. C. and Thornton, E. N. (1910) 'Native Syphilis in the Northern Districts: Its Menace to Public Health', *Transactions of the SA Medical Congress 12th Meeting, Cape Town, 31 October–5 November 1910*, Cape Town: Townshend, Taylor, Snashall, pp. 160–72.

McArthur, D. C. and Thornton, E. N. (1911) 'Native Syphilis in the Northern Districts: Its Menace to Public Health', *South African Medical Record*, vol. 9, pp. 18–30.

McNeil, K. B. A. (1935) 'Are We Making the Best of Our Future Citizens in South Africa from the Time of Conception?', *South African Medical Journal*, vol. 9, pp. 741–54.

Melle, G. J. M. (1935) 'Letter: Epidemic Syphilis', *South African Medical Journal*, vol. 9, p. 56.

Millar, J. G. (1909) 'A Medical Aspect of the Native Labour Question', *South African Medical Record*, vol. 7, pp. 163–5.

Miller, Roberta Balstad (1993) 'Science and Society in the Early Career of H. F. Verwoerd', *Journal of Southern African Studies*, vol. 19, no. 4, pp. 654–61.

Miller, Roberta Balstad (1994) 'Science, Sociology and Social Engineering: South Africa in the 1930s', paper presented at the Journal of Southern African Studies conference on 'Paradigms Lost, Paradigms Regained? Southern African Studies in the 1990s', University of York, September 1994.

Mitchell, J. A. (1921) 'The Problem of Venereal Disease. Address Given at Annual Conference of the Transvaal Branch of the National Society for Combating VD, Johannesburg, 24 February 1921', *South African Medical Record*, vol. 19, pp. 122–4.

Moodie, T. Dunbar (1983) 'Mine Culture and Miners' Identity on the South African Gold Mines', in Belinda Bozzoli (ed.), *Town and Countryside in the Transvaal*, Johannesburg: Ravan Press, pp. 176–97.

Moodie, T. Dunbar (1988) 'Migrancy and Male Sexuality on the South African Gold Mines', *Journal of Southern African Studies*, vol. 14, no. 2, pp. 228–56.

Moroney, Sean (1982) 'Mine Married Quarters: The Differential Stabilisation of the Witwatersrand Workforce, 1900–1920', in S. Marks and R. Rathbone (eds), *Industrialisation and Social Change in South Africa. African Class Formation, Culture and Consciousness, 1870–1930*, London and New York: Longman, pp. 259–69.

Morris, Alan G. (1988) 'Comments on Baker and Armelagos', *Current Anthropology*, vol. 29, no. 5, pp. 723–4.

Mort, Frank (1987) *Dangerous Sexualities: Medico-Moral Politics in England Since 1830*, London and New York: Routledge and Kegan Paul.

Mostert, N. (1992) *Frontiers: The Epic of South Africa's Creation and the Tragedy of the Xhosa People*, London: Cape.

Murray, Colin (1981) *Families Divided. The Impact of Migrant Labour in Lesotho*, Cambridge: Cambridge University Press.

Murray, J. F. (1957) 'Endemic Syphilis or Yaws? A Review of the Literature from South Africa', *South African Medical Journal*, vol. 31, pp. 821–4.

Murray, J. F., Merriweather, A. M. and Freedman, M. L. (1956) 'Endemic Syphilis in the Bakwena Reserve of the Bechuanaland Protectorate: A Report on Mass Examination and Treatment', *Bulletin of the World Health Organisation*, no. 15, pp. 975–1039.

Nicolson, M. (1988) 'Medicine and Racial Politics: Changing Images of the New Zealand Maori in the Nineteeth Century', in David Arnold (ed.), *Imperial Medicine and Indigenous Societies*, Manchester and New York: Manchester University Press, pp. 66–104.

Odendaal, A. (1984) *Vukani Bantu! The Beginnings of Black Protest Politics in South Africa to 1912*, Cape Town and Johannesburg: David Philip in association with the Centre for African Studies at the UCT.

O'Malley, C. K. (1940) 'Syphilis in South Africa', *South African Medical Journal*, vol. 14, p. 459.

Oosthuizen, O. J. (1929) 'On Biological and Economic Concepts', *Journal of the Medical Association of South Africa*, vol. 3, pp. 131–5.

Packard, Randall M. (1987) 'Tuberculosis and the Development of Industrial Health Policies on the Witwatersrand, 1902–1932', *Journal of Southern African Studies*, vol. 13, no. 2, pp. 185–209.

Packard, Randall M. (1989) *White Plague, Black Labour: Tuberculosis and the Political Economy of Health and Disease in South Africa*, Berkeley and Los Angeles: University of California Press.

Palmer, Mabel (1931) 'The Economic Position of the Native', *The Natal Missionary Conference Annual Report, 1931*, p. 49.

Panos Dossier (1988) *AIDS and the Third World*, 3rd edn, London, Paris and Washington: Panos.

Parnell, Susan (1987) *'Council Housing for Whites in Johannesburg, 1920–1955'*, MA thesis, University of the Witwatersrand, Johannesburg.

Parnell, Susan (1988) 'Public Housing as a Device for White Residential Segregation in Johannesburg, 1934–1953', *Urban Geography*, vol. 9, no. 6, pp. 584–602.

Parnell, Susan (1989) 'Shaping a Racially Divided Society: State Housing Policy in South Africa, 1920–1950', *Environment and Planning C: Government and Policy*, vol. 7, pp. 261–72.

Parnell, Susan (1993) 'Creating Racial Privilege: The Origins of South African Public Health and Town Planning Legislation', *Journal of Southern African Studies*, vol. 19, no. 3, pp. 471–88.

Parry, Richard (1983) 'In a Sense Citizens, But Not Altogether Citizens.... Rhodes, Race and the Ideology of Segregation at the Cape in the Late Nineteenth Century', *Canadian Journal of African Studies*, vol. 17, no. 3, pp. 377–91.

Parsons, Rosy (1988) 'Social Implications of Sexually Transmitted Diseases in South Africa in the First Half of the Twentieth Century (with Special Reference to Natal)', MA thesis, Institute for Commonwealth Studies, University of London.

Perine, P. L., Hopkins, P. R., Niemal, P. L. A., St John, R. K., Causse, G. and Antal, G. M. (1984) *Handbook of Endemic Treponematoses: Yaws, Endemic Syphilis, and Pinta*, Geneva: World Health Organisation.

Perks, W. (1925) 'Die Sosiale Probleem van Vrouearbeid', *Die Huisgenoot*, vol. IX, no. 168, pp. 32–3.

Philip, Howard (1987) 'The Local State and Public Health Reform in South Africa: Bloemfontein and the Consequences of the Spanish 'Flu Epidemic of 1918', *Journal of Southern African Studies*, vol. 13, no. 2, pp. 210–33.

Philip, Howard (1990) *'Black October': the Impact of the Spanish Influenza Epidemic of 1918 on South Africa*, Pretoria: Government Printer.

Phillips, Ray E. (1938) *The Bantu in The City. A Study of Cultural Adjustment on the Witwatersrand*, Cape Town: The Lovedale Press.

Pijper, A. (1919) 'Damaged Goods', *South African Medical Record*, vol. 17, pp. 323–5.

Pijper, Adrianus (1921) 'Syphilis Among the Coloured Population of Pretoria: A Record of 500 Wassermann Reactions', *South African Medical Record*, vol. 19, pp. 302–5.

Pitje, G. M. (1950a) 'Traditional Systems of Male Education Among Pedi and Cognate Tribes, Part II', *African Studies*, vol. 9, pp. 105–24.

Pitje, G. M. (1950b) 'Traditional Systems of Male Education Among Pedi and Cognate Tribes, Part III', *African Studies*, vol. 9, pp. 194–201.

Pollak, Hansi (1932) 'Women in Witwatersrand Industries: An Economic and Sociological Study', MA thesis, University of the Witwatersrand, Johannesburg.

Porter, Charles (1920) 'The Municipal Treatment of Venereal Diseases', *South African Medical Record*, vol. 18, pp. 153–5.

Porter, Dorothy (1991) ' "Enemies of the Race": Biologism, Environmentalism, and Public Health in Edwardian England', *Victorian Studies*, vol. 34, pp. 159–78.

Porter Mathew G. (1920) 'Woman's Responsibility to the Health of the Nation' (presidential address to the Eastern Province Branch of the BMA), *South African Medical Record*, vol. 18, pp. 109–11.

Posel, Deborah (1991) *The Making of Apartheid 1948–61. Conflict and Compromise*, Oxford: Clarendon Press.

Proctor, André (1979) 'Class Struggle, Segregation and the City: A History of Sophiatown, 1905–1940', in Belinda Bozzoli (ed.), *Labour, Townships and Protest: Studies in the Social History of the Witwatersrand*, Johannesburg: Ravan Press, pp. 49–89.

Purcell, F. W. F. (1940) 'Syphilis in South Africa', *South African Medical Journal*, vol. 14, pp. 453–6.

Rauch, J. H. and Saayman, L. R. (1938) 'Native Syphilis', *South African Medical Journal*, vol. 12, p. 885.

Redding, Sean (1987) 'The Making of a South African Town: Social and Economic Change in Umtata, 1870–1950', PhD thesis, Yale University.

Rich, Paul (1980) 'The Origins of Apartheid Ideology: The Case of Ernest Stubbs and Transvaal Native Admininstration, c. 1902–1932', *African Affairs*, vol. LXXIX, no. 315, pp. 171–94.

Richardson, P. and van Helten, J.-J. (1980) 'The Gold Mining Industry in the Transvaal, 1886–99', in P. Warwick (ed.), *The South African War. The Anglo-Boer War, 1899–1902*, Harlow: Longman, pp. 18–36.

Richardson, P. and van-Helten, J.-J. (1982) 'Labour in the South African Gold Mining Industry, 1886–1914', in S. Marks and R. Rathbone (eds), *Industrialisation and Social Change in South Africa. African Class Formation, Culture and Consciousness 1870–1930*, London: Longman, pp. 77–98.

Ricono, M. (1911) 'Syphilis and Yaws', *South African Medical Record*, vol. 9, pp. 215–16.

Ricono, M. (1916) 'Yaws and Similar Diseases in South Africa', *South African Medical Record*, vol. 14, pp. 83–9.

Rothmann, M. E. (1932) 'Sociological Report b). The Mother and Daughter in the Poor Family', in *Report of the Carnegie Commission. The Poor White Problem in South Africa. Part V*, Stellenbosch: Pro Ecclesia.

Rothschild, Bruce, Rothschild, Christine, Henneberg, Maciej and Henneberg, Renata (1996) 'Clarification of the Endemic Non-Venereal South African Treponematosis: Osseous Evidence for Yaws', unpublished paper.

Roux, Edward (1948) *Time Longer than Rope. A History of the Black Man's Struggle for Freedom in South Africa*, London: Victor Gollancz.

Russell, Bertrand (1988) *Marriage and Morals*, London: Unwin (first published 1929).

Russett, Cynthia Eagle (1991) *Sexual Science. The Victorian Construction of Womanhood*, Cambridge, Mass. and London: Harvard University Press.

Sax, S. (1952) 'The Introduction of Syphilis into the Bantu Peoples of South Africa', *South African Medical Journal*, vol. 26, pp. 1037–9.

Schapera, Isaac (1933) 'Premarital Pregnancy and Native Opinion. A Note on Social Change', *Africa*, vol. 6, pp. 59–89.

Schapera, Isaac (ed.) (1934) 'The Present State and Future Development of Ethnographical Research in South Africa', *Bantu Studies*, vol. VII, pp. 219–342.

Schapera, Isaac (1947) *Migrant Labour and Tribal Life*, London, New York and Cape Town: Oxford University Press.

Schreuder, D. M. (1976) 'The Cultural Factor in Victorian Imperialism: A Case-Study of the British "Civilising Mission" ', *Journal of Imperial and Commonwealth History*, vol. IV, no. 3, pp. 283–317.

Scott, C. J. (1933) 'Yaws', *Proceedings of the Transvaal Mine Medical Officers Association*, vol. XIL, no. 139, pp. 41–61.

Scott, C. J. (1939) 'Yaws. A Further Report on the Robinson Deep Occurrence', *Proceedings of the Transvaal Mine Medical Officers Association*, vol. XVIII, no. 206, pp. 151–5.

Scott, F. P. and Lups, J. G. H. (1973) 'Endemiese Sifilis', *South African Medical Journal* , vol. 47, pp. 1347–50.

Searle, G. R. (1976) *Eugenics and Politics in Britain, 1900–1914*, Leyden: Noordhoff.

Segal, Lauren (1989) 'Mines, Migrants and Women: Strike Action and Labour Unrest on the Witbank Collieries from 1940–1950', BA dissertation, History Department, University of the Witwatersrand.

Shillington, Kevin (1982) 'The Impact of the Diamond Discoveries on the Kimberley Hinterland', in Shula Marks and Richard Rathbone (eds), *Industrialisation and Social Change in South Africa. African Class Formation, Culture and Consciousness, 1870–1930*, London and New York: Longman, pp. 99–118.

Shropshire, D. W. T. (1970) *Primitive Marriage and European Law. A South African Investigation*, London: Frank Cass (first published 1946).

Simkins, C. (1981) 'Agricultural Production in the African Reserves of South Africa, 1918–69', *Journal of Southern African Studies*, vol. 7, no. 2, pp. 256–83.

Simons, H. J. (1968) *African Women. Their Legal Status in South Africa*, London: C. Hurst.

Simons, Jack and Simons, Ray (1983) *Class and Colour in South Africa, 1850–1950*, London: International Defence and Aid Fund for South Africa.

Soloway, Richard Allen (1982a) *Birth Control and the Population Question in England 1877–1930*, London: University of North Carolina Press.

Soloway, Richard (1982b) 'Counting the Degenerates: the Statistics of Race Deterioration in Edwardian England', *Journal of Contemporary History*, vol. 17, pp. 137–64.

Sontag, Susan (1988) *AIDs and Its Metaphors*, London: Penguin.

Stals, E. L. P. (ed.) (1986) *Afrikaners in die Goudstad. Deel 2 1924–1961*, Pretoria: HAUM Opvoedkundige Uitgewery.

Stepan, Nancy (1982) *The Idea of Race in Science: Great Britain 1800–1960*, London: Macmillan.

Stepan, Nancy Leys (1991) *The Hour of Eugenics. Race, Gender and Nation in Latin America*, Ithaca and London: Cornell University Press.

Steyn, Maryna and Henneberg, Maciej (1995) 'Pre-Columbian Presence of Treponemal Disease: A Possible Case from Iron Age Southern Africa', *Current Anthropology*, vol. 36, no. 5, pp. 869–73.

Stocking, George W. (ed.) (1984) 'Radcliffe-Brown and British Social Anthropology', in *Functionalism Historicised. Essays on British Social Anthropology*, Wisconsin and London: University of Wisconsin Press, pp. 131–91.

Stoler, Ann Laura (1989) 'Rethinking Colonial Categories: European Communities and the Boundaries of Rule', *Comparative Studies in Society and History*, vol. 31, pp. 134–61.

Stoler, Ann Laura (1991) 'Carnal Knowledge and Imperial Power. Gender, Race and Morality in Colonial Asia', in Micaela di Leonardo (ed.), *Gender at the Crossroads of Knowledge. Feminist Anthropology in the Postmodern Era*, Berkeley, Los Angeles and Oxford: University of California Press, pp. 51–101.

Stone, Mitchell S. (1993) 'The Victorian Army: Health, Hospitals and Social Conditions as Encountered by British Troops During the South African War, 1899–1902', D.Phil thesis, University of London.

Streak, Michael (1974) *The Afrikaner as Viewed by the English, 1795–1854*, Cape Town: C. Struik.

Swanson, Maynard (1977) 'The Sanitation Syndrome: Bubonic Plague and the Urban Native Policy in the Cape Colony, 1900–1909', *Journal of African History*, vol. XVIII, no. 3, pp. 387–410.

Swanson, Maynard (1983) '"The Asiatic Menace": Creating Segregation in Durban, 1870–1900', *International Journal of African Historical Studies*, vol. 16, no. 3, pp. 401–21.

Swartz, Sally (1995) 'The Black Insane in the Cape, 1891–1920', *Journal of Southern African Studies*, vol. 21, no. 3, pp. 399–416.

Taylor, A. B. (1931) 'Medical Needs in Urban Areas', *The Natal Missionary Conference Annual Report, 1931*, pp. 53–6.

Taylor, W. N. (1954) 'Endemic Syphilis in a South African Coloured Community', *South African Medical Journal*, vol. 28, pp. 176–8.

Tobias, J. M. (1944) 'The Problem of Venereal Disease in the Transkei', *South African Medical Journal*, vol. 18, pp. 142–4.

Tonkin, Dorothy (1926) 'Welfare of Girl Workers', *The Social and Industrial Review*, vol. 2, no. 6, pp. 414–7.

Towers, Bridget (1980) 'Health Education Policy 1916–1926: Venereal Disease and the Prophylaxis Dilemma', *Medical History*, vol. 24, pp. 70–87.

Trapido, Stanley (1980) 'The Friends of the Natives: Merchants, Peasants and the Political and Ideological Structure of Liberalism in the Cape, 1854–1910', in Shula Marks and Antony Atmore (eds), *Economy and Society in Pre-Industrial South Africa*, London and New York: Longman, pp. 247–74.

Turner, G. A. (1915) 'Circumcision Amongst Natives', *Medical Journal of South Africa*, vol. 10, pp. 133–8.

Turrell, Rob (1987) *Capital and Labour on the Kimberley Diamond Fields, 1871–1890*, Cambridge: Cambridge University Press.

van Beukering, J. A. (1965) 'Endemic Extravenereal Treponematosis in the North of the Cape Province', *Tropical and Geographical Medicine*, vol. 17, no. 1, pp. 40–4.

van Heerden, Petronella (1925) ''n Moederskapleergang Op Ons Universiteite', *Die Huisgenoot*, vol. X, no. 191, pp. 35, 37, 43.

van Heyningen, Elizabeth (1984) 'The Social Evil in the Cape Colony 1868–1902: Prostitution and the Contagious Diseases Acts', *Journal of Southern African Studies*, vol. 10, no. 2, pp. 170–97.

van Heyningen, E. B. (1989) 'Agents of Empire: The Medical Profession in the Cape Colony, 1880–1910', *Medical History*, vol. 33, pp. 450–71.

van Heyningen, Elizabeth (1991) 'Poverty, Self-Help and Community: The Survival of the Poor in Cape Town, 1880–1910', *South African Historical Journal*, vol. 24, pp. 128–43.

van Niekerk, Andrea (1988) 'The Use of White Female Labour by the Zebedelia Citrus Estate 1926–1953', MA thesis, University of the Witwatersrand.

van Onselen, Charles (1982a) *Studies in the Social and Economic History of the Witwatersrand 1886–1914. Vol. 1. New Babylon*, Johannesburg: Ravan Press.

van Onselen, Charles (1982b) *Studies in the Social and Economic History of the Witwatersrand 1886–1914. Vol 2. New Nineveh*, Johannesburg: Ravan Press.

Vaughan, Megan (1991) *Curing Their Ills. Colonial Power and African Illness*, Cambridge: Polity Press.

Vaughan, Megan (1992) 'Syphilis in East and Central Africa: The Social Construction of an Epidemic', in Terence Ranger and Paul Slack (eds), *Epidemics and Ideas: Essays on the Historical Perception of Pestilence*, Cambridge: Cambridge University Press, pp. 269–302.

Venter, A., Pettifor, J. M., Exposto, F. da L. M. P. P. Sefuba, M. (1989) 'Congenital Syphilis – Who Is At Risk? A Prevalence Study at Baragwanath Hospital, Johannesburg, 1985–1986, *South African Medical Journal*, vol. 76, pp. 93–5.

Walker, Cherryl (ed.) (1990) *Women and Gender in Southern Africa to 1945*, Cape Town and London: David Philip and James Currey.

Walker, P. H. (1911) 'Gcushuwa, Syphilis or Yaws', *South African Medical Record*, vol. 9, pp. 182–3.

Walkowitz, Judith R. (1980) *Prostitution and Victorian Society. Women, Class and the State*, Cambridge: Cambridge University Press.

Wallace, Marion (1993) 'Urban Control and the Compulsory Examination of Women in Windhoek, 1915–1940', Institute of Commonwealth Studies postgraduate seminar or Health and Empire, 12 March 1993.

Warren, James F. (1990) 'Prostitution and the Politics of Venereal Disease: Singapore, 1870–98', *Journal of Southeast Asian Studies (Singpore)*, pp. 360–83.

Warwick, P. (1980) 'Introduction', in P. Warwick (ed.), *The South African War. The Anglo-Boer War, 1899–1902*, Harlow: Longman, pp. 12–17.

Warwick, P. (1983) *Black People and the South African War, 1899–1902*, Cambridge: Cambridge University Press.

Watney, Simon (1987) *Policing Desire. Pornography, AIDS and the Media*, London: Methuen.

Webb, Douglas (1995) 'The Social Epidemiology of HIV and the Development of AIDS Prevention in Southern Africa', D.Phil thesis, University of London.

Weeks, Jeffrey (1977) *Coming Out. Homosexual Politics in Britain from the Nineteenth Century to the Present*, London: Quartet.

Weeks, Jeffrey (1985) *Sexuality and its Discontents. Meanings, Myths and Modern Sexualities*, London: Routledge and Kegan Paul.

Weindling, Paul (1993) 'The Politics of International Co-ordination to Combat Sexually Transmitted Diseases, 1900–1980s', in Virginia Berridge and Philip Strong (eds), *AIDS and Contemporary History*, Cambridge: Cambridge University Press, pp. 93–107.

Welgemoed, N. C., Mahaffey, A. and van den Ende, J. (1986) 'Prevalence of Neisseria Gonorrhoea Infection in Patients Attending an Antenatal Clinic', *South African Medical Journal*, vol. 69, pp. 32–4.

Wells, Julia C. (1982) 'The History of Black Women's Struggle Against Pass Laws in South Africa 1900–1960', D.Phil. thesis, Columbia University.

Wells, Julia C. (1983) 'Why Women Rebel: A Comparative Study of South African Women's Resistance in Bloemfontein (1913) and Johannesburg (1958)', *Journal of Southern African Studies*, vol. 10, no. 1, pp. 55–70.

Wells, Simpson (1919) 'Some Problems of Maternal and Antenatal Pathology' (presidential address to the Cape of Good Hope branch of the BMA), *Medical Journal of South Africa*, vol. 14, pp. 388–394.

West, R. P. H. (1933/34?), *Facts About Ourselves for Growing Boys and Girls*, Johannesburg: Johannesburg Public Health Department and South African Red Cross Society (Transvaal).

White, Luise (1990) *The Comforts of Home. Prostitution in Colonial Nairobi*, Chicago, Ill.: University of Chicago Press.

Wilcocks, R. W. (1930) 'Psychological Observations on the Relation between Poor Whites and Non-Europeans', *The Social and Industrial Review*, vol. 9, no. 53, pp. 237–42.

Wilcocks, R. W. (1932) 'The Psychological Report', in *Report of the Carnegie Commission. The Poor White Problem in South Africa. Part II*, Stellenbosch: Pro Ecclesia.

Willcox, R. R. (1951) 'Njovera: An Endemic Syphilis of Southern Rhodesia', *Lancet*, vol. 1, pp. 558–60.

Willcox, R. R. (1960) 'Evolutionary Cycle of the Treponematoses', *The British Journal of Venereal Diseases*, vol. 36, pp. 78–91.

Willcox, R. R. (1979) 'Venereal Diseases', in G. M. Howe (ed.), *A World Geography of Human Diseases*, London, New York and San Francisco: Academic Press, pp. 201–35.

Willcox, R.R. (1980) 'Venereal Diseases in the Pacific Islands', *British Journal of Venereal Diseases*, vol. 56, pp. 277–81.

Williams, Brian and Campbell, Cathy (1996) 'Mines, Migrancy and HIV in South Africa – Managing the Epidemic', *South African Medical Journal*, vol. 86, no. 10, pp. 1249–51.

Williams, Raymond (1985) *The Country and the City*, London: Hogarth Press.

Wilson, Monica (1981) 'Xhosa Marriage in Historical Perspective', in Eileen Jensen Krige and John L. Comaroff (eds), *Essays in African Marriage in Southern Africa*, Cape Town and Johannesburg: Juta, pp. 133–47.

Woods Hutchinson (1897) 'Prostitution as a Factor in Progress', *South African Medical Journal*, vol. V, no. 50, pp. 133–5.

Worboys, Michael (1988) 'Manson, Ross and Colonial Medical Policy: Tropical Medicine in London and Liverpool, 1899–1914', in Roy MacLeod and Milton Lewis (eds), *Disease, Medicine and Empire. Perspectives on Western Medicine and the Experience of European Expansion*, London and New York: Routledge, pp. 21–37.

Worger, William H. (1987) *South Africa's City of Diamonds. Mine Workers and Monopoly Capitalism in Kimberley, 1867–1895*, New Haven and London: Yale University Press.

World Health Organisation (1983) *Apartheid and Health,* Geneva: World Health Organisation.

Zwi, Anthony and Bachmayer, Deborah (1990) 'HIV and AIDS in South Africa: What is an Appropriate Public Health Response', *Health Policy and Planning,* vol. 5, no. 4, pp. 316–36.

Zwi, Anthony and Cabral, Antonio Jorge R. (1991) 'Identifying "High Risk Situations" for Preventing AIDS', *British Medical Journal,* vol. 303, pp. 1527–9.

Index